KUNO MEYER

1858 - 1919

A Biography

*'I hope to be able to take up the study of the Irish language and
literature as the principal object of my life's work'*

(KUNO MEYER TO WHITLEY STOKES, 11 JUNE, 1882)

Seán Ó Lúing

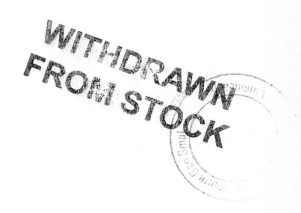

Published in Ireland by
Geography Publications
Kennington Road
Templeogue, Dublin 6W

ISBN 0 906602 17 3

Front Cover photograph of Kuno Meyer, reproduced
by kind permission of Rolf Baumgarten

Cover Design and Typesetting by Phototype-Set, Drumcondra, Dublin 9
Printed by Colour Books, Baldoyle Industrial Estate, Dublin 13
Bound by Museum Bookbindings, Dublin 2

I ndil - chuimhne
ar mo bhanchéile ró-ionmhain

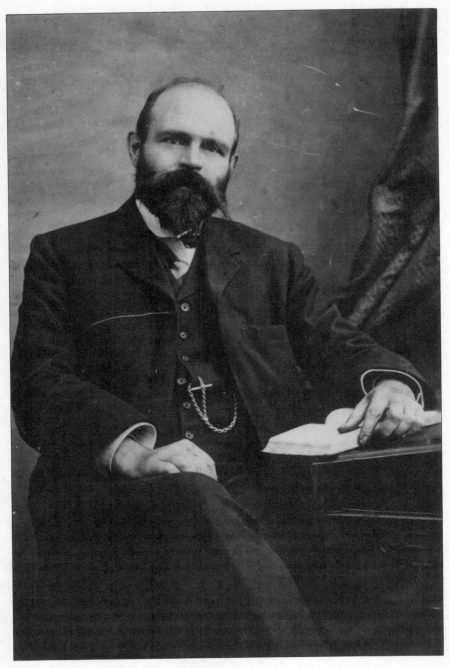

Kuno Meyer (photograph by Messrs. Bassano, London). Copy courtesy of the National Library of Ireland.

Contents

Acknowledgements

I should like firstly to record my obligation to the Council of Trustees of the National Library of Ireland for their kind permission to quote extracts from materials in the Library for the purposes of this biography. The major part of my research was carried out in the National Library, for the assistance and unfailing courtesy of whose staff, throughout many years, I am profoundly grateful.

To the staff of the Manuscripts Department of Trinity College Dublin, and in particular to Stuart Ó Seanóir for much valuable help, I wish to record my sincere feelings of obligation.

I owe a special word of thanks to Douglas Sealy, who readily and kindly gave me permission to make use of correspondence of his grandfather Dúbhglas de h-Íde.

To the staff of the Royal Irish Academy my thanks are due for their constant attention and services, and especially to Mrs. Bridget Dolan, whose ever ready help and kindness, in this as in other projects, it is an obligation and a pleasure to acknowledge.

I should like to express my sincere thanks to Adrian Allan, the Assistant Archivist of the University of Liverpool, who provided me with copies of relevant material in the University Archives which has been most useful, besides bringing to my attention some indispensable publications, likewise for the photograph of Kuno Meyer and his wife which appears in this book. His ready cooperation and interest call for a special word of appreciation.

I have profited from research in the Bodleian Library, Oxford, whose kind permission to use and quote from the Gilbert Murray papers and Kuno Meyer's letters to Wallace Martin Lindsay I gratefully acknowledge. And I sincerely appreciate the kindness of Alexander Murray who gave his ready permission to quote from the papers of his grandfather Gilbert Murray.

In the course of my researches I have had communication with Kuno Meyer's nephew, Hans Eduard Meyer of Berlin. I have reason to be grateful for his help and interest, for a copy of his father's essay on Kuno Meyer which appeared in *Irische Korrespondenz* and for the photograph of his aunt, Antonie, Kuno Meyer's sister, which is included with the illustrations. A survivor of the 1914-18 war, in which he was severely wounded, he makes a brief appearance in the following pages. It is with a keen sense of regret that I record his death which took place at the end of 1983. *Requiescat*.

I am grateful to Dr. Christhard Hoffmann, of Technische Universität Berlin, the biographer of Eduard Meyer, for his helpful replies to my queries on details of the Meyer family and for a copy of his essay on Eduard Meyer in *Classical Scholarship, a biographical encyclopedia* (1990).

For assistance in shaping the Bibliography and many useful

suggestions I am grateful to Gearóid Ó Lúing. Helen Meany read the proofs and gave sound advice thereon, an office for which I am sincerely in her debt. Rolf Baumgarten of the Dublin School of Celtic Studies very kindly provided the portrait of Kuno Meyer which adorns the dust jacket.

To the ever-constant support and encouragement of William Nolan of Geography Publications I can gratefully testify.

Retrospectively, I wish to pay tribute to the memory of Cormac Ó Cadhlaigh, Professor of Modern Irish in University College Dublin, who in his lectures first introduced me to the great name of Kuno Meyer, and to a knowledge of many others in the field of Celtic scholarship.

By way of elucidation, it may be pointed out that in the following pages Alice Stopford Green is identical with Mrs. John Richard Green, as is Toni Meyer with Antonie Meyer, John MacNeill with Eoin MacNeill or Eoin Mac Néill, and the Hungarian health resort Pöstyén with Pistyan, all these forms deriving from the correspondence in which they appear.

Whilst every reasonable effort has been made, it has not been possible to trace some copyright holders. Apologies are offered to anyone who may have inadvertently been omitted, and any such omissions will be rectified in future editions.

For any errors I take full responsibility.

Seán Ó Lúing,
Blackrock,
Co. Dublin.

Chapter 1

AT the beginning of the twentieth century in Ireland there was in progress a language and literary movement in which three streams flowed side by side. One was the Gaelic League, the popular nationwide movement for the revival of the Irish language; along with it, and deriving from it, was the literary movement, expressing itself in English, of which W.B. Yeats and Lady Augusta Gregory were representative; the third stream was the Celtic-Irish scholarly movement of which Kuno Meyer was leader and chief personality. Much has been written about the first two streams. Little attention has been given the third, the scholarly movement which was, in effect, also a product of the Gaelic League.

Kuno Eduard Meyer was born in Hamburg on 20 December 1858. He was the son of Eduard and Henriette Meyer and the second child in a family of four, Eduard, Kuno, Antonia and Albrecht. It was a cultivated household where classical German poetry and ancient literature predominated, Goethe being central to the family's poetical studies. Kuno's earliest education was in the Siemsenschen Privatschule after which he entered the Johanneum, the Classical School where his father taught and at which his attendance is recorded as 1868 to 1879.[1] The Johanneum was pre-eminent as an educational centre. Its influence on Kuno Meyer's brother, Eduard, who became one of Germany's greatest classical historians, has been acknowledged by Victor Ehrenberg and Christhard Hoffmann.[2]

Kuno Meyer left school suddenly. Irish friends who knew him later thought he ran away from school, impelled by a love of adventure, the feel of a boat and the salt smell of the sea. There was wanderlust in the family's veins. Kuno's younger brother, Albrecht, had travelled into the fastnesses of Yucatan, there to die of fever at the age of twenty-one. Kuno and Eduard travelled far and wide in their time. For Kuno on this occasion it was travel with a purpose, to acquire a practical knowledge of the English language in Edinburgh, as he relates in the only half page of autobiography he ever wrote.[3] Two years (1874-76) in Edinburgh as amanuensis and reader to a blind German scholar, whose temper was none too serene, gave him a perfect command of English both written and spoken. While in Scotland he came into contact for the first time with Gaelic speech on the Isle of Arran and gained a knowledge of Ossianic literature.[3a] He returned to the Johanneum to complete his school course. He was the life of his school, his teachers being the object

1

of sallies in German and Latin verse, later collected under the title *Musarum Munuscula*, these being, as he expressed it, with youthful exuberance, 'poems sublime soothing joyful melancholy festive plaintive raging maledictory', a seventy-four page collection published in Hamburg by his friend Ferdinand Schlotke, anno 1879, with the inscription, original in Latin:

> Kuno dedicates this little volume to his congenial circle of fellow-students, with whom for many years things good and bad were shared in common, as a token of remembrance for departing companions and a monument to pleasant times

which, true to Johanneum tradition, shows him to be a competent Latinist and, amongst other things, an admirer of Kaiser Wilhelm to whom he dedicates a poem written in gratitude for the Emperor's recent delivery from peril:

> Raise high your cups and voices, friends!
> Let us give thanks to God
> Let us sincerely sing
> The triumphal praises of Caesar,

ending the little volume with a translation, after Catullus, of that most untranslatable of all couplets, *Odi et amo*:

> Ich hasse und liebe.
> Warum? magst Du fragen.
> Was weiss ich's zu sagen.
> Ich fühle die Triebe
> Und muss es ertragen.

In 1879 he entered the University of Leipzig where his elder brother Eduard had gone as privatdozent. Through his reading he must have become attracted to Celtic studies, for besides pursuing Germanic languages and comparative philology he began the study of Celtic languages and literature under a teacher for whom he was to acquire the deepest respect, Ernst Windisch. Professor Windisch, whose main study was Sanskrit and Indo-European Philology, had also gained distinction in the field of Celtic learning, encouraged through his friendship with Standish Hayes O'Grady and Whitley Stokes. There were two further interruptions to Kuno Meyer's academic career. He broke off his studies for a year, 1880-1881, to act as Hauslehrer for the Arnold family in Lowestoft. With his interest in Celtic studies now active, he wrote from there in August 1881 to the editor of the *Revue Celtique*[4] to ask if space might be found for his recently copied text of *Macgnimartha Find*, explaining that David Comyn's faulty text was uncritically based on an unreliable transcript by Euseby Cleaver. Meyer's text duly appeared in *Revue Celtique*, his first contribution to Celtic studies.[5]

Very early in his career Meyer had corresponded with Whitley Stokes, man of two crafts, Macc Da Cherdda, as he styled himself, who left his mark on the history of India by codifying the Anglo-Indian laws, a vast undertaking and, in his capacity as philologist, produced an impressive array of Irish language material. Meyer may have written to him while he was still in India, for we find Stokes writing to the young student from Simla in 1881, 'I am much flattered that you have been reading my Irish publications, and I hope that you have been doing so very critically, for they are full of mistakes, I am sorry to say'.[6] Shortly afterwards Stokes came back from India, where he had spent nineteen years, and had occasion to help his admiring apprentice in many ways. From Ireland he forwarded the transcript of a poem to Meyer who was then putting in his term of military service as a one-year volunteer, a duty for which his enthusiasm is not evident. He apologised for the delay in acknowledging the poem, explaining that he was now, as a poor private soldier, in the midst of very trying exercise and drill. 'For I am serving my military year as a so-called Einjahrig-Freiwillinger, and whilst I always managed to find two or three hours leisure for private work in winter, it is now almost impossible for me even to decently keep up the little correspondence I have. This will last till the end of September when I shall be a free man again, and then I hope to be able to take up the study of the Irish language and literature as the principal object of my life's work, although it will be difficult to turn it to practical purpose either here or in England. Let me again thank you, Dear Sir, for your kindness towards me.'[7]

Thus was the purpose of his life declared, at the age of 24. He renewed his university course, achieving his doctorate in 1883, not forgetting to record his gratitude to his teachers, especially Zarnke and Windisch, in his doctoral thesis published the following year under the title *Eine irische version der Alexandersage*. He was now qualified to seek employment and had not long to wait. A vacancy occurred in University College Liverpool for a lecturer in German owing to the departure for Marburg of Dr. Wilhelm Viëtor who in fact had been the first person to hold the post as Lecturer in Teutonic Languages and Literature. Viëtor had favoured more modern methods of language teaching than prevailed and in his later career achieved marked distinction. Kuno Meyer applied and was appointed as having the necessary qualifications in Germanic studies. His application was supported by John Rhys, Professor of Celtic in Oxford, in a letter which was probably helpful. It reads:

Dear Sir,

I understand that my friend Dr. Kuno Meyer is a candidate for the post of reader of German at the University College in Liverpool, and it gives me very great pleasure to say a word for him. Though I have been chiefly brought in contact with him as an excellent and most promising Celtic Scholar I can testify to his being in all respects a superior man, of high general culture, of most gentlemanly and fascinating manners and altogether eminently qualified, so far as I can judge, for the post which he is now seeking.

Believe me
Yours very truly
John Rhys M.A.
(Fellow of Jesus College, Late Fellow of
Merton Coll. Professor of Celtic in the
University of Oxford).[8]

3

An excellent and most promising Celtic Scholar he was to be. It is true that in his capacity as Lecturer on Teutonic Languages he did teach German, and with his Latin colleague Herbert Strong published *Outlines of a history of the German language* (London 1886), a German Grammar for Schools (London 1887) which ran into several editions, and a selection of German readings for beginners (Leipzig 1888) after which his productions, if not his interest, in German came to an end. He had become possessed by a passion for Celtic studies.

He adapted himself readily to his environment. University College Liverpool was a new institution, having received its primary charter in 1881. It was part of a wider educational movement which saw the rise of the civic universities, as distinguished from the older establishments of Oxford and Cambridge and was part of the radical reform and reconstruction of education that followed in the wake of the industrial revolution. Liverpool in the latter quarter of the nineteenth century had developed into an important industrial and shipping centre, forming communications with all parts of the world, and its claim to a university which would reflect and serve its commercial prosperity was acknowledged. The applied sciences were given the premier position in its curriculum. Sister institutions received their charters during the same period and in the industrial region of central and northern England the new University Colleges of Manchester (previously Owens College), Sheffield, Leeds, Birmingham and Nottingham were established.

Liverpool was a new university, untrammelled by conservative traditions, liberally endowed by the city's great industrialists, with freedom to develop its own capacities. Its character might be summed up in Kuno Meyer's words, as uttered later in the light of his experience:

> Two things, above all, we put upon our programme. The first was that it should be a real living University, in touch with the life of a great nation and with scientific progress all over the world; that all knowledge was to be its province; that its function was not to be confined to the communication of already established knowledge, but to include the continual investigation of unexplored fields; that it was to be a factory as well as a market of learning. And the second feature was that the University was to provide efficient training for all the professions that call for scientific attainments, that it should not confine itself to the professions of the old world, but that it would be a workshop where students should be trained on scientific methods for all the innumerable new professions and departments of science and learning which have been called into being by the changed conditions of modern life. These pledges we have faithfully begun to carry out. New and fast-growing schools have sprung up in the most varied departments of science and learning – schools of ancient and mediaeval archaeology, of philology, anthropology, local history, palaeography, of tropical medicine and research, biochemistry, bacteriology, the last Chair that is just being created being one for parasitology and arachnology. To fill these posts men of eminence have been invited; and others, men of worldwide fame, like J.G. Frazer, the author of 'The Golden Bough', have left the older seats of learning to come among us, attracted not by larger salaries, but by the prospect of a large field of activity and the freer atmosphere of our young university.[9]

Into such a context as this Meyer settled happily. He enjoyed his Liverpool years and English life generally. Gregarious and popular, a good talker who was at home in the company of his fellows, he entered with zest into the university's social life and formed many friendships amongst his colleagues. He was a founder member of the University Club and its President in 1897-98. He joined the Bachelors Club. He was on the publication committee of *Otia Mersiana,* the learned journal of the Arts Faculty, of which four issues appeared between 1899 and 1904, and contributed Irish language items to it, including his exquisite translation of Cailleach Bhéara, the Old Woman of Beare. In a science-oriented university its early demise was to be expected and Meyer's friend, Walter Raleigh, celebrated in verse Meyer's fruitless attempts to obtain finance for it from 'The Man of Business' who, it appears, was 'Great Professor Woodward'.[10] The editor, John Sampson, sent round a circular seeking contributions for its support, to no avail, and 'this ill-starred periodical', Raleigh's description, collapsed after four issues.[11]

Meyer was not long appointed when he introduced Celtic studies to the University, taking classes in Welsh and Irish. His student and disciple, J. Glyn Davies, recorded the following memories of him:

> I came into contact with Kuno Meyer at the end of 1885 when he had already become known as a freak German who could speak Welsh and as a sort of colleague to the Welsh-speaking negro seaman Gymro Du. It was known to a few emancipated Welshmen that he was prepared to give instruction in Welsh and to deliver patriotic addresses, concerned with Taliesin, Owen Glyndwr and other mysterious and meaningless names that never failed to bring down the house. In October 1885 he addressed the Welsh National Society on the Study of Celtic Languages and Literature, a scholarly address that failed to open the eyes of the antiquaries in his audience. If he had instead sung the ballad of Mochyn Du he would have leapt into fame.
>
> The address at the Welsh National had one result – it put him in touch with the Welsh community in their week-day frame of mind.[12]

The credit for introducing Welsh as part of the Celtic studies course to the curriculum belongs wholly to Kuno Meyer. He took a particular interest in forwarding the career of J . Glyn Davies, advising and coaching him towards his appointment as Lecturer in Welsh in 1908. He took a keen interest in the music and poetry of Wales and sought finance for the study of Welsh and the development of Welsh archaeology. The University of Wales was to honour him with a Doctorate. He was on terms of acquaintance, if not actual friendship, with David Lloyd George, in propitious times before the shadows of war darkened. John Rhys, who should know, being a native of Wales and an eminent Celticist, paid Meyer the tribute of being a Celtic scholar 'who had approved himself to my countrymen .... he succumbed to the touch of the magic wand, and since then he has become practically a Welshman. I think I cannot pay him any greater compliment.'[13] As a first step towards instruction in Welsh, Meyer edited *Peredur ab Efrawc*, a thirty-nine page text and had it privately printed as a class book.

Regarding his Irish classes, Glyn Davies goes on to say:

> I have a vague impression that these were attended by three or four at first, but the classes dwindled down to an attendance of two again - O'Donovan, a brilliant and

mature scholar, and myself, newly bitten by the attraction of a language that was reputed to be like Welsh.... Modern Irish was a new and wonderful world to me and I needed no spur to keep me pegging away at this most difficult language. But Kuno Meyer was intent on Middle Irish.... He had the scholar's dislike for slipshod Irish, and the book that I liked – a collection of folklore by Douglas Hyde, – must have been, as I can well see now, very irksome to him....

It was not Kuno Meyer's fault that the classes dwindled down in Welsh and in Irish - he was a university lecturer, and Liverpool failed to supply him with an audience sufficiently well equipped. He started with Middle Irish and Mediaeval Welsh, his own familiar ground .... his method was scholastically right for a German teaching Germans; it was right for a scholar reading with scholars. But the teaching was wrong for attracting permanent students from non-University ranks.'[14]

Brilliant though Glyn Davies was he did not have a degree, but was closer to the heart of his countrymen than the formalities of learning could make him. The O'Donovan who attended the Irish classes was Richard, son of the famous John O'Donovan who edited the Annals of the Four Masters. It is interesting to note from Glyn Davies' account that Meyer was more at home in the earlier forms of Irish. Nevertheless, Meyer spared no effort in trying to learn spoken Irish and visited Achill and other parts of the west of Ireland for that purpose. With his sister, Antonie, he spent some weeks on the Aran Islands in the autumn of 1889, eager to acquire a knowledge of the modern language at its source. His Aran letter to Whitley Stokes brought back nostalgic memories to the senior scholar. Meyer wrote him on 27 August:

Dear Dr . Stokes,

We are very happy here, having found most comfortable lodgings and being so far favoured by fine weather. We had to give up the idea of staying on Inis Meadhon, but having a boat at our disposal, we shall go there often. The priest here, Father O'Donohue, is most kind towards us. Mr. Quinn from Liverpool is here also, struggling bravely with the language. I am taking down as many words, phrases, etc. as I can pick up. They certainly use fewer English loan words here than in Achill .... We shall stay here for about a fortnight.[15]

Meyer found that Heinrich Zimmer's visit was still remembered in Aran. 'He once addressed a Land-league meeting, and almost had a row with the agent.'[16] Some encounter that, the Celtic savant and scion of a Castellaun landworker, in conflict with the landlord's henchman, which did not surprise Stokes.[17] Zimmer would have earned the approbation of Father Michael O'Donohoe,[18] champion of Aran's rackrented parishioners, of whose kindness Meyer speaks .

Meyer's news from Aran brought back the past to Whitley Stokes who had been on Inis Meadhon in 1858, along with Charles Petrie, Frederick Burton, Samuel Ferguson, Eugene Curry and his father, William Stokes, F.R.S. 'There were as many folksongs and folk melodies as wild flowers', he recalled. 'You must be very happy in Ara na Noib, if you have fine weather. I think that, on the whole, the happiest ten days of my life were spent there in 1858. I hope that Fräulein Meyer imitates her brother and takes down some of the tunes, of which there were then hundreds in existence'.[19] Stokes had some suggestions to offer on the edition of *Aislinge Meic Conglinne* which Meyer was planning. Meyer wrote back a letter which, as a record of the island, deserves to be reproduced in full:

Kilronan
Aranmore

Dear Dr . Stokes,

I was delighted to get such a long and interesting letter from you. It had been much delayed in transmission, and was marked 'Liverpool', 'Greystones' (where?) &c. We are leaving for Dublin and home on Wednesday next, and shall be back in Liverpool on Sunday week. Though we have not been able to carry out half our plans, mainly owing to the state of the weather, we have on the whole spent a very happy time, and would gladly prolong it. I am seriously thinking of coming back to Inis Meadhon before long, as it offers such unique opportunities for learning Irish. Scarcely anybody knows English there, and they talk the Irish very clearly and purely. It is a dreadfully poor place, though, and one would have to provision oneself well. We could get nothing but bláthach – Queen Medb's favourite drink – and a horrible kind of cake. There exists a satire on Inis Meadhon by a modern Mac Conglinne, some Connemara man, they say, which I must get hold of before I go. The beginning is

Inis Meadhón

Tír gan arán

Inis gann gortach.

My sister and I fully endorse this sentiment. I am very glad to have made the acquaintance of a young priest from Mullingar, called O'Growney, who is now spending his vacation on Inismaan to improve his knowledge of Irish. I believe this man will one day be a very thorough Irish scholar. He possesses now a remarkable knowledge of the modern language in all its dialects, having lived in Munster, Mayo and Donegal, and is very anxious to become better acquainted with the older language. He strikes me as of a very scholarly bent and instinct. By the bye, he told me that most of O'Curry's MSS and copies are in Clonliffe College, Drumcondra. I shall have a look on my way back. I have set Quinn to copy the *Duanaire Finn* from the Franciscan MS. I am anxious to see what he will make of it.

I have not been able to get at the meaning of the curious words you mentioned in your last letter. They seem to have but few old plant-names here. There is, as you say, no mill in Aran. O'Growney knew mol 'a mill-shaft', but none of the other words.

Your suggestions about an edition of the *Aislinge Meic C*. almost entirely agree with the plan I had formed myself. If Andrew Lang could be induced to write the Introduction, the book would be sure to sell. I could scarcely do justice to the subject, beyond pointing out a few things, but no one could do it better than he. I think I shall write to him about it.

I wish we could write down the tunes they sing here. But neither my sister or I are able to do it. I am afraid they are not as numerous now as they were when you were here. Too many modern songs have come in and crowded them out. I am disgusted with the state in which all antiquities are left here. The old churches and oratories are little better than stables for all sorts of animals, as far as they are not filled with nettles, briars, &c. The inscribed stones are most of them quite covered up. We had to work hard before we could unearth the inscription Oroit ar Scandlan in Eany's Church. Something ought to be done by the Government or by private subscriptions. The dúns are much better off. They have appointed caretakers to look after them.

With many kind regards
Yours always
Kuno Meyer[20]

In the milieu of his Celtic studies, he made many friends and contacts. His circle of correspondents widened. His text of the Irish Odyssey, *Merugud Uilix maicc Leirtis*, a uniquely slim adaptation of the original, was marked by messages from appreciative recipients. Reinhold Köhler, writing from Weimar on 16 April 1886, thanks him for his Erzählung von Ulixes[21] and the celebrated classicist Ulrich von Wilamowitz-Moellendorff wrote him from Göttingen to acknowledge 'ihrer inschriben Odyssee'.[22] Stokes, who sent a short notice of it to the *Academy* XXX (1886) 108-9, wrote in a friendly vein of criticism – 'Though I cannot think you right in normalising the spelling, and though I consider it a mistake to make "critical editions" of texts in any language like Irish, where there never was any *one* pre-eminent dialect, or writer, or period of literary cultivation, I am grateful for the book, and hope it will do good. ... I hope you will do some more of these refracted rays of classical literature and I conclude my notice by saying so',[22a] and this tells us much about the approach of Stokes to the Irish language, which was different from what Meyer's developed to be, the elder's one of honest, clinical, searching dedication, the younger's ardent and evangelistic while no whit less bound to the strictest canons of accuracy. Inevitably his studies led him to acquaintance with Robert Atkinson, a scholar with an undeservedly bad reputation amongst Irish language students due, as Meyer said, to 'the unfortunate remark which in the heat of controversy escaped from the lips of one who has himself done so much to make Irish literature accessible, the remark that Irish literature, when not religious, is either silly or indecent.'[23] While Meyer did not hesitate to criticise institutions for being neglectful of Irish he did not censure individuals. Atkinson welcomed him to Dublin. 'I need not tell you that I shall be glad to see you, and that I shall do all in my power to facilitate your study here during your short leisure.'[24]

Other correspondents were the voluminous writer, Sabine Baring Gould of Lew Trenchard, Devon, who wanted to know where and what had Meyer written relative to the Irish invasions of Wales and expressed his certainty that there were large Irish colonies in Devon and Cornwall, of whose presence many proofs existed.[25] Walter William Skeat, the Anglo-Saxon scholar, wrote about word meanings.[26] An ever helpful and admiring correspondent was Seaghan Pléimion, editor of the *Gaelic Journal,* who looked after Meyer's order for copies of the periodical and explained Irish words to him.[27] He valued Meyer's advice. 'As soon as convenient, look through the Irish articles and the notes on them and say what more I can do best to help Irish learners. It is really a pity we did not know each other sooner. Ach níl neart air .... Your meeting with Father O'Growney I look upon as a good augury for the old tongue.'[28] O'Growney, a full account of whose labours we lack, and Kuno Meyer became firm friends in their devotion to the language and we can document their mutual interest through a handful of O'Growney's letters from his address of Ballinacargy, Co. Westmeath.[29]

His great teacher Windisch was a regular correspondent, while Thurneysen, Zimmer, Ludwig Christian Stern and Sophus Bugge kept faithfully in touch. As text after text of his came off the printer's press so Meyer's reputation grew and his mail increased. Testimony to the significant appreciation he was gaining for Irish literature appears from letters of the brilliant Greek scholar, historian and biographer of St. Patrick, John B. Bury. The first, quoted here, relates to Meyer's edition of *King and Hermit*, a tenth century poem detailing a colloquy between King Guaire and his hermit brother, and an item about the death of Niall of the Nine Hostages from *Stories and Songs from Irish MSS*.[30]

> Bodafon
> Llanbedr
> Merionethshire
> July 10th [1901]
>
> My dear Meyer
>
> ....Thanks many times for the Opuscula, which I have been reading – not merely dipping into – with much interest. I am specially pleased to have the text of the *Orcuin Néill*; the traditions about this King have a bearing on some Patrician questions with which I am concerned.
>
> I enjoyed the sylvan atmosphere of the Marbán poem ever so much, reading it under a tree – an oak of course ('Manrglas darach'), for nearly every tree is an oak tree here – and watching little 'bric' (if this means trout) jumping at flies. This is just the place for an 'úarboith' for a modern hermit with Marbán's woodland tastes. He could get lots of 'dercna fróich', but alas! 'for a 'logg di subuir' he would have to send to Barmouth.
>
> It is clearly of the greatest importance that the scattered historical material, of which your Expulsion of the Dessi is a sample, and all the genealogical and chronological documents, should be edited. It would be a great step if the numerous MSS. in London, Dublin and Oxford, were fully catalogued. I wish we could induce some of the clever young men in Trinity, who have had a classical training, to turn their attention to Celtic; but they rightly think it does not pay, and *chrémata, chrémat' anér* is eminently true in Ireland.
>
> I have already read about thirty chapters in the Welsh N.T., and am beginning to get into the language. I find it much easier than Gaelic, but don't think I shall like it quite so well.
>
> Tomorrow, I expect, History Preliminaries will arrive, to interrupt me for a day or two.
>
> Very sincerely yours
> J. B. Bury.[31]

From TCD Common Room on 7 July [1902] Bury wrote: 'My dear Meyer, I have not yet thanked you for the charming story of Liadain and Curithir which you have brought to light. It is a pity that one has to guess so much between the lines. I am awaiting with much interest your promised edition of the *Cáin Adamnáin*,' and goes on to discuss, but not to accept, the Windisch-Stokes explanation of a term in the Codex Ardmachanus.[32]

It must have been sometime in 1891 that Meyer, on his way home from a lecture, was followed by a young man who deferentially introduced himself as John Sampson. They talked of Shelta, the Gypsies' tongue. It was a turning point in Sampson's life, for Meyer, recognising the youth's talent and the value of his work, became his friend and introduced him to the brilliant circle of kindred spirits who were winning distinction for the University of Liverpool. Sampson, whose life up to then had been a hard struggle, was assigned to the staff of the University, of which he later became its distinguished Librarian, and an expert in the structure of old manuscripts. He was Irish, out of Corcach Mór, so Meyer tells us, and now happily joined the little band of comrades who loved to roam the Welsh hills and valleys in their romantic attachment to the freedom of the wilds. They camped out on the Welsh hills and sought the society of the wandering gypsies. A member of the group recalled how Kuno returned one evening to their camp-fire near Bala, with a Gypsy harper for company, to enliven their proceedings with Welsh melodies, or with the harmonies of penillion singing at which Meyer himself excelled.[33] The adventure and camaraderie of those care-free days are commemorated by Meyer in the dedication of his *King and Hermit,* the marvellous little collection of nature poetry which he translated from the Irish. The dedication is dated at Liverpool March 10, 1901, but refers to events of some ten years earlier, and addresses his comrades -

Damer Harrison
John MacDonald
Walter Raleigh
John Sampson

as follows:

Kamlé pralalé,
When, a few years ago, we five, like Marbán the Hermit, exchanging for a while the flockbed of civilisation for the primitive couch of the earth, went agypsying into Wales, and every evening pitched our tent now by a murmuring brook, now upon the shingle of the sea, then again among the heather on a mountainside, or in some woodland glade, where the hundred-throated chorus of birds awoke us at dawn, and the hooting owl startled us out of our slumbers at night, – some of you, town-born and bred like myself, felt for the first time that exquisite charm of an intimate intercourse with nature which has found such beautiful expression in the verses of a nameless Irish poet. In memory of those happy times I dedicate this little book to you.

Tumaro pral shom
K . M .

His pupil J. Glyn Davies, Welsh to the core in spirit and language, who later became Meyer's colleague in the Welsh department, was but little impressed with their genuine knowledge of nature, considering that neither Meyer nor Sampson actually knew 'a trout from a flounder, nor a blackbird from a starling.' Whether so or not, the wind on the heath was exhilarating. But at some point Kuno Meyer must have been careless of his health because from camping in the foggy Welsh hills he contracted rheumatism, which developed into painful arthritis, invading the muscles of his head and neck, causing him to become bent and subject to frequent pain, in contrast to the splendid physique which he previously enjoyed and was remarked by friends who had admired him in military uniform. Yet he never complained. His ailment dated from 1892 and in

10

that year his sister Antonie (Toni) and his mother came over permanently from Hamburg to look after him. But for the rest of his life his rheumatism proved a handicap, for which he was to seek remedy or alleviation in many clinics throughout Europe. He sought treatment for it at an early stage, which did not greatly improve his condition as he wrote to Stokes from Smedley's Hydropathic Establishment, Matlock, on 26 July:

> Dear Dr . Stokes,
>
> I am still very far from a complete recovery. My mother and I came here about a fortnight ago. Since then we have had the worst weather so that I, like all other patients here, have made but little progress. The treatment here is very severe. The food which I am allowed is of truly Mac Conglinnian simplicity, as the poet says:
>
> > Is é mo chuit - mor in bét -
> > ro ordaig dom in liaig án:
> > corca bruithte, ordu éisc,
> > lemnacht acus tur arán,[34]

comparing his diet to that provided for the wandering scholar in the ancient wonder tale, by which he was restricted, as medically ordered, to cooked oatmeal, fish, fresh milk and dry bread, healthy but Spartan. Besides, he was not allowed to smoke, or to work, but was to lie on his back all day. He broke the regime to sit up a while and write letters. Do take care of yourself, advised Stokes, haunted by the dread that death stalked the path of Celtic studies ever since it claimed his young mentor Siegfried at thirty-three. Some improvement must have taken place as he sent better news to Eugene O'Growney from whom we find a sympathetic message welcoming him back to activity:

> A chara dhílis
>
> Fáilte romhat ar t'ais chugainn . Is maith liom do sceula ar fheabhas do shláinte, agus tá súil agam nach sáróchair thú féin arís leis an iomarcaidh saothair. .... Fáilte uaim do'n mháthair agus do'n dheirbhshiair!
>
> > E. Ó Gramhna. [35]
>
> (My faithful friend
>
> Welcome back to us. I am glad to have news from you of your good health, and I hope you will not exhaust yourself again with overwork.
> .... My greetings to your mother and sister!)

Meyer's teacher Ernst Windisch had occasion to deplore the attacks made by Celtic scholars on each other. Kuno Meyer was to have early experience of the stings and arrows of Irish language controversy. His edition of the *Cath Finntrága*, or Battle of Ventry, was the occasion of one of those full scale onslaughts which Celtic scholars took joy in inflicting on their fellows. The Battle of Ventry has the character of a popular folktale and was a favourite recital of West Kerry storytellers.

But the manuscript from which Meyer had to work presented him with many problems and while engaged on it he discussed its difficulties with his friend, Whitley Stokes, making the sensible observation that – 'One has, however, quite made up one's mind to the fact that for a long time to come all work in Celtic Philology can be done but incompletely'.[36]

11

No doubt with the intention of doing Meyer a good turn, Whitley Stokes suggested to Standish Hayes O'Grady, friends as they were then, that he might review it. O'Grady, who spoke Irish from his boyhood in County Limerick and had edited an important Irish text for the Irish Archaeological Society before having to traverse the globe in his profession of engineer, from the Yukon to Australia, put pen to paper as Irish scholar after a lapse of thirty years and contributed to a learned journal an extensive and unnecessarily destructive review which he ended by saying:

> What has been said above will not, I trust, be thought too severe; something of the kind appeared to be called for in the interest not only of the future learner, but of the Editor himself. A little diffidence is not unwholesome, and from beginning to end of the book there is not a word tending to disarm criticism, on the contrary the tone is throughout quite magisterial.[37]

With reason Meyer complained to Stokes:

> I cannot help being greatly annoyed at the tone which he has used, but much more by the unfairness of his criticism. I am of course very glad to have his valuable remarks upon doubtful passages of the text, and many things he has said are of great interest and importance, but anybody who looks at the length of his paper and does not really enter into the subject must think that I have brought out a most useless and blundering edition, in fact an Elendes Machwerk - which is not the case. .... I am however satisfied that those who care to look into the matter will find out the unfairness of his criticism. What he says about my magisterial tone, and my not having tried to disarm criticism, I do not understand. I like his jokes well enough, and whatever is just in his remarks I am the first to acknowledge and be thankful for, but why he, with his great knowledge of Modern Irish and of Irish literature, should thus try to do serious harm to a beginner who has had the bad luck to get at a text of such difficulty, without one word of acknowledgement or encouragement, I do not comprehend. I consider it a very unfortunate thing that he should have broken his long silence in this manner.
> I wonder whether I ought to answer him. He has made many mistakes himself which would be worth correcting.[38]

Very different was the reception given to his labours by the celebrated folklorist Jeremiah Curtin who sent him a friendly word recording his pleasure in reading *Cath Finntrága*.[39] When O'Grady published his text and translation of *Silva Gadelica* in 1892 Meyer availed of the opportunity to reply in kind and, aided by Whitley Stokes, to broadcast a comprehensive three part list of errors in *Revue Celtique* XIV and XV, 1893-4. It is only fair to say that he was never one to keep alive a quarrel. He gave just dues where deserved and had words of courtesy and appreciation for O'Grady on many occasions such as when in 1901 he praised him to the Pan-Celtic Society in these terms:

> Standish Hayes O'Grady, most learned of all native Irish scholars.... Would that he might also continue the catalogue of the Irish MSS in the British Museum.... It is as I have had occasion before to say, not only the first reliable printed catalogue of any large collection of Irish MSS, but the editor's fine translations and curious notes make it one of the most important as well as the most delightful Irish books ever published – nor is there any scholar living now who can interpret for us the style and the spirit of bardic poetry in so masterly a manner.[40]

12

In the summer of 1894 Kuno Meyer was visiting Halle when he was asked why was there no specialist German journal to cater for the increasing needs of Celtic studies. He expressed himself as doubtful if such would pay or even if a publisher for it might be found but he was persuaded that Niemeyer in Halle would agree to the project. Thus was the distinguished name of Max Niemeyer, publisher, introduced to the realm of Celtic studies, who by his impact, and that of Ehrhardt Karras, printer, on the production of learned works in the Celtic languages, attained special prestige for the excellence and despatch of their printing and publishing. The letter below gives the genesis of the *Zeitschrift für celtische Philologie*. In it Meyer tells of the main reason for his being in Germany, which was to fulfil a long cherished wish and visit as an act of pilgrimage the grave of the most revered of Celtic scholars and founder of Celtic Philology, Johann Kaspar Zeuss. The letter was to Whitley Stokes, by now a close confidant.

Probstxella,
den 12 tn August 1894

Meininger Hof
E. Zimmermann

My dear Dr . Stokes,

Here I am in a small Thuringian village waiting for a train to take me to Kronach, the place where Zeuss was born and died. I intend to stay there at least one day and get from two surviving cousins – [.i. Heinrich and George Zeuss: *written over line*] old men they must be now – biographical data and, if possible, a picture of their celebrated kinsman. I also mean to have his grave photographed. This has long been a favourite wish of mine, and it is just possible that I may secure some interesting and valuable MS., perhaps a diary, or the like. For I suppose that all Irish books &c. were sent to Ebel for the 2nd edition of the *Grammatica C.* If I get any new and interesting data I shall put them together in an article, which will fitly open a publication of which you will be surprised, and I am sure glad, to hear. At the Halle festivities I was recently asked why there was no German Celtic Fachblatt or Zeitschrift, and when among other things I replied that it would not pay and no publisher for it be found, I was told on all sides that Niemeyer in Halle would almost certainly consent to publishing it. I at once went to see him and after a good deal of talk we agreed to try to start an International Celtic Review or Journal, provided we can get you, Windisch, Thurneysen, Strachan and a few others as Mitarbeiter. Windisch, whom I visited in Leipzig a day before he left for the Schwarzwald, was greatly interested, but in his loyal way was afraid of hurting the susceptibilities of Darby of Ballyjubbin. But I tried to show to him that there is room for two such Reviews, and that one has to wait a long time at present to get an article printed in the *Rev. Celtique*. He finally gave the undertaking his blessing, but will not have anything to do with the Redaktion, as he has his hands full with the *Morgenländische Zeitschrift*. Niemeyer insists that it is necessary to have a German Redacteur [. i . residing in Germany], and I have written to Thurneysen asking him to take the post. But as he is no doubt away on his holidays it may be some time before he answers. Meanwhile you will be so good as to tell me what you think of the idea, and whether you would be inclined, in case the thing comes off, to support it by occasional contributions. Niemeyer thinks of a six monthly issue – each heft to cost 5 or 6/- and to be had separately by non-subscribers for a little more. There would be no pay for contributors, at least not at first, but they would get 15 tirages à part. He thinks if he could get 120 subscribers, he would not be out of pocket. That strikes me as a

13

number which it should be possible to attain. I would of course write to Darby explaining the state of affairs, as soon as we see our way a little more clearly. As to my own part in it, I should not be wanted as a Redacteur, but to urge Irish, Scotch and Welsh scholars to contribute as well as to subscribe – though at present I can think of very few only whose contributions would be welcome. I shall send off this letter from Kronach tomorrow, when I hope to be able to add an account of my success there.

[The following note is added in pencil]

Kronach

The results of my pilgrimage are not quite what I expected, though I do not regret having come. I saw the 2 nephews – not cousins – who were children at the time of Zeuss' death. One of them possesses a capital oilpainting of Z., which I am having photographed. But beside some diplomas, medals, &c, there are no documents. All MSS and most books seem to have gone to Glück. Some priests also took their share. I went to the grave on which there is a statue of Z., very poorly executed, and then to Vogtendorf, where I saw the house in which he was born and in which he died. A tablet on the wall commemorates these facts. This house also I am having photographed. At Vogtendorf I saw quite a clan of Zeusses – a delightful old blacksmith, his nephew, who told several characteristic traits of his uncle and who strongly expressed his opinion that the 'professor', as he called him, was not quite right in his mind, founding this among other things on the fact that he neither drank beer or wine (only milk), nor smoked. He used to have his pockets full of sweets which he ate as he walked up and down in the garden, or in his room. I shall try to get more information from two priests who were friends of Zeuss and who I hear are still alive.[41]

Darby of Ballyjubbin was none other than Henri d'Arbois de Jubainville, whose impressive name and locality were, it seems, the subject of a private joke between Stokes and Meyer. He was editor of the *Revue Celtique*, established in 1870 and going strong, a journal of outstanding merit. Meyer wrote to D'Arbois, who replied on 23 August 1894 to thank him for the information about the forthcoming Celtic Zeitschrift.[42] Thurneysen, whom Meyer hoped would be redacteur or editor resident in Germany, was unable to accept and Stokes expressed regret at the disappointing news. 'I thought of L. C. Stern'.[43] Ludwig Christian Stern it was who became redacteur and joint editor with Meyer of the *Zeitschrift für celtische Philologie*, the first issue of which appeared in 1896 and was to be cited in its abbreviations of ZCP or CZ as the source of many a learned contribution. A prospectus issued in February 1896 by the publisher David Nutt, The Strand, London, announced that No. 1 was nearly ready and a list of its contributors included the great names of Celtic scholarship, Thurneysen, Strachan, Stokes, Wallace Lindsay, Gaidoz, Loth, Rhys, Zimmer, Meyer, Stern along with some lesser lights. It stated that although published in Germany the new journal would at all times be conducted in view of the fact that the majority of Celtic students lived in the English speaking world.

Stokes found all about Zeuss very curious. They had preferences in common. 'I wish I resembled him more than in my love for milk and sweetmeats'.[44] Zeuss's grave stands just inside the gate of the carefully tended city cemetery of Kronach. To this day he is honoured by the city

14

as one of its most distinguished sons and is commemorated by an impressive modern school, the Kaspar-Zeuss Gymnasium, and by a bronze statue in the city park, erected in May 1990, showing him in studious pose holding an open book. There is an avenue named in his memory but it is proposed to give his name in due course to one of the important city streets. His birthplace, now demolished, in the nearby village of Vogtendorf is denoted by a plaque on the house next to where it stood.[45]

In the early years of the twentieth century Kuno Meyer was a harbinger of optimism and unity of hearts in a land to which faction was no stranger and could impart a message of such enthusiasm as this:

> I have never yet known the Irishman or Irishwoman who were not in their heart of hearts proud of their beautiful native land, and loved it with a far-brought love, a love out of the storied past; who were not proud of their men and women; who did not think of them as every patriot ought, the best and noblest and fairest in the world. From that love will spring a wider and a greater Ireland, than an island of party and faction. I do not despair that even Professor Mahaffy, whose brilliant wit and ready satire too often give the lie to his true Irish heart, will be a contented citizen of that greater Ireland, and that a time will come when he and men like him will be proud of that precious inheritance of their nation, their great and noble literature, which is the envy of other nations and in which, with its history, its poetry and all its associations, a basis of union will be found for all Irishmen of whatever race and creed.[46]

He said this is the course of a survey of Celtic Studies delivered in the Antient Concert Rooms in Dublin on 23 August 1901. It was one of the important events of the Pan-Celtic Congress held during August 19-23, a colourful occasion with pageantry, pipe-music, the wearing of the kilt and fraternal association between delegates from the Celtic nations. Speakers who followed Meyer included Lord Castletown, W.B. Yeats and the formidable Heinrich Zimmer, the Tiger of Greifswald, the hard steel of whose criticism was felt by many an eminent celtologue. The Celt has reason to be grateful to him, for all that. No scholar has better contradicted Mommsen than he. His contribution was to the point – There was, he said, in modern times, no literature more beautiful than the Celtic literature, but there must be something done to make known this literature to the Celt himself, and to make the people of the Continent aware of its existence; to compile a bibliography of Celtic literature was a necessity.

The distinguished Greek scholar, John P. Mahaffy, who seemed to enjoy rubbing people the wrong way and was at the centre of much controversy, learned and otherwise, was later found on the Continent to be posing as an Irish nationalist, which might tend to confirm Meyer's surmise.[47] Meyer gave his impressions of the Congress to his correspondent, Mary Hutton, later that year:

> Dear Mrs Hutton,
>
> Your letter of the 13th August has remained unanswered too long – but I have led a roaming life ever since. I was a week in Wales, a week in Dublin and a fortnight with Mr. Whitley Stokes in Cowes whence I have just returned. You will have read all about the Pan-Celtic or Pankiltic, as scoffers called it, Congress. It

was very picturesque, there was some excellent music, one met a large number of interesting people, but the lasting result is not apparent. I was particularly interested in making the acquaintance of Professor Zimmer who afterwards paid me a visit here and met Professor Strachan of Manchester. We buried the war-hatchet and smoked many pipes of peace together. I was particularly struck with his marvellous knowledge of the modern languages. Welsh especially he speaks with absolute fluency and correctness. I suppose you have heard that he has been made Professor of Celtic at Berlin – the first chair of the kind in Germany. He talked much about a new book of his – 'Pelagius in Irland' – shortly to appear which will throw unexpected light on Irish Christianity of the 5th and 6th centuries. ...

    I am now engaged on a very curious and pretty love-story called *Comrac Liathaine agus Cuirithir* . ...[48]

Douglas Hyde said that Kuno Meyer called the attention not only of the world, but what was perhaps harder, the attention of Irishmen themselves, especially those of them who regretted that they were Irish, to the value of Irish literature in the evolution of Western European thought from the sixth century onward.

Hyde remembered how, when the Gaelic League was just six years old, and beginning to turn the corner, some of its enemies, led by the Provost of Trinity College, made an attempt to stem the tide by assuring a Viceregal Commission which sat to inquire into Intermediate Education in Ireland, that Irish literature was either religious, silly or indecent and that this being so, the Irish language should have no place in any such education. Hyde wrote for support on behalf of Irish to Zimmer, Windisch, Holger Pedersen, Georges Dottin, York Powell, L.C. Stern, Owen Edwards, Alfred Nutt and Eleanor Hull, names to which the devotees of Irish language and literature have reason to be grateful, for they sent powerful answers in support of it. Meyer's own letter of support was gratefully acknowledged by Hyde for being 'all that could be desired. It will greatly strengthen the hands of the Gaelic League to have it'.[49] Though shorter than most of the others, it put succinctly and effectively the claim for having Irish included in the education programme. Written from his Liverpool address, 57 Hope Street, and dated 24 January 1899, it acclaimed Irish Literature as a marvellous manifestation of the human spirit and, in its form and genius, in prose and in poetry, as a true and unique literature. Describing its value in a system of education he made four points - (1) To refrain from teaching it to Irish youths who spoke it as their mother tongue would be a grotesque educational blunder. (2) The Irish language, well taught, he regarded as a first-rate means of mental training. (3) Why, he asked, in their education for life and all it meant, deprive Irish youth of such intimate touch with the literature of their past? (4) What material would you provide for your university professors of Celtic studies if you freeze the fountain at its spring?

Answering the charge that modern Gaelic was a degenerate daughter of Old Irish, he affirmed that, far from being such, the modern Gaelic language, as used by educated speakers and writers, was a natural and healthy development of the Old Irish, remarkable alike for the raciness and wealth of its vocabulary and for its idiomatic construction, affording therefore an excellent means of linguistic training.

'Wishing you every success in your endeavour to combat such false and ignorant charges against a literature to the study of which I have devoted my life'.[50]

'But it was perhaps Kuno Meyer who in the end won us our victory' said Douglas Hyde. It came about in this way, taking up the story from Hyde himself. Dr. Salmon, who was Provost of Trinity College at that time and a member of the Commission, was anxious not to have a mere Irishman examining in Celtic, and looked around for a learned foreigner, because he was profoundly suspicious of us all, explains An Craoibhín, and imagined (quite wrongly of course) that the Irish examiners were marking too high. So an expert was brought in against whom the Gaelic League could not cavil, and Kuno Meyer, whom none of the Trinity College people suspected of any fondness for Irish, except a philological one, was invited to overlook the examinations for the Intermediate Board. There was a good deal of angry comment at the time on the introduction of a foreigner to examine over the heads of native Irish scholars. 'Have you heard' wrote Meyer to Mary Hutton 'that I have been appointed Intermediate Examiner in Irish: an appointment which will cause much dissatisfaction (and rightly so) in Ireland.... I am composing Irish exam. papers for the Intermediate Board. For I am the wicked foreigner to whom the *Claidheamh* alludes in its last number. The good cause will not suffer at my hands, whatever the intentions of those who appointed me may have been'.[51]

Dr. Michael P. O'Hickey in particular was bitterly annoyed at Meyer's appointment and wrote rather furiously. In the face of this Meyer had hesitated about accepting the invitation, but Douglas Hyde urged him strongly, for he suspected what the upshot would be, and wrote to Dr. O'Hickey and others asking them not to publicly object. It was in the context of these events that Hyde wrote to Kuno Meyer this interesting letter which, among other things, shows what an uncomprising fighter for his cause Douglas Hyde was:

Ratra
Frenchpark
Co. Roscommon
n.d.

My dear Dr. Kuno Meyer

A thousand thanks for your friendly letter. Of course I knew all about your appointment and can tell you the whole history of it when I see you. I am so glad it is not Zimmer who has been appointed. The idea of the Gallda party on the Board, who are in the majority, was that Irish is waxing too powerful and I know for certain this year that it is being far more widely taught in the Catholic schools than ever before. They don't like to see Gaelic Leaguers like Dr. O'Hickey, John Mac Neill or myself appointed as examiners, first because they grudge us the emolument, second, because they profess to believe that we undermark the papers, to make matters unduly easy for students taking up Irish.

Mahaffy's idea, I am nearly sure, was, that if he could get a German professor with a high standard, and of University ideas, to examine, he would mark so low

17

and pluck so many of the students that the Catholic colleges in disgust and despair would next year either drop the teaching of Irish altogether or restrain it within narrow limits. If Zimmer had been chosen (I believe he was, but found himself unable to act) this might have taken place to some extent. With you it is different. You have taught Irish to English-speaking people yourself, you know how hard a language it is for fourteen year old boys and girls to master, and you are in complete sympathy with the general movement.

If I might venture to make a suggestion to you, it would be to get the papers set for the last 5 or 6 years and make your own of equal difficulty ...

Dr. O'Hickey, who should in the ordinary course have been reappointed this year (as each examiner has always been reappointed for a second year,) is of course desperately offended at the slur cast on his character and bona fides, and when the Gaelic League learns that a stranger has been appointed there will be an indignant protest at the national insult. No outside examiner was ever imported to examine in classics or German or mathematics, only in Irish, as a deliberate slap in the face to us. [*Written in over line*. N.B. in order to get hold of a stranger, they raised the salary this year, for the first time, from about £40 to £100, this was done with a purpose]. It is a studied impeachment of our honour, because we have a plethora of competent Irish examiners at home, even of University standing like Father Dineen, P. Pearse, Miss O'Farrelly, O'Neill, etc, etc, and the action of the Commissioners is as much as telling the public that we cannot be relied upon!

Now please don't be in any way put out or distressed if an outbreak of the first magnitude occurs, as soon as your appointment is publicly made known. Nothing is intended, nothing will be hinted, against you. The attack if made (and I am convinced that it cannot be avoided) will be directed solely against the Commissioners. It is no use my attempting to prevent such an attack, I would be over-ridden. If then it breaks out and I take part in it as President of the League, you will understand exactly what is taking place, and why.

I need not say that you personally have earned the gratitude of every Irishman, and I have the most absolute confidence in you, but the Commissioners must be checked.

Now I have written absolutely frankly to you, and I know you do not mind, and will understand what is behind the scenes so far as we are concerned. I hope to be in Dublin before the end of this week but I fear you will be gone by that time. I do hope you shall be able to pay me a visit in March. It would be a great pleasure.

Mise
do chara
An Craoibhín

Do not understand from what I have said that I shall not try to check the outburst of anger which I foresee. I shall try, but, I fear, in vain.[52]

One cannot withhold a feeling of sympathy for Drs. Atkinson and Mahaffy. Distinguished scholars as they were, they had no notion of what a subtle antagonist they were facing in Douglas Hyde who was, in the traditional phrase, trí chor den bhóthar rómpu – three turns of the road in advance of them. The result was what he had foreseen.

Kuno Meyer's marks were even higher than those of the Irish examiners and more than justified the standards which they had been setting. The hostility of the scholars who had opposed any status for the language was thoroughly subdued. Douglas Hyde believed that this action of Kuno Meyer's saved the language from being crushed and elbowed out of the Intermediate Examination.

Meyer was an interested spectator at the performance of Douglas Hyde's *An Tincéar agus an tSidheog* in George Moore's garden, 4 Ely Place, on May 19, 1902, using a galley print of the text to follow the play.[53] Moore, a friend, albeit a mercurial one, invited him to be his guest when he should be in Dublin in June to mark the Intermediate papers. Meyer had evidently sent him his text and translation of the Song of the old woman of Beare and Vision of Laisrén.[54] Moore's invitation reads:

4 Upper Ely Place,
Dublin,
May 27th

Dear Dr. Kuno Meyer

I had a presentiment that your letter would be an interesting one and I looked forward to hearing from you; and your letter, which arrived on Sunday, suggests so many things that I think you had better stay with me when you come to Dublin in June for the examinations. You will be engaged all day with examination papers and may find relaxation in talking literature with me in the evening. I shall be glad if you will stay here instead of going to an hotel for your conversation will be of great interest and advantage to me. The stories you send to me are strange relics of an ancient civilisation – I like the old woman the better of the two; but Villon's version of the last years of her who has been loved by many men is more clear and explicit. The Irish poem is dim and vague as the Book of Kells. The French poem is like sculpture – the Irish mind does not seem to have passed from the stage of arabesques to that of sculpture.[55]

In his Preface to the love story of *Liadain and Curithir*, dated 12 January 1902, Meyer foreshadowed the steps he was to take in the following year to have the manuscript content of Irish literature scientifically edited and published. He pointed out that early Irish literature, in its full extent and variety, was known to none as yet. No one could speak with authority on it as yet. It was unexplored and unknown. Of the large body of tales and poems in manuscripts only a relatively small number were published with translations and very few of these in such a form as to appeal to the general reader, 'for the public will not take much interest in Irish literature until men arise to do for it what Dasent has done for the Old Norse sagas, or what Rückert and Schack did in Germany for Oriental poetry'. *Liadain and Curithir,* an Irish love-story of the ninth century, was acknowledged by Augusta Gregory:

Coole Park
Gort
Co. Galway
June 7 (1902)

A great many thanks for the 'love-story' – very charming and will be a framework for poets – how much you have done for Irish; I do think Trinity is silenced for ever. That is a beautiful verse 'Ceol caille - etc.' I hope W. Yeats will take some texts from it.

I have been speaking a good deal of time with your old grey men and women, looking for legends of the Fianna. I have got some, and a great many other stories, and a few versions of the Sons of Usnach. It is in cottages and workhouses here we find the really cultivated classes!

Always sincerely yours
Augusta Gregory.[56]

Meyer had been to dinner with Lady Gregory and W. B. Yeats. Stokes hoped he enjoyed it but Yeats did not fit into his pattern of merit. 'That minstrel's work I *cannot* enjoy. His verses seem to me as emasculated as Burne Jones' Knight, whom I always long to kick',[57] Stokes having a poor opinion of what he called the rant and incoherence of the so-called Celtic revivalists and a preference for Samuel Ferguson above all Irish poets.

University College Liverpool was in the beginning not an independent institution but a constituent college of Victoria University which was a federation of Manchester, Liverpool and Leeds colleges. With its progress and expansion there was a demand and a need for independence and this was granted by Charter of 15 July 1903 after which it became Liverpool University. It was a development watched with keen interest by Meyer. Writing to J. Glyn Davies in May 1901 he mentioned that strong moves were being made to found a Liverpool University and that he had hopes for a Celtic Chair. In October 1903 he told Glyn Davies that the Celtic Chair was almost pledged. The year 1902 was marked with important decisions on his part and developments in his favour. His health had improved as a result of changing to New Brighton in Cheshire where he benefited from the better air, although the disease which affected him, which he told Mary Hutton gloried in the name of rheumatoid arthritis, glossed as *crithgalar,* had taken a hold which could not be shaken off, yet his general condition was so good that he could afford to ignore it.[58]

In the summer he received an invitation to take up a Chair of Teutonic Languages in the University of London, about which he had correspondence with Sir Edward Lawrence, Chairman of Council, University College (two letters), and Principal Dale (three letters).[59] His staff colleagues, apprehensive that he might leave, and appreciating that his services could be retained if his devotion to Celtic studies were recognised in tangible form, submitted a printed Memorial to the Council of the University suggesting that a Chair of Celtic be established for the period of his tenure. Nineteen members put their names to it. It was successful. As a preliminary step Meyer was appointed Reader in Celtic. At a dinner organised to mark the occasion at which Meyer was the guest of honour, John Rhys, Professor of Celtic in Oxford, took the Chair and reviewed Meyer's learned contributions to Celtic scholarship, with special emphasis on his talent for the discovery of literature and poetry. How to reward his work could best be achieved by establishing for him a Celtic Chair in the University. The proposal was acclaimed by Frederick York Powell, Professor of History in Oxford, 'the ardent champion of Irish learning', and faithful supporter of Kuno Meyer, in an eloquent speech.

Kuno Meyer gracefully acknowledged the kindness of the speakers and audience on the occasion of his appointment to the Readership and of his having given up the idea of exchanging Liverpool for London. In the course of his speech he pointed to the necessity of giving those born

20

to a native knowledge of the Celtic tongues a 'Scientific and methodical teaching in their own language and in the history of that language'.[60]

By the end of 1902 Meyer had produced a body of work in Celtic studies that earned for him a special authority in the field. Having founded the *Zeitschrift für celtische Philologie,* and taken on the duty of editing it jointly with Ludwig Christian Stern, he had set it on a fair way to becoming a major influence in Celtic learning; with Whitley Stokes he had established in 1898 and conducted the *Archiv für celtische Lexicographie,* a compendium of Celtic glossaries, word collections and idioms, culled and supplied by various contributors, parallel with which he was, on his own part, assembling and publishing since 1898 instalments of his own *Contributions to Irish Lexicography* as being a preliminary step towards the creation of an Irish dictionary, which was the basic need in Irish studies. Not to speak of his numerous other contributions, texts, translations, and poems which appeared in a variety of publications every year since 1881, making in all an impressive corpus of work. In the course of his talk at the Liverpool dinner in his honour, John Rhys had singled out for special praise his edition of the wonder-tale *Aislinge Meic Conglinne,* the Vision of Mac Conglinne. A wonder-tale it was indeed, dedicated to Whitley Stokes, with acknowledgement for his assistance and thanks to friends including Eugene O'Growney whose scholarly knowledge of the modern language was the source of many suggestions.

Whitley Stokes, much pleased, had written - 'Mac Conglinne has arrived .... It is a first rate performance, in my opinion'[61] which was praise from Stokes, though he was aware enough of Meyer's integrity in scholarship to say that he would rather receive corrigenda than compliments. And for the fascinating text *The Voyage of Bran,* volume 1 of which appeared in 1895 in the Grimm Library series, with an essay by Alfred Nutt on the Irish vision of the happy otherworld, Stokes had words of high welcome, 'I am delighted with Bran',[62] which reminds us that Stokes, 'Son of two Crafts', was also a folklorist of a considerable order.

Commendation from him alone would suffice as tribute to Kuno Meyer. At the end of 1902 Meyer wrote to Mary Hutton:

> I have had a very restless life lately. I was on the point of accepting a post in London, but they have kept me here by the promise, among other things, of a Chair of Celtic. It is hoped that the Welsh, Irish and Scottish colonies here will collect the necessary endowment. Meanwhile, I have not been idle. I hope to send you shortly another green book containing some more Lyrics; and I have undertaken the edition of *Cáin Adamnáin,* a most difficult task, for the Clarendon Press. Professor Strachan will bring out an Irish Grammar and Reader as soon as he has finished the second volume of the *Thesaurus* with Stokes. That will place Irish studies on quite a different footing. If the same were done for modern Irish the beginner would then have little more to complain of.[63]

His decision to stay in Liverpool for the foreseeable future, and therefore within easy distance of Dublin, might be said to have important consequences. It might well have had a bearing on his proposal to launch formally his scheme for a School of Irish Learning soon after. The extraordinary success of the Gaelic League offered him a milieu and he chose its chief event of the year, the Oireachtas, as the occasion to announce his project.

NOTES

1. *Das Johanneum* (Hamburg) Heft 15, Juni 1931, 71-5.
2. Victor Ehrenberg, *Aspects of the Ancient World* (Oxford 1946) 221; Christhard Hoffmann, 'Eduard Meyer', in *Classical Scholarship, a biographical Encyclopedia* (New York and London 1990) 264-5.
3. Cf *Vita* in Kuno Meyer, *Eine irische version der Alexandersage* (Leipzig 1884).
3a. At a lecture given by Meyer in Belfast on Early Irish Literature, the Chairman, Dr. J. St. Clair Boyd, told the audience that Dr. Meyer came to take an interest in Celtic studies from the fact that as a boy he spent a couple of months on the Isle of Arran, off the coast of Scotland. He went to lodge with his friends in a farmhouse where the farmer and his family were Scotch-Gaelic speakers. This was his first acquaintance with the Gaelic and it excited his interest to hear those people speaking it. *Irish News* (Belfast), *News-Letter* (Belfast) 26 March 1902.
4. Letter of 4 Aug. 1881, from 4 High St., Lowestoft. TCD. Ms No 10085 (15).
5. *Revue Celtique* V, 195-204. Contribution dated Leipzig Oct 1881.
6. Quoted in R.I. Best: 'Whitley Stokes (1830-1909). A memorial discourse, 1951'. *Dublin Magazine* Vol. 32, No. 2, 5-18.
7. Meyer to Stokes, 11 June 1882, from Leipzig, Münzgasse 18. TCD Ms No. 10085 (16).
8. Letter of 2 Feb. 1884 from Jesus College Oxford. TCD Ms No. 4222.
9. 'The new universities' in *Freeman's Journal* (Dublin) 6 July 1908.
10. Walter Raleigh, 'Sestina Otiosa' in *Laughter from a cloud* (London 1923) 222-3.
11. Walter Raleigh, *Letters,* 2 vols (London) 1926. Vol 1, 236.
12. J. Glyn Davies: Celtic in University College and University of Liverpool. University of Liverpool Archives, Box 159, Page 1. Xerox copy supplied through the kindness of Mr. Adrian Allan, Assistant Archivist, 20 July 1983.
13. *A Celtic Chair for Professor Kuno Meyer*. Liverpool University Club 1903, p. 4.
14. J. Glyn Davies: Celtic in University College and Univ. of Liverpool. Univ. of Liverpool Archives, Box 159, pp. 3-5. Another account says the Irish class consisted of eight or nine students and a letter of Meyer's, dated 18.9.1889, shows his keen interest and readiness to accommodate learners of the language. *Irisleabhar Muighe Nuadhad*, Féile Pádraig, 1913, 7-8.
15. TCD Ms 10085 (23).
16. *Ibid.*
17. 'I am not surprised at Zimmer's Land-league propaganda' said Stokes, some of whose comments suggest a feeling of impatience with Zimmer, with whose social views he was out of sympathy. Stokes to Meyer, 30 Aug. 1889, from St. Giles, Oxford. TCD Ms No. 10085 (24).
18. For Father O'Donohue's career, cf An tAth. Mártan Ó Domhnaill, *Oileáin Árann* (B.Á.C. 1930) 267-274.
19. Stokes to Meyer, 30 Aug. 1889. TCD Ms No. 10085 (90).
20. Meyer to Stokes. TCD Ms No. 10085 (25).
21. TCD Ms No. 4222 (5).
22. Letter of 21 June 1886. TCD Ms No. 4222 (4).
22a. Stokes to Meyer, 30 March 1886, from 15 Grenville Place, London. TCD Ms No. 10085 (18).
23. Meyer, *Liadáin and Curithir* (1902) 7.
24. Robert Atkinson to Meyer, 4 Feb. 1889. TCD Ms No. 4222 (9).
25. Letter of 19 June 1899. TCD Ms No. 4222 (58).

26. Letter of 5 Dec. 1890, from 2 Salisbury Close, Cambridge. TCD Ms No. 4222 (28).
27. Letter of 4 Oct. 1889. TCD Ms No. 4222 (10).
28. Seaghan Pléimion to Meyer, n.d. TCD Ms No. 4222 (10).
29. Eugene O'Growney to Meyer. TCD Ms No. 4222 (15) to (20).
30. *Otia Merseiana* II (Liverpool 1901) 75-105.
31. J.B. Bury to Meyer, letter of 10 July (1901). TCD Ms No. 4222 (81). Dercna fróich = berries of health. Logg di shubuir = a dish of strawberries. The Greek quotation, from Pindar, Isthmian II, 17, means 'Money, money, makes the man.'
32. Bury to Meyer, 7 July (1902). TCD Ms No. 4222 (88).
33. Cf. 'John Sampson (1862-1931)' by Andreas in *Journal of the Gypsy Lore Society* (XI) 1932, pp 3-4.
34. Meyer to Stokes, 26 July 1892. TCD Ms No. 4224 (2).
35. E. Ó Gramhna to Meyer, 26 Feb. 1893 from St. Patrick's College, Maynooth. TCD Ms No. 4222 (22).
36. Meyer to Stokes, 30 Oct. 1883, from Hamburg, Abendrothsweg 37. TCD Ms No. 7970 (180).
37. Standish H. O'Grady, 'Remarks on the Oxford edition of the Battle of Ventry' in Philological Society *Transactions* (1884) 619-646. Quotation from p. 647.
38. TCD Ms No. 7970 (182).
39. Jeremiah Curtin to Meyer, 26 Sept. 1893 from 18 Torrington square, W.C., London. TCD Ms No. 4222 (26).
40. *The Gael* (New York) Oct. 1901, p. 299.
41. Meyer to Stokes. TCD Ms No. 10085 (32).
42. TCD Ms No. 4222 (33).
43. Stokes to Meyer, 21 Sept. 1894, from London. TCD Ms No. 10085 (81).
44. *Ibid.*
45. Details noted by the present writer and John Marin of the Deutsch-Irische Gesellschaft, Bonn, on the occasion of visiting the grave of Zeuss in Kronach on 28 May 1990.
46. *The Gael* (New York) Oct. 1901, p. 301; reprint in *Celtia* Nov. 1901, 167-9.
47. Meyer to R.I. Best, p.c. 8 Aug. 1909 from Segesvár, quoting paragraph from *Wiener Freie Presse* showing Mahaffy posing publicly as Irish nationalist. NLI Ms No. 11002.
48. Meyer to Mary Hutton, 23 Sept. 1901, from 6 Montpelier Crescent, New Brighton, Cheshire. NLI Ms No. 8616 (1).
49. Douglas Hyde to Meyer, 26 Jan. from Ratra, Frenchpark, Co. Roscommon. TCD Ms No. 4222 (82).
50. *Intermediate Education (Ireland) Commission,* Appendix to the Final Report of the Commissioners. Part II. Miscellaneous Documents. Dublin 1899. pp. 70-71.
51. Meyer to Mary Hutton, Tullyroe, Deramore Park, Belfast. Extract from two communications, 18 and 23 Feb. 1902. NLI Ms No. 8616 (2).
52. Hyde to Meyer, n.d. TCD Ms No. 4222 (92).
53. The galley proof is in NLI Ms No. 11002 with a note in the hand of R.I. Best, also present.
54. *Otia Merseiana* I (Liverpool 1899) 119-28.
55. George Moore to Meyer, 27 May (1902) from 4 Upper Ely Place, Dublin. TCD Ms No. 4222 (109).
56. Augusta Gregory to Meyer, 7 June (1902) from Coole Park, Gort, Co. Galway. TCD Ms.
57. Stokes to Meyer, 16 Feb. 1902. TCD Ms No. 10085 (81).
58. Meyer to Mary Hutton, 21 Jan. 1902, from 6 Montpelier Crescent, New Brighton, Cheshire. NLI Ms No. 8616 (2).
59. Correspondence 8 July-20 Oct. 1902. University Archives, Liverpool 66/7. Details courtesy of Mr. Adrian Allan, Assistant Archivist, University of Liverpool, communicated to writer 20 Oct. 1980.
60. *A Celtic Chair for Professor Kuno Meyer*. Liverpool University Club 1903. p. 11.

Meyer's tenure of appointments on the staff of University College Liverpool (later the University of Liverpool) comprised: Lecturer in German 1884-94, Professor of Teutonic Languages 1894-1903, Reader in Celtic 1903-08, Professor of German 1903-1911, Professor of Celtic 1908-1914. (Details from the University Archives, Liverpool, courtesy of Mr. Adrian Allan).

61. Stokes to Meyer, 2 Nov. 1892 from 15 Grenville Place, London, S.W. TCD Ms No. 10085 (29).

62. Stokes to Meyer, 29 Oct. 1895 from 15 Grenville Place. TCD Ms No. 10085 (34).

63. Meyer to Mary Hutton, 27 Dec. 1902, from 6 Montpelier Crescent, New Brighton. NLI Ms No. 8616. Early in April of that year Meyer had a visit from York Powell with whom he arranged for the Clarendon Press to publish *Cáin Adamnáin*, the Law of Adamnán which exempted women from military service. It did not appear until 1905 and sadly, York Powell, champion of Irish language and learning, did not live to see it. He is commemorated in the touching dedication.

Chapter 2

THE ideas that led to the establishment of a scientific School of Irish Learning had been articulated in the latter quarter of the 19th century, deriving their origin from the progress made on the European continent by German and other scholars in the scientific study of the language. Johann Caspar Zeuss of Bavaria, author of the celebrated *Grammatica Celtica* (1983), had been the pioneer in the exposition of Celtic grammar, to be succeeded in the same field by his disciple Hermann Ebel, who revised and republished his master's book in the light of more advanced knowledge. Others followed. Ernst Windisch, Heinrich Zimmer, Ludwig Christian Stern and Rudolf Thurneysen opened up the riches of Irish literature with critical and scientific editions of Early and Middle Irish Texts. The question began to be asked 'what are native Irish scholars doing?' which query would borrow the candid view that what they were doing was not being done well.

The columns of the literary weekly *The Academy* provided a forum for much important discussion and controversy. In a letter to *The Academy* of 13 August 1881 Kuno Meyer had critical things to say about the text of 'The youthful exploits of Finn' edited by David Comyn, while indicating that he hoped soon to be able to publish the whole of that valuable text, a matter which drew a reply from Comyn (*Academy* 10 Sept 1881) in explanation and defence of his work. Joining in the discussion, David Nutt, in a contribution of 20 August, touched on a point which was becoming increasingly sensitive. After hailing the recent appearance of Heinrich Zimmer's *Celtische Studien* as marking a new era in Irish philology he expressed the hope that henceforth they might be rid of the uncritical slovenliness which had been the curse of Celtic studies. 'And I trust', he went on, 'that Irish scholars will be roused to the scandal and shame of allowing Germans to annex the whole of their rich and precious literature, while they stand idly by, and content themselves with publishing at rare intervals garbled scraps'. (*Academy* 20 Aug 1881).

A sense of rivalry, even betimes of veiled hostility, developed between the scientific philologists and the native traditionalist scholars. Amongst those who approached the study of Irish from the philological side was Whitley Stokes, who had no native knowledge of the language but was possessed of immense linguistic and etymological learning. It was a reference of his to 'the corrupt dialects of modern Irish' in the *Academy* of 1 December 1888 which drew an extensive comment from the editor of

25

the *Gaelic Journal*, John Fleming, in two letters to the *Academy* under the heading 'Old Irish and the spoken language'.[1]

Coming from a scholar of such reputation, said Fleming, the words would naturally convey to prospective students the notion that modern Irish was worthless for philological purposes, whereas the currently spoken tongue was really the only key to the understanding of innumerable passages in the earlier language. This might easily be proved by showing how scholars of old and middle Irish, who were ignorant of the modern speech, fell into egregious mistakes from which a knowledge of modern Irish might have saved them. Taking Stokes himself as such an example, and a contribution of his to *Revue Celtique* of May 1886 as text, Fleming went on to illustrate his argument by citing errors of Stokes therein 'from which a knowledge of the despised modern Irish would have saved him'. Caught offside, Stokes, who was a great controversialist, did not reply, wisely, for Fleming could be formidable, but the discussion was further developed in correspondence from John Rhys, Standish Hayes O'Grady, Alfred Nutt, Tomas O'Flannaoile and others, and included an important intervention by Kuno Meyer in the *Academy* of 28 September 1889.

Objective in his views and sympathetic to all sides, a friend of Stokes and held himself in the highest regard by Fleming, Meyer's approach was constructive and clear-minded. Defending scholars of the older language, he pointed out that they were handicapped by the lack of published materials in modern Irish, 'for modern Irish has no literature', nor, except for the *Gaelic Journal* (founded 1882), were there any papers or prints in the vernacular, nor any handbooks, grammars or dictionaries to represent the living language which might serve as an aid to scholars. Having posed the question of who were called on to supply these wants, Meyer offered the reply:

> Surely those alone who can do it, and from whom for many decades it has been expected. And so long as they neglect to fulfil this just expectation, they should not lightly censure those who, in the face of great difficulties, attempt to accomplish another task - a task which properly belongs to Irishmen too, but which they have long completely handed over to foreigners - the editing and translating of their great and unique mediaeval literature. If the spirit of nationality, which is at present re-asserting itself in Ireland, has any vitality in it, it cannot surely long remain indifferent to a heritage to which at least it can lay undisputed claim.[1A]

Later in more specific vein, Meyer lamented to the historian Alice Stopford Green that the holders of Celtic chairs in Ireland either could or would not do their duty in the fact that not one of them had founded a school.[2] Meyer probably had the matter under consideration when he was invited by the National Literary Society to lecture on Ancient Irish Literature and the claim has been made for the Society that his lectures, delivered on 22 January 1900 and 10 December following, resulted in the setting up of the School of Irish Learning.[3]

Stimulus came with the influence of the Gaelic League, founded 1893, the success of which gave Meyer the milieu in which he could with confidence make a public appeal for a School of Irish studies to go hand in hand with the popular movement. On Thursday 14 May 1903, under the auspices of the Oireachtas of the Gaelic League, he delivered a lecture in the Concert Hall of the Rotunda in Parnell Square on the subject of 'The necessity of establishing a School of Irish Literature, Philology, and History', the chair being occupied by the President of the Gaelic League, Douglas Hyde, who introduced the speaker. Chairman and speaker were indeed old friends, knowing each other's ways and views, having cooperated with subtle sympathy and understanding to uphold the status of Irish at the Intermediate Education inquiry of 1899.

Meyer began by pointing to the Gaelic revival as one of those almost elemental phenomena, the suddenness and force of which seemed to carry everything before it, astonishing nobody more, perhaps, than those who started it. Nor could the calmest and most sceptical onlooker remain indifferent, for the object at stake was the salvation of a nationality at the eleventh hour. In the course of a comprehensive address, which reviewed the resurgence of the Irish and Welsh languages, Meyer expressed the hope that nothing would be done to discourage the dialects, these being the rich source from which a literary language would develop. But it was necessary to bring the movement into direct and intimate relations with scholarship, to provide an avenue for every student of Irish to the higher regions of study and research, to crown the whole edifice by a revival of native scholarship, and thus to bring about a second golden age of Irish learning. (Meyer, too, was an idealist). Having surveyed the achievements of O'Donovan and O'Curry, he came to the heart of his message:

> Now it is absolutely necessary, if there is to emanate from Ireland work of first-rate importance in history, philology, literature, archaeology, that there should be established a school in which the foundation for these studies would be laid by a study of the Irish language and literature. Without a knowledge of the Irish language in all its stages - old Irish, middle Irish, modern Irish - no real advance in our knowledge of the various subjects mentioned above is possible, because the sources, the documents, are written in Irish. I need not here again dwell on the wealth and variety of Irish literature in all its branches, or reiterate what I have said elsewhere, that no one is in a position to speak with authority of it as a whole. The facts are not yet before us. But let us consider for one moment the magnitude of the task that has got to be accomplished. Let me begin with the language. To trace the history of the language from the oldest available records to modern times, to establish the laws which govern it, to follow its changes from period to period, from dialect to dialect, then, when all this has been done, to date and locate every piece of prose or poetry with exactness - these are some of the tasks which await the student of Irish philology. As to literature, the amount and variety of the work to be done is even greater. Here is the oldest vernacular poetry and prose of western Europe - handed down in hundreds of manuscripts, very few of which have been edited, many of which have hardly been opened for centuries, while the majority have only been hastily glanced at. What a task for generations of students! Who can say what revelations await us, what revolutions in our knowledge may be in store here? Every new publication comes as a surprise. The general reading public and the majority of the learned would almost refuse to credit the wealth, the age, the beauty, of this literature.... It would take me too long to continue this sketch of the work awaiting the hand of the historian, archaeologist and

27

topographer. I will say once more that, whatever the foreign student may achieve, he cannot hope to cope with its difficulties so successfully as the native student. It is a task which must be accomplished by Irishmen and Irishwomen essentially.[4]

Ending his address with an impassioned appeal, Meyer declared his own willingness to make a start on the morrow, given a room, blackboard and students. The journey from Liverpool was short and he could come often. All that was needed for a beginning was to hire a room or two in the centre of Dublin and install a working library. His scheme was not Utopian. There were, he believed, hundreds of young people eager to respond to it and equip themselves for research in the early literature of their language. He would leave the matter there in the full conviction that he had not spoken in vain. (For text of address, see Appendix, pp 240-46).

Amongst those who applauded Meyer's address was Father Peter O'Leary, greatest modern Irish writer of the day. Writing in the *Weekly Freeman* he agreed the plan was not Utopian but practical, bold and imbued with exactly the sort of daring which from the start had characterised the work of the Gaelic League. Noting Meyer's comment on the importance of the living Irish speech and its dialects, he would like to hear him call on the native speaker to participate, because there was not the remotest possibility that anything could be done without him. Dr. Meyer, he observed, was astonished at the strength and virility of the Gaelic League. 'I can tell him where the strength and virility originated. The native Irish speech has been from the start permeating the movement, carrying its "vulgar" vigour into the framework of the movement, in spite of the prejudices of your "scholarly" people'.[5] This was an echo of what John Fleming had said years earlier. Father O'Leary stressed that it must be the duty of the Gaelic League to supply the motive source of energy. Father O'Leary's influence in the language revival made certain that heed would be given to his voice. Kuno Meyer was a sympathetic listener.

Within six weeks of Meyer's Oireachtas address the School of Irish Learning took practical shape. He wrote to his Belfast correspondent Mary Hutton on 22 June:

> I am crossing to-night to open the little Summer School of Irish studies by an address to-morrow. Professor Strachan is going to hold the first course in July, Old-and Middle-Irish. Will you be able to attend? Even a few attendances if you could not take the full course would be of great advantage.[6]

He gave his address next day in the Aula Maxima of University College, St. Stephen's Green, made available through the good offices of Dr. William Delany, S.J., whose support throughout was warmly appreciated by Meyer.

In a full discourse he set out the objects and system of the school in greater detail than his Oireachtas lecture had permitted and his two addresses taken together form one of the most important statements in the history of Celtic scholarship. They are basic documentation for the

28

character of the School and have a bearing on all subsequent developments in Irish language studies.

Having read carefully all that appeared on the subject in the newspapers following his Oireachtas lecture, Meyer thanked the Dublin press for its support and spoke with special appreciation of Father O'Leary's letters. He proposed to set out exactly what they planned to do in 'this Summer School which will be opened in July.' In his view nothing was more important or necessary for the advance of native Irish scholarship than a thorough acquaintance with the older stages of the language, without which no genuine progress could be made in the study of Irish literature, history and archaeology, nor indeed was it possible to obtain a scholarly knowledge of modern Irish without an acquaintance with its older forms. For this purpose they had been fortunate in securing the services of John Strachan, Professor of Greek at Owens College, Manchester, who would devote part of his Summer vacation to the great cause which he and all the promoters of the scheme had at heart. Meyer went on to discuss the details of the scheme, which was the establishment of a permanent School of Irish Studies, under the heads of organisation, funds, housing, staff, students and teaching methods.

The School he envisaged would accommodate native speakers, those whose modern Irish was acquired orally or from books, students of literature, history and archaeology, students of classical or modern languages who wished to know Irish for literary or philological purposes, all of whom should find in the School what they wanted.

For the basic principle which would guide the School in its teaching methods, Meyer took as text the canon proposed by his Liverpool colleague Walter Raleigh, that the increase of knowledge was the faith by which men of learning lived, the creed that united students and teachers in a common aim, and inspired them to work together, so that the students would advance in the feeling that they were in contact with knowledge in the making and would acquire those habits of careful enquiry and independent judgement that were the only guarantees of human progress.

Closing his address with his belief in what the school should envisage as its ideal, Meyer revealed himself as a man of tremendous faith: 'For its object is and motto should be: increase of scholarship, advance of knowledge and learning, for the benefit of mankind, for the Glory of God'.[7]

A similar aspiration had been uttered in an earlier era by Michael O'Clery.

In the discussion which followed approval for Meyer's enterprise came from Dr. Cox, Patrick Weston Joyce, Edmund Hogan, S.J., John MacNeill, T.W. Rolleston, Dr. Delany, S.J., and Douglas Hyde, great names in their time, all of whom stressed the advantages that would accrue to the Irish language from such a foundation.[8] The first of Dr. John Strachan's lectures was announced to take place in the Aula Maxima of University College on the 6th of July. Hard hitting but not unhelpful criticism came once again from Father O'Leary, who took exception to Meyer's view that without a thorough acquaintance with Old Irish no genuine progress in Irish language learning was possible, a process he compared to climbing a tree by beginning at the top. In denouncing it, he put forward with vigour his own conviction that it was impossible for any person to interpret our old language without a thorough knowledge of the living speech, that one must work backwards from the present, stage by stage, to a comprehensive knowledge of Irish, modern, middle and early, and in the attempt to demolish Meyer's theory he took up one and a half closely printed columns of the *Weekly Freeman*.[9] For all the vigour of his criticism, Father O'Leary warmly approved of the project and became a strong supporter of the school and one of Meyer's well-respected friends.

Criticisms notwithstanding, Meyer lost no time. The School was set up, and the first session held in July 1903 in the Aula Maxima of University College, St. Stephen's Green, lent for the purpose through the kindness of the President, Dr. Delany, who is praised in private correspondence of Kuno Meyer, along with Alice Stopford Green and Lord Castletown, as one of the School's best friends.[10] The opening session has been documented by the methodical Richard Irvine Best, whose bound notebook of 137 closely written pages of neat miniscule records his notes of 'Professor Strachan's Lectures on Old Irish Grammar delivered at University College, Dublin July 6th to July 31st 1903',[11] evidence of how earnest and careful a learner he was. At a very early stage Best became Secretary of the School and to all intents and purposes its historian. The long association between himself and Meyer, beginning at that time, is important for the result that the correspondence between them traces the vicissitudes of the School, of its students and teachers, of its fortunes, good and bad.[12]

John Strachan lectured on Old-Irish grammar for four weeks, two hours daily, using Whitley Stokes' edition of the Würzburg Glosses as textbook and for paradigms Windisch's Old-Irish Grammar of which two English translations were available. For these lectures forty students enrolled, coming from Galway, Cork, Waterford, Belfast and Sheffield, nearly all of whom were more or less conversant with modern Irish. Amongst them was Patrick Pearse. Professor Strachan also held a morning class for more advanced students, with *Táin Bó Cúalgne* for text, in Edward Gwynn's rooms in Trinity College.[13]

In September Kuno Meyer held classes in Irish palaeography and manuscript reading for three weeks, one and a half hours daily, with twelve students in attendance. Photographic reproductions of Irish manuscripts of various ages were read and studied and instruction was given in methods of cataloguing and editing. Dr. Henry Sweet (known to later acquaintances as 'Bitter Sweet' for his disappointment in academic prospects) held a class in practical phonetics with special reference to Modern Irish, the object being to give students such knowledge of speech-sounds and pronunciation as would enable them to investigate the history of the language and record the Modern Irish dialects phonetically. Twelve students attended. A successful beginning had been made.[14]

Even before the first session opened Meyer and Best had being busy with preliminary details. According to the very earliest item of what was to become a lifetime correspondence between them, a postcard dated 27 June 1903, Meyer hoped for a good number of gifts for the School library and was asking friends to send any such to Best at 37 Molesworth Street, while he told Best to order O'Grady's Catalogue of the Irish MSS in the British Museum.[15] From David Nutt of London Meyer ordered Zeuss' *Grammatica Celtica*, Sarauw's *Irske Studier* and what was up to then published of Holder's *Altceltischer Sprachschatz*; Nutt promised some from his own list; Meyer himself donated the series *Zeitschrift für celtische Philologie* and *Archiv für celtische Lexicographie*.[16] The Council of the Royal Irish Academy presented some valuable books, as did Whitley Stokes, Edward Gwynn, Professor E. Kuhn and others. 'Could you help with a subscription? Above all things a library is needed', begged Meyer of Mrs Hutton[17] and two days later acknowledged the prompt and generous response of Mr Hutton and herself to his 'somewhat importunate request'.[18] Funds were accumulating. W.P. Ker of University College London sent £10 towards the Library, T.W. Rolleston £5, C.H. Oldham £5 for 5 years and Meyer had no fear about having all that was necessary for a good start.[19] He was delighted to hear of Mrs. Hutton's project to attend Professor Strachan's classes. 'You will be his best pupil', and he would give her a training not to be equalled by anybody except perhaps Thurneysen.[20]

By 23 July a sum of £24 was available for book purchase with hopes that it would increase to £50 and Meyer sent a list to Best of necessary books which might be bought cheaply secondhand in Dublin. 'Then we must really look for a flat large enough to house us. Unfurnished of course, so that we can get the suitable furniture.'[21]

He would like to have Sir Antony MacDonnell on the School's Board of Governors. Meyer was not averse to titled names, not from snobbery, but for the practical reason that they could be the agency of benefits for his project. Sir Antony, a native of Co. Mayo, now permanent Under-Secretary at Dublin Castle after a distinguished career in the Indian Civil Service, would be a valuable presence on the Board as giving an impression of official approval and might be a useful lever towards getting much needed finance. Meyer wrote to him and while waiting for an answer gave way to a doubt whether he would accept, as 'it might not be approved of in high circles', Sir Antony's own words as expressed.

But when the first Report of '*Sgoil Árd-Léighinn na Gaedhilge*/School of Irish Learning' appeared, coming from 27 Clare Street, Dublin and dated November 1903, the name of Rt. Hon. Sir A.P. MacDonnell, P.C. duly appeared amongst the distinguished list of Governors of the School, of which Kuno Meyer was announced as Director, R.I. Best as Secretary and J.G. O'Keeffe as Treasurer.[22]

27 Clare St., the first location of the School, was central and conveniently close to the National Library, Trinity College and the Royal Irish Academy. Its rental and furnishings were paid for through the kindness of Thomas Kelly of the New York legal firm of Kelly and Gatty and in all the subsequent reports of the School acknowledgement is made to Mr. Kelly's continued support. The hand of modern progress has not (yet) levelled the undistinguished looking building, although many external features of it have changed. 'I hope you will agree that we must not bother about attacks, criticism, etc.' wrote Meyer to Best on 6 November 1903. 'We have been so incredibly successful that I think we may say without vanity that we have set about it in the right way. We know what we want and we are fortunately strong enough to get it. Besides, whatever you do is criticised in Ireland. So we must just put up with it.' [24]

> I wish I could tell you all about the School, (wrote Meyer to Mary Hutton). The chief news is that Sir A. MacDonnell has promised us a grant of £100 for purposes of publication - but this must not at present go any further. Then we shall take a whole house as soon as possible. Mrs. Green is collecting money and has herself given another £25. Lord Castletown has promised £50. Both Dr. Sweet and I were greatly satisfied with our classes. I took the best students to the Academy to teach them to catalogue and copy, and they are eager to go on by themselves. We shall soon begin to publish... [24]

John Sampson, Librarian of Liverpool University, was expected to arrive the following March to advise on cataloguing methods, on which he was an expert, having produced catalogues that set an example to the British Museum, knowing besides a great deal about Irish manuscripts, 'the only scholar who has ever reconstructed the original Leabhar na hUidhre from its fragments ... not English, but Irish, a native of Corcach Mór.'

Sampson, large of frame, topped by a splendid dome, was a well-known figure in Liverpool, the friend of gypsies and no enemy to a bottle of gin. He had a talent for witty and accomplished verse with which he would entertain his friends. In the event he could not come to Dublin, detained by his great edition of Blake.

It was time for Meyer to turn his attention to the publications which would represent the School. One of these was to become the first ever journal in Ireland devoted to the scientific study of the Irish language. There was to be a companion volume devoted solely to the printing of texts with translation. He explained his design to Mary Hutton:

> I am seriously thinking of two publications in connexion with the School;
>
> (1) a periodical to be called *Éire*, on the model of the *Zeitschrift*, but for Irish philology and literature only.
> (2) a series of Irish texts with English renderings, on the model of Windisch's *Irische Texte*. I am at a loss for a good title for this latter publication. Perhaps you can suggest one. I hope you will contribute to both. The texts may be printed in Irish or Roman type as the contributors think best. I have already quite a number of contributions... [25]

Coming to the end of the year he had words of praise for Richard Best who deserved them if ever man did, for 'all your work in connection with the School. I don't know how we should and could have got on without you?'[26]

NOTES

1. *The Academy*, 24 August and 14 September 1889.
1a. Stokes wrote to Kuno Meyer on 28 Sept. 1889. 'The only fault I find with your letter in today's *Academy* is that it does not go half far enough. You might well have said that you and your countrymen could teach Fleming and his lot far more than they can teach you – that a dialect may be "corrupt" without ceasing to be instructive – a student may learn anatomy from a putrefying body – that the real reason why the Celtic Irish don't publish their literature is 'because they are afraid of having their inevitable blunders exposed.' (This, *I know*, is the reason for O'Grady's inactivity.)' TCD Ms No. 10085 (24).
2. Meyer to Alice Stopford Green, 22 May 1900, in R.B. McDowell, *A passionate historian* (Dublin 1967) 79, giving source as 'Wakeling papers'.
3. National Literary Society, 6 St. Stephen's Green. Reports and Balance Sheet 1916-17. Souvenir of Number Six ... Dublin 1918, pp 13-14 'It was the Society that invited Meyer to deliver two lectures on Ancient Irish Literature and as a result of his visits the School of Irish Learning was founded.' The lectures were entitled 'The Oldest Period of Irish Literature', 22 Jan. and 'Ancient Irish Poetry', 10 Dec. 1900. NLI Pamphlets 953.
4. The full text of Meyer's address is printed in *Celtia* May-June 1903, 82-86.
5. *Weekly Freeman* (Dublin) 30 May 1903.
6. Meyer to Mrs. Mary A. Hutton, Belfast, 22.6.1903, from 6 Montpellier Crescent, New Brighton, NLI Ms No. 8616 (3).
7. *Celtia* July-Aug. 1903, 99. The full text of Meyer's inaugural address is printed in this issue, pp 93-99.
8. *The Irish Daily Independent and Nation* (Dublin) 24 June 1903 gave an extensive report and supported the venture in its sub-leader 'Irish Learning'.
9. *Weekly Freeman*, 18 July 1903.
10. Dr. Delany's support is indicated in the following letter:

> Aug. 5, '03
> University College,
> St. Stephen's Green,
> Dublin
>
> Dear Dr. Meyer
> Many thanks for your kind letter. It was a very great pleasure to help in any way the excellent project initiated of establishing a School of higher study in Irish and I congratulate you heartily on the great success of Professor Strachan's course of lectures. You may count on me with confidence as eager to support in every way I can the further developments of the Scheme. Our Hall shall be at the disposal of the lecturer in September or at any other time during the year for *Evening Lectures* and for morning Lectures during the College vacations .... I shall gladly give the use of the Hall for the Lectures in Irish.
> Wishing you a pleasant holiday
> believe me
> yours sincerely,
> William Delany

T.C.D. Ms No. 4222 (90)
11. NLI Ms No. 11,008. Best's address then was 32 Upr. Baggot St.
12. They first met in 1903 at a dinner party in George Coffey's house, when Best told Meyer of his difficulties in acquiring a knowledge of Old Irish. Meyer volunteered

to help him on his flying visits to Ireland, if a room and blackboard were provided and a few serious students to make up a class. Best promised this, but meanwhile Meyer's lecture at the Gaelic League Oireachtas had taken place, to be followed by the Summer School in the Aula Maxima – Details from brief typewritten notes about Meyer, by Richard Irvine Best, among small collection of Eoin MacNeill's papers in Archives Dept. of University College Dublin.

13. First Report of 'Sgoil Árd-Leighinn na Gaedhilge/School of Irish Learning' 27 Clare Street, Dublin, November 1903. Copy in Eoin MacNeill Papers, NLI Ms. No. 10882.
14. *Ibid.*
15. NLI Ms No. 11,002.
16. Meyer to Best, by postcard 29.6.1903. NLI Ms No. 11,002.
17. Meyer to Mary Hutton 22.6.1903. NLI 8616 (3).
18. Meyer to Mary Hutton 24 July [*recte* June] 1903 on notepaper of Standard Hotel 81 & 82 Harcourt St., Dublin. NLI Ms No. 8616 (3).
19. *Ibid.*
20. *Ibid.*
21. Meyer to Best, 23 July [1903], from 6 Montpellier Crescent, New Brighton. NLI Ms No. 11,002.
22. The personnel of the School was as follows:

SGOIL ÁRD-LEIGHINN NA GAEDHILGE
School of Irish Learning

Governors:

Sir William Butler, KCB	Rev. E. Hogan, S.J. Litt.D.	John MacNeill, B.A.
Mrs. J. R. Green	Douglas Hyde, LL.D.	Whitley Stokes, D.C.L.
Edward Gwynn, M.A.	The Rt. Hon. Sir A. P.	John Strachan, LL.D.
	MacDonnell, P.C.	

Director:
Kuno Meyer, Ph.D.

Trustees:

Lord Castletown	Rev. W. Delany, S.J., D.D.	W.P. Geoghegan

Students' Committee:

R.I. Best	Miss M. Byrne	J.G. O'Keeffe
P. Bradley	Miss M. O'Kennedy	E. O'Naughton
J. H. Lloyd		Eamonn O'Neill

Secretary:
R.I. Best

Treasurer:
J.G. O'Keeffe

Bankers:
The Hibernian Bank, Dublin.

23. Meyer to Best 6.11.1903 from New Brighton. NLI Ms No. 11002.
24. Meyer to Mrs. Hutton 24 Sept. 1903, from Standard Hotel, Dublin. NLI Ms No. 8616 (3).
25. Meyer to Mary Hutton 18.10.1903 from Standard Hotel. NLI Ms No. 8616 (3).
26. Meyer to Best 23.12.1903 from New Brighton. NLI Ms No. 11,002.

Chapter 3

My thoughts often go back to the first days of the School of Irish Learning – that bleak stormy autumn, the days and nights of rain, the in and out of trams in the dripping tempests on your devoted way to lectures and classes, our one open restaurant, dinner of the unfailing "chop", and back in the rain to the hotel, where in the empty smoking-room you lay on the sofa and had your first rest and warmth. How vividly I remember your patience and fortitude. You were alone in believing a Dublin School could be formed. You rode down all doubts and criticism. And you carried through your work triumphantly.

Alice Stopford Green to Kuno Meyer 28 January 1915

NLI Ms No 11,001(2)

K UNO Meyer was a man possessed by a vision. This was to establish in Ireland a School that would reveal to the world the wealth and importance of Celtic, especially Irish, literature. *Volvere volumina Hiberniae,* to unroll to the witness of the world the contents of Ireland's ancient manuscripts, was a phrase he echoed in his writing.[1] As teacher, with a gift of communication that came from the love of his subject, he inspired the devotion and activity of his students. One of the School's alumni who became a distinguished scholar, Eleanor Hull, has written that the stimulating force of Meyer's teaching made itself felt over a whole generation of Irish and English students. 'He was a born teacher, vitalising, inspiring, encouraging, as no other teacher we have known has been.'[2] He envisaged for Irish studies a place on the curricula of the great universities of Europe and America. Time and time again he insisted that it was Ireland's duty to produce and publish the treasures hidden in her historic codices and that the proper way to do this was by the industry of her own scholars.

If native Irish scholars did not carry out the task, those of other nations would, and the disgrace would be Ireland's. Meyer did not allow his missionary zeal to be curbed by his painful arthritis. He appealed from platform and press, enlisted the support of friends and colleagues, negotiated for government aid, cajoled the great and wealthy to subscribe, stopping short at Carnegie who 'only cared for popular causes', and wrote innumerable letters. Here is one, which embodies the message he gave to all. The recipient was C.T. Hagbert Wright, LL.D.

Old Waverly Temperance Hotel
42-46 Princes Street
Edinburgh
6.2.1904

Dear Sir,
    In answer to your questions let me once more put the whole case briefly before you.
    Dublin should be the centre of Irish studies and publications. As neither the Royal Irish Academy nor Trinity College have made it such a centre, I founded the School of Irish Learning with the support of the best Irish scholars, many enlightened friends of Ireland and the Gaelic League. The two chief objects are to train young native scholars in Irish philology, and to publish Irish literature. If something is not done in Ireland now, the work of publication will go wholly to Germany, just as before the founding of the early English Texts Society the work of editing the older English Literature was almost entirely done by German scholars. I founded with the greatest ease two periodicals in Germany entirely devoted to Celtic studies. There is none in Ireland.
    Such an appeal as we are now making is of course quite new, and to many the word 'Irish' suggests a discreditable political agitation instead of a highly creditable growth of serious scholarship, little understood by the wealthy classes in Ireland.
    As we have begun so well, and found such ready support in various quarters, I feel confident that we shall soon set a standard of work for any future efforts in this branch of studies and higher education generally. Everything, as you know, is done with extreme economy, scholars like Professor Strachan, Mr. John Sampson and others are ready to devote their leisure to the School at a very trifling remuneration, but for purposes of publication a more substantial support than we have yet had is necessary. Sir Antony MacDonnell held out the hope of a grant from the Treasury and has repeatedly urged it upon them, but apparently without success. But even here £100 or £200 per annum would enable us to start at once with the publication of catalogues, editions and translations.
    I write in some hurry and confusion as I am on a journey.

Believe me,
Yours very faithfully
Kuno Meyer[3]

A modest flow of subscriptions began to arrive. It was great news to Meyer that Lord C. (Castletown presumably) had 'at last paid his first instalment'. A cheque for £5 came from Lord de Freyne, 'an Tiarna', French Park, Roscommon (was some subtle persuasion of Douglas Hyde at work?). The archaeologist R.A. Stewart Macalister sent his cheque from Jaffa. A telegram from Sir Antony raised hopes by announcing the grant from the Treasury, hopes that were deferred presently, and remained in doubt from time to time, until finally, after much to do, the grant materialised in the shape of £100 per annum, no great wealth but useful, until withdrawn after five years. Impatient at the wait for it, Meyer decided to rely on private subscriptions and to go ahead with printing the journal which would be called by the old nominative *Ériu* following John Strachan's preference. 'We must make a try with the first number. If you can get a good design for the title-page, do so; but it must be really good'.[5] To Best's fine eye for the aesthetics of print is due the excellent standard of typography begun and maintained by the journal. Some minor things did not go smoothly. James George

O'Keeffe of Ballintubber, Co. Cork, the hardworking secretary, was upset, and had to be consoled by Meyer who expressed sorrow that 'our impetuous friend Mrs. G. has written you an annoying letter. If it is any comfort to you to know that you have fellow-sufferers, let me tell you that she has written me several such.'[6] Is it possible in the context to think of anyone other than Mrs. Green, who was the School's most generous friend? But O'Keeffe had been ill, for which Meyer was sorry. His own health was very indifferent. To his natural wanderlust was added the necessity of going to health and treatment centres throughout Europe seeking relief from his racking arthritis. He never went anywhere without taking work with him. Following a course of baths at Pöstyén in Hungary, where he felt the better of the lovely climate but 'rather forlorn and lonely amongst these Magyars of whose language I understand nothing', most polite and kind though they were, we find him in mid-August 1904, after much more wandering, at Bad Cudowa, Germany, where he received the first issue of *Ériu* with which he was very pleased. The history of the Hungarian movement which he had been studying gave him some new ideas as to the Gaelic movement and these he put down in writing. As he was leaving Cudowa for Leipzig a letter from Best arrived with the news that Osborn Bergin had got a scholarship. This had been provided from the generous purse of Alice Stopford Green who wrote to Professor Strachan on June 8 that in order to secure the immediate progress of the School, she would guarantee a scholarship of £100 a year for two years and for a third if it proved desirable and necessary. A note by Best on her letter[7] confirms that the scholarship was for Bergin to study in Berlin under Heinrich Zimmer and Freiburg in Breisgau under Rudolf Thurneysen. Meyer was glad, having great hopes of Bergin, and considered that a year each with the two great German masters would be adequate, 'for I understand that he is already far advanced'.[8] He was glad too to hear that Mrs. Green was going to America and was sure she would not return empty-handed. A few hundred a year would set them up. Best, holidaying in Anascaul, Co. Kerry, was envied by Meyer, who never forgot his own fascinating excursion of earlier years to Corkaguiney. 'When you get back to Dublin ... you must send a copy of *Ériu* to Mr. Wyndham. I will write to him. Dr. Stokes is delighted with *Ériu*'[9] Nobody was held in higher esteem than Whitley Stokes by Meyer and to have the approval for the School *Journal* from a scholar and critic of his standing was achievement indeed.

Not long after his return from Hungary Meyer delivered an address to the Liverpool branch of the Gaelic League, on 26 October 1904, in which he outlined certain ideas he had developed during his stay in Hungary. Having referred to the series of 'brilliantly written and instructive' articles on Hungary (the work of Arthur Griffith) in the columns of the *United Irishman* Meyer, speaking as one who wished well to the Gaelic movement, pointed to the movement for the revival of the Hungarian language and literature which he had studied, as something that contained fruitful lessons for Ireland that were never more opportune than at the present moment. 'I desire most earnestly to promote the cause of the Gaelic Movement which, from its inception, has had my heartfelt sympathy and, so far as I have been able to give it, my co-oper-ation'.[10]

There being no further news of the promised government grant, his hope and trust now centred solely in Mrs. Green.[11] At this early date he had already noted the excellence of Osborn Bergin, who met him in Liverpool on his way to Berlin. 'There is no doubt that he is a wonder-fully gifted man and will be a great credit to the School'. Bergin was very keen on making the best of his stay in Germany. He had sent Bergin's paper on the modern Irish verb to be printed. What a fine piece of work Dinneen's dictionary was! They must order a copy for the Library.[12]

The indefatigable proponent of Irish studies, Alice Stopford Green, who had been to America to take soundings of support for the School, sent Meyer lists of people and institutions to whom circulars might use-fully be forwarded. It was hard, she advised him, to realise how ignorant they were that there was any literature at all 'except what Mr. Yates told them last year and he stopped at about 200 A.D.'[13] But she found their interest very ready to be aroused and the Catholic University at Washington was extremely anxious for co-operation. She offered to see Meyer anywhere convenient and give him details. Following their meet-ing Meyer addressed a letter to the Archbishop of New York, a draft of which in the Best papers provides a good example of Meyer's talent for persuasion. It was probably written at the end of 1904 and reads:

Most Reverend Archbishop

Mrs. J.R. Green has just given me the particulars of her work in America for the spread and advance of Celtic Studies among the Irish sections of the commu-nities and among the Universities there. She has told me of the great interest you take in the matter and asks me to supplement her statements by an account of what we are doing in Dublin and by a programme of work in America.

It was in the first instance the fact that any one who wished to study Irish or Celtic philology and literature, archaeology and history had to resort to the German or French Universities that first made me conceive the idea of founding a School of Irish Learning in Dublin. It met with generous support on all sides, and within a year and a half of its existence it has already trained more than a dozen young scholars who now continue to work under the direction of Professor J. Strachan of Manchester University, and myself. It has brought out the first num-ber of a learned periodical devoted entirely to Irish philology and literature and it has mapped out work.

But more workers are urgently needed. With the spread of the interest in Irish studies the time is not far distant when well-trained scholars will be needed all over the country for the most important posts, as professors at universities and colleges, teachers in the higher schools, librarians, and above all for the purpose of carrying on the work of editing and translating Irish literature. The general public and the learned world are only gradually beginning to realise the enormous amount of work to be done. As a student of Irish literature for over 25 years I do not hesitate to say that there is no other branch of learning - except, perhaps, the Oriental ... where so much remains to be done, where the wealth of material is so great, where the results to be achieved are more far-reaching, for the whole history of the middle ages, for the origins of mediaeval and modern literature.

Now, in the great work at the beginning of which we assist, America, and especially the American universities, should naturally cooperate. A country which has in the last decade or two developed so rapidly in ancient and modern research, where famous schools of Oriental, classical, romance and Teutonic studies have arisen, cannot continue any longer to exclude Celtic from its programme. We expect a great accession of strength from it. Mrs. Green was much impressed by the fact that it had hardly been realised as yet how the Irish and the Universities might work together and help each other in furthering this work.....

The simple organisation proposed by her to start the work would greatly strengthen our hands in Dublin ..... Mrs. Green has drawn up a short statement (which I enclose) on the first steps necessary towards such an end.

May I add one word more as to the real immediate needs of our School. It is not large sums of money that are wanted, but men to work, and organisation.

If we could get such a sum as £200 a year we could develop our work, both in teaching and editing, and our sole expenses, which have hitherto been borne by such friends of the movement as Mrs. Green, are the professional fees and printing and the founding of one scholarship. The increase of the latter is the very first need of the School....

The support and sympathy of America at the outset would react most favourably upon Ireland herself. One of our chief difficulties is that the wealthy people of Ireland set themselves against any movement that would restore to the Irish the memory of their history and language. It would also be a very great advantage if during the time the School is in session at Easter or in the long vacation (July-August) some students from America could take part in the work of the School.[14]

While it was Meyer's observation to Best that Mrs. Green had brought nothing back with her from America except promises,[15] this view must be qualified by the fact that from America presently came one of the School's most brilliant and imaginative alumni, Gertrude Schoepperle.

Meyer had personal worries. His mother was seriously ill with bronchitis and heart trouble. She was living with him in Liverpool, having come from Germany with her daughter Antonie when Meyer was stricken with arthritis. She got better as the year drew to a close, but the improvement was temporary. In the spring they both sought the warmer climate of Italy and there she died on 7 April 1905, at Battaglia. Meyer sent the news to Best: 'Early this morning my dear old mother died in my arms, after but a few days illness. Her old trouble, bronchitis acting on a weak heart, was the cause of her death'.[16] He asked Best to let John Strachan know. Best sent him words of consolation, for which Meyer was grateful. 'My mother was a woman such as one rarely meets now.'

NOTES

1. At the end of his lecture 'Learning in Ireland in the Fifth Century' delivered on 18 Sept. 1912 and published in Dublin 1913, p. 20.
2. 'Kuno Meyer' by a pupil. *Irish Book Lover* (XI) Dec. 1919, No. 5, 35.
3. NLI Ms No. 11,002. The name of C.T. Hagbert Wright, LL.D. appears in the list of donations and subscriptions to the School of Irish Learning in *Ériu* V for £6-6-0. He was once on the staff of the National Library.
4. Meyer to Best 28.2.1904 from New Brighton, NLI Ms No. 11,002.

5. Meyer to Best 10.2.1904. NLI Ms No. 11,002.
6. Meyer to James G. O'Keeffe 17.2.1904 from New Brighton. NLI Ms No. 2113.
7. Alice Stopford Green to John Strachan 8.6.1904 from 36 Grosvenor Road, Westminster. NLI Ms No. 15122.
8. Meyer to Best 28.8.1904 from Leipzig, Flossplatz 13 II p. adr. Frau Streiner. NLI Ms No. 11002.
9. *Ibid.*
10. Dated but unidentified presscutting in NLI Ms No. 11002.
11. Meyer to Best, postcard 30.9.1904. NLI Ms No. 11,002.
12. Meyer to Best, postcard 13.10.1904 addressed to Best at 37 Molesworth Street, Dublin. NLI Ms No. 11002. This was the first and smaller edition (1904) of Dinneen's Irish-English Dictionary.
13. Alice Stopford Green to Kuno Meyer 25.11.1904 from 36 Grosvenor Road, Westminster. NLI Ms No. 11002.

    In an interview with the *Westminster Gazette* of 24 December 1904 Mrs Green gave an outline of the work of the School:

> My scheme is the School of Irish Learning which was recently founded in Dublin by a small group of people, among them Dr. Whitley Stokes, whose subscriptions were devoted to the object of inviting two of the first professors in England to give vacation classes in Dublin for students of Old and Middle Irish. Dr. Kuno Meyer, from Liverpool University, is now head of the School, and Professor Strachan, of Manchester University, shares his work. The Irish school can now claim to offer opportunities that can be found nowhere else in the world. Its classes would be an honour to any German university ...
>
>   The school is worked on much the same plan as the École des Chartes at Paris, which was started sixty-four years ago for the editing of newly discovered MSS and for historic criticism ... Now the Irish school follows the same course of studies with smaller numbers, but with no less scholarly conscience. I have watched a class at work with the greatest interest, where the Professor gave to his pupils the photographs of an unedited Irish manuscript, which they have to decipher, copy and translate, and by the end of their studies the manuscript is practically edited, with the help of Dr. Kuno Meyer's corrections, and the students gain a first-class training in the process. The work of the School is regularly published, and the first number of the journal *Ériu* showed the high character of the work done.

14. NLI Ms No. 11002.
15. Meyer to Best 19.12.1904 from New Brighton. NLI Ms No. 11002.
16. Meyer to Best 7.4.1905 from Hotel des Thermes, Battaglia. NLI Ms No. 11002.

Chapter 4

IN a circular of 25 August 1905 issued by the School over the signatures of O'Keeffe and Best a brief outline was given of the School's progress, and an appeal made for funds to carry its work a step further. The School, it said, was founded for the purpose of training native scholars to investigate the great mass of literary and historical documents which had come down in the Irish language. During the three years of its existence it had published important material in *Ériu*, now recognised by competent authorities as the foremost Celtic Review. In the training of scholars also successful work had been done. But so far instruction had to be given from outside, by means of short summer courses. In the case of one or two of the best scholars, it was felt that this training should be continued for a longer period, and the means afforded them of acquiring a knowledge of the kindred Celtic tongues and the methods of philological research.

An Honours School in Celtic Languages had just been established at Manchester University under the direction of Professor John Strachan and it was hoped an Irish scholar could be sent over to take advantage of the instruction to be given there. Such a scholar was available, a graduate M.A. of the Royal University who had been a regular attender at the School and was considered by Strachan to be suitably qualified. As his own means were insufficient an appeal was being made on his behalf. A sum of £150, spread over two years, would meet the expense and of this £25 had already been promised. Subscriptions were invited, to be sent to Lord Castletown of Doneraile Court, Mrs. J.R. Green, 36 Grosvenor Road, Westminster or to the Secretary or Treasurer. A note in R.I. Best's handwriting on the margin of the printed circular tells us that the candidate for instruction was Joseph O'Neill. He was a student of much promise and a contributor to *Ériu* but caused Meyer deep disappointment when he presently withdrew from Celtic studies, for which he had been trained, to take up a post as Inspector under the Department of Education.

By July 1906 the School was well established and Meyer's draft report, dated 27 July 1906,[1] outlined its progress, noting that the third session just ended had been in every respect a success. As in previous years two courses were held, one of a fortnight's duration at Easter, another extending over a month in July. The Easter course, conducted by Meyer, on Old-Irish metrics and the study of poetry, was attended by twelve students. It was opened by a public lecture on Old-Irish Poetry attended by a large audience, Lord Castletown presiding. The July double course for beginners and advanced students, conducted by John Strachan, was attended by twenty who came from Ireland, England, Wales and America, the subjects being Old-Irish Grammar and the study of various Old- and Middle-Irish texts. A well- attended public lecture on Ogam was delivered in April under the auspices of the School by Principal Rhys of Jesus College Oxford.

Mrs. John Richard Green's generosity had enabled Osborn Bergin to continue and finish his studies in Germany with Professor Zimmer in Berlin and Professor Thurneysen in Freiburg. He had just obtained his degree of Ph.D. *magna cum laude* at Freiburg on the subject of 'Palatilisation in Irish,' which was an important contribution to the history of the language. The liberality of Lord Castletown and others had enabled Joseph O'Neill to spend a year with Professor Strachan at Manchester University and to proceed to Freiburg to continue his studies there. At the centenary of Johann Kaspar Zeuss, the founder of Celtic Philology, celebrated at Bamberg in Bavaria on July 31st, the School, together with many Universities and Academies, was represented by the Director, Kuno Meyer, who deposited a laurel wreath in the name of the School on the grave of Zeuss at Kronach.

Since the School was now about to enter on a further development more funds were urgently needed. It was proposed that Osborn Bergin should come to live in Dublin as a permanent Professor of the School, at a salary of £120 a year ['initial salary of £80' overwritten in pencil], to conduct classes in Irish, particularly Old- and Middle-Irish, from October to July. It was hoped he could take up residence on the premises of the School which had now moved to 33 Dawson Street.

Mrs. John Richard Green had promised to continue her contribution of £100 for scholarships. The thanks of the School were due to her as to many other benefactors, notably Lord Castletown, Douglas Hyde who had collected £55 from citizens of New York, the Secretary R.I. Best and the Treasurer, J.G. O'Keeffe, for valuable services freely given.

The report was signed by Kuno Meyer, who sent it to Best with a letter asking him to amend or add where necessary. 'How do we stand financially? No so bad, I think. £100 from the Government, £100 from Mrs. Green, £55 from Hyde, £? from subscriptions. Have the books sold fairly well? All this O'Keeffe will work out. Could the back rooms in Dawson St. be possibly made habitable for Bergin? He has his exam tomorrow. Thurneysen told me he is of course sure to pass with flying colours'. Such was the position of the School at the end of July 1906.

'Dear Mr Best', wrote Strachan, 'I think *Ériu* is going to flourish. The first volume need not fear comparison with any other Celtic periodical and it should get better and better.[2] The *Journal* of the School of Irish Learning, *Ériu*, John Strachan's choice of title, first issued in 1904, was 'Devoted to Irish Literature, History and Philology'. With the appearance of Volume V a four page folder was circulated describing its range and purpose with a view to attracting more subscribers. It was issued

42

from the School's new premises, 122A St. Stephen's Green, corner of York Street, opposite the Royal College of Surgeons. The names of its editors are long familiar to students of Irish: Meyer and Strachan, Vols I-III, Meyer and Bergin, Vol. IV, Meyer and Marstrander, Vol. V. Established for the publication of scholarly editions and translations into English of the manuscript materials preserved in the Irish Language and illustrating the Literature, History, Religion and Social Life of ancient and mediaeval Ireland, also investigations into the history of the Irish Language from the earliest times to the present, its range of interest accorded with the German notion of *Altertumswissenschaft* which Meyer introduced to Irish studies.

These manuscripts dated from the eighth to the early nineteenth century, and their contents might be classified under the heads of (1) *Religious Literature* and documents bearing on the history of the Early Irish Church, such as Lives of Saints, Visions, Homilies, Commentaries on the Scriptures, Monastic Rules, Hymns, Religious Poetry, etc; (2) *Prose Epics* of which a great number remained yet to be edited and translated; (3) *Bardic Poetry*, of which practically nothing had been published; (4) *Brehon Laws*; (5) *History*, consisting of Annals, Tribal Histories, Genealogies and Semi-historical Romances; (6) *Learning*: Treatises on Latin and Irish Grammar, Glossaries, Metrical Tracts, Astronomical, Geographical and Medical Works, the value of which for the history of Irish Learning in the early centuries, and in the Monastic schools, could not be exaggerated; Selections from Classical and Mediaeval Literature such as Lucan's *Pharsalia*, Heliodorus' *Aegyptiaca*, numerous Arthurian Romances, Chansons de Geste, etc; (8) a vast amount of anonymous and popular Poetry, mainly lyrical, of which hardly anything had yet been edited.

Such was the prospectus of work envisaged by the School. Until these documents were published and made the subject of critical study, no proper History of Ireland, her language or institutions, was possible. The *Journal* could claim with truth to be 'absolutely indispensable to all students of ancient Irish history and Celtic civilisation'.

The second periodical for which Meyer had proposed *Irische Texte* as a model and invited Mary Hutton to suggest a title, never developed into anything like the sumptuous *Irische Texte* series. In fact it took its title *Anecdota from Irish Manuscripts* from the contributions Meyer had earlier been printing in the *Gaelic Journal*. Meyer's initial design for it was over-ambitious. The *Irische Texte* series edited by Whitley Stokes and Ernst Windisch and published in Leipzig, was comprised of impressive tomes of which the first numbered over 800 pages. The editorship of *Anecdota* was shared between Bergin, Best, Meyer and J.G. O'Keeffe, it was printed by the expert hand of Ehrhardt Karras, Halle a.S. and published jointly by Max Niemeyer of Halle and Hodges Figgis of Dublin, the first number of 80 pages appearing in 1907. The Preface stated that this was the first instalment of hitherto unedited Irish texts, undertaken with the object of furnishing fresh material for investigation to the increasing number of workers to whom the original manuscripts were inaccessible and with the hope that it would provide handy textbooks for students.

It was hoped to issue a volume every six months to serve as a useful auxiliary to *Ériu* but as things turned out only five volumes in all appeared between 1907 and 1913, each with an 80 page or so content. In the general curtailment of learned activities caused by the European war of 1914-18 it ceased to appear.

The names of Max Niemeyer, publisher, and Ehrhardt Karras, printer, are inseparable from any account of Celtic studies of the time and must be accorded an honourable mention for their standards, skill and overall cooperation. Their names appear again and again in correspondence in terms of approval.

Despite his physical handicap, Meyer travelled a great deal. While much of this was due to his pursuit of health, which obliged him to travel to various clinics and resorts for treatment of his arthritis, there was in his nature a restless questing urge that drove him to old cities and centres of Europe whose repositories might yield a Celtic gloss, manuscript or poem, for his peregrinations had for their constant object the enrichment of knowledge, especially of the Celtic kind. 'J'admire votre ubiquité'[3] said Gaidoz.

Ubiquitous he was. One of many journeys found him on New Year's Day 1907 in Seville, where at his hotel table a guest who was obviously not Spanish sat down to breakfast. An exchange of greetings revealed that he was Irish. 'An bhfuil tú Connachtach?', enquired Meyer, whose modern Irish was not quite perfect, to be answered 'Táim go deimhin', his acquaintance proving to be a Lynch of Galway, with no other business than to see the world. In Cordoba Meyer found no manuscripts but picked up a lot of old and curious books. On the *S.S. Africa*, off Tagus mouth on 8 January, in perfect weather with a sea blue and calm, he passed the morning reading Cervantes' *Rinconete y Cortadillo*, a delightful picaresque story of two charming young scoundrels.

A great new project now occupied his mind, which was to cost him much thought and concern during the years ahead. This was the long-projected Dictionary of the Irish Language, which in this year of 1907 had fallen to his responsibility. Many ideas about it came to his mind, one of which was that it was altogether premature and should be dropped for the present, another that the scale might be reduced, as for instance that John Strachan might produce a dictionary to the *Thesaurus Palaeohibernicus* and other Old-Irish texts.

A comprehensive dictionary was long felt to be necessary if real progress was to be made in Irish language studies. Such a work was projected in 1852 under the auspices of the Irish Archaeological Society and was entrusted to Ireland's leading scholars John O'Donovan and Eugene O'Curry, but death struck both of them early, leaving only preliminary collections from their hands for the great work. Little was done until 1880 when Robert Atkinson became editor, holding the responsibility for twenty seven years, making limited progress because, excellent though he was in many respects, this task was really beyond his abilities. Whitley Stokes was always critical of his capacity for it and, if we know his mind, approved hugely when Atkinson retired in 1907.[4] Meyer succeeded him as overall director of the project, with Bergin as editor. The project was henceforth under the aegis of the Royal Irish Academy, the venerable institution of learning and science situated in 19 Dawson Street Dublin.

Meyer's qualifications for the task were obvious. He had an established connection with the Royal Irish Academy since 1904 when he was elected Todd Professor in the Celtic Languages, an appointment accorded to a Celtic scholar of first rank with the duty of giving and publishing lectures on suitable Celtic themes as a memorial to the 19th century scholar James Henthorn Todd. His reputation as a lexicographer had been long and widely acknowledged. With Whitley Stokes he had been engaged since 1898 in publishing collections of Celtic glossaries and allied material in the *Archiv für celtische Lexikographie,* completing the third volume in 1907, added to which was the related work *Contributions to Irish Lexicography A - DNO,* a collection excerpted from Irish books and manuscripts in the course of his wide reading. The expression *Contributions* occurs quite often in the context of the Dictionary discussions in the sense that the meanings of words given therein were to be not discursive but brief, concise, exact.

There was another factor to be considered which was later to affect the production of the Dictionary but for the present remained in the background as not being urgent. The Reverend Maxwell Henry Close, a great champion and supporter of the Irish language, who died in 1903, left a bequest of £1000 to the Academy to go towards the expenses of printing an Irish dictionary, on the specific condition that if some portion of the dictionary were not in print within ten years of his death the bequest would lapse. This meant that portion of the dictionary was to appear by August 1913 to be exact. It was 1907 and there was as yet no need for alarm on that score.

For the present, Meyer enjoyed his voyage back to England, passing Finisterre, the 'Críoch na Cruinne' of Irish literature, with the Bay smooth as glass, wondering whether George Moore was in Dublin, but preferring to stay with Best as they had much to talk over. 'I want to give a little dinner party at Jammet's on Saturday evening, to which I hope you and your wife, Bergin, Gwynn, and if he cares, Moore will come'. He employed the leisure of the voyage to write to them.

In London he would stay at the Thackeray Hotel, Great Russell Street, opposite the British Museum, where he worked frequently, although finding its draughty, ill-lighted manuscript room a strain, on which he blamed a near-serious eye ailment which beset him in 1910. On these occasions he would lose no opportunity of seeing Alice Stopford Green, who lived at 36 Grosvenor Road and the Irish scholar whom he admired over all else, Whitley Stokes.

45

'I saw Whitley Stokes last night, wonderful well and active.' Stokes was editing *In Cath Catharda*, the Civil War of the Romans, a redaction of the first seven books of Lucan's *Pharsalia*, whose rhetoric appealed to the mediaeval Irish writer and was cast by him into the form of the *scél* or story. Stokes had it nearly ready for press, having worked out a huge glossary to it. This was no doubt a satisfaction to Meyer, for glossaries could go to swell the Dictionary. He was also happy to find a new vellum manuscript in the Museum, lately bought, full of interesting things, especially versions of the shorter *Táins* which were by way of being satellites to the great epic tale *Táin Bó Cúalgne* or Cattle Raid of Cooley.

A discussion about the Dictionary with the Royal Irish Academy Committee was not a success. He was far from being happy with the Committee, since most of its members had not the remotest notion of what work the Dictionary entailed. Meyer wanted a special Dictionary Subcommittee of experts to include Best, Bergin, Hogan, Westropp, Gwynn, John MacNeill, perhaps Louis Claude Purser, and Douglas Hyde. 'One cannot waste one's time and strength over such absurd scenes as that of yesterday.'[5] Lloyd Praeger could represent the official element on such a committee. He put his ideas into writing and sent a report and suggestions in a formal letter to the President.[6] On 10 July he left for Berlin, where he used to stay with his brother Eduard at Mommsenstrasse 7. He spent several hours at the Egyptian Museum to see how work was progressing on the Egyptian Dictionary. 'It made my mouth water to see the long series of rooms, all with iron walls and doors, the large number of workers and the way in which the work was being done'. Director Erman explained it all to him and he learned a great deal. They had pretty much the same difficulties as they had in Dublin with the Irish Dictionary as regards the scientific part of the work, badly edited texts, much unpublished material 'though not nearly as much as we have', difficulties of interpretation etc., but then they were partly supplied by the government, partly by scholars and institutions all over the world with all that was necessary to overcome their difficulties. They practically transcribed every text afresh and correctly, and thus revised the whole of the existing structure, which would then be published. 'It made me realise once more that the R.I.A. do not understand the task upon which they have embarked, and that I have to work with wholly insufficient means.' Meyer proposed to remedy this, with the new Committee as the first step.

Praeger and Falkiner were bothering him about a statement of probable expenses, as if this were the moment to talk of that. He hoped Maud Joynt would come to Liverpool in October to learn the trade of dictionary making; Marstrander had other plans and was doubtful. Meyer saw that if he wanted further assistance he would first have to train students. Perhaps Bergin might discover one or two for him. Meyer was off to Pöstyén on the morrow.[8] But by the end of the year he had still not arrived at a firm decision about the worrisome problem of the Dictionary. He unburdened himself to Best:

> As to Dictionary matters I know not what to think, or write, or do. What with the state of my health, my endless and evergrowing work here - I have not been able to sit down for real work ever since October - Bergin's slow though excellent and indispensable methods, the necessity of embodying the vocabulary of the glosses both in single words and phraseology, the lack of assistants - what can one suggest? MacClelland says go on with the Contributions. But what would the Council say to that? They can hardly be called a Dictionary. The truth is none of these gentlemen understand the difficulties of the task, and I do not understand their interpretation of the bequest. They would have been glad to have had a Dictionary from Atkinson on the 'concise' plan. After all a Dictionary is a Dictionary whether it contains numerous illustrations or not. Ask Praeger's advice. I trust greatly in him.[9]

On July 22nd[10] Meyer set out for one of his favourite resorts, Pöstyén, in Hungary, for the improvement of his health but with no desire to separate himself from work. A letter and proofs from Best reached him on the 28th and Meyer had no good to say of the Dublin University Press which had failed to send him proofs of the Reader of Poetry which was to be included with his Primer of Irish Metrics. 'Mo mallacht forru!' The Bests were going to 'Sunset View' Kilkee on holiday and his sister Antonie had arrived in Bruges.[11]

Kilkee sounded pretty to Meyer, who had travelled little in Ireland despite his immersion in its literature. In Pöstyén his window faced the sunrise. Every morning he was up at 5, was driven to the bath, returned at 6.30 to go to bed again for an hour, then washed and took breakfast in a flood of sunshine by an open window. Then he generally worked for two hours doing an index to the three volumes of the Archiv but it was hard to get through the rest of the day for want of company. He strolled, sat around, spent some time on the river and went to bed about 9. Antonie was touring up the Rhine with a niece and was due at Coblenz. He hoped Best would not work too much in Kilkee. Strachan's Welsh book would be a great boon and might cause the Welsh at last to take up their ancient language at the University.[12]

He read Tauchnitz novels, 'awful rubbish'. Unfortunately they had stopped the German Theatre where he was. They only played in Hungarian now. He wished he could send the Bests some of the delicious peaches and melons which were to be had for almost nothing in Pöstyén. Even Doctor Johnson could have eaten his fill. He had written Atkinson to come to Hungary. 'They actually cure cases like his here, as I have seen myself. What do doctors know! The humbugs.' He was delighted that Best was so pleased with Kilkee. It looked a magnificent coast and were he not so rheumatic he would like to imitate (for a while) Senan and other old Irish saints in spending some time on those rocks and inlets.

A melancholy card had arrived from poor O'Keeffe who was tortured by toothache. Meyer himself had been feeling wretched recently with all sorts of pains brought on by the baths. Still he hoped it was a good sign.

The weather at Pöstyén continued monotonously fine, one day like another, a proper climate for invalids.[13]

Moving on, he arrived in Gossensass, Austria, on 26 August, where he lodged in Villa Männer, having sailed up the Danube from Budapest to Vienna, a delightful trip. That same morning he had sent off proofs, work never taking second place. He wished he could transplant Best to where he was; next year Best must holiday on the continent. 'Let me have *Betha Adamnáin* and further proofs'.[14] Meyer had begun to walk again and even to climb a little. If only his thumbs were not so swollen. He could not hold the pen without difficulty and pain. The neighbourhood swarmed with old Celtic names which he supposed were all in Holder's great work *Altkeltischer Sprachschatz,* and he amused himself speculating on their etymology.[15]

The Bests were leaving Kilkee on 3 September, 'much refreshed I hope both of you by your holiday.' His own monotonous life in Gossensass was pleasantly interrupted the previous night by quite an Irish evening.

He had found William O'Brien and his wife staying at a nearby hotel, had introduced himself to them, discovered that they knew all about him and spent several hours with them. They were on their way home from Palestine and he regretted very much that they were leaving on the morrow. He was quite astonished to find out how much modern Irish O'Brien knew and how much of the older literature he had read in translation. His wife was a very charming little French lady, who worshipped her husband. Altogether it was a very pleasing recollection. They talked politics and Meyer was struck with the moderation and sanity of his views.

Addressing himself as ever to the duties of scholarship he planned for tasks ahead with an air of urgency, like an earnest schoolmaster. Miss Annie Scarre must utilise her time well and bring home some historical prose or poetry to work at. They must now think of *Anecdota II.* He hoped Best and Bergin and O'Keeffe would all contribute. He had just heard from Stokes who promised 27 quatrains ascribed to St. Moling.[16] He was pleased to hear from Best of George Moore's good opinion of his style and to learn about Mrs. O'Brien's wealth, wherefore she should certainly contribute to the School funds,[17] Meyer not being one to lose an opportunity of getting help for the School from any source that might offer. One wonders if Best was not mistaken in supposing that Sophie O'Brien was wealthy. Not in her later years certainly, when she lived in poverty in Paris, aided by a modest subvention from the Irish government. She survived to a great age, widow of many decades.

Meyer was going to Bregenz in Austria for the next ten days. This was the ancient Celtic Brigantium, a beautiful place on Lake Constance. Columbanus had preached Christianity there. From there he would visit St. Gall which he had never seen.[18]

On 22 September Meyer sent news to Best from Schweizer Hof, Basel, where he had just arrived, having spent two days in Freiburg with

Thurneysen, who had not seen *Anecdota* but was delighted with it when Meyer showed him a copy. 'I was astonished to find that he had the ogam craze, sanest of Celtologists as he is, and would like to see every stone in situ. Another thing, he is a great pigeon-fancier and has any number of these creatures, and rare kinds.' Thurneysen had heard that O'Malley, Tomás Ó Máille, who was in Manchester studying under Strachan, was standing for some post, which suggested he might be leaving. Meyer was concerned that Strachan would be left without any students in Manchester. He had a pleasant long letter from Praeger to whom he wished to be remembered. In his Basel hotel he found Meredith's *One of our Conquerors,* (1891), the first decent book that came his way in a long while.[19] Meyer was an avid reader of English literature, amongst his favourite authors being Jane Austen, some book by whom he is said to have taken with him always on a journey.

A postcard arrived from Hermann Osthoff who was coming to attend the philologists' congress due to be held in Basel. Osthoff had learned his Irish in Aran and was turning his attention to Celtic studies with eagerness and the talent of the great philologist that he was.

> Tá áthas mór orm go bhfeicfead-sa arís gan mhoill thú. Tiocfaidh mo bheanchéile do dtí tionól na dteangeolaithe i n-éinfheacht liom, agus gheobhamuid lóistín i dtigh ósta a bhfuil ainm Métropole air.... Go raibh tú slán......[20]

For Meyer, the wandering scholar, time was not unpleasant and hard work and good results were making life worthwhile despite the persistent painful arthritis. The philologists' congress was the kind of function he could enjoy and he looked forward to its congenial company and learned discussion.

All unpresaged, tragedy struck.

NOTES

1. Meyer to Best 27.7.1906 from Krug's Hotel, Sonneberg i Th., NLI Ms No. 11002.
2. Strachan to Best 12.2.1905 from Thorndale, Hilton Park, Prestwich. NLI Ms No 13336.
3. Henri Gaidoz to Meyer 21.8.1905 from Evian (Hte Savoie). TCD Ms 4223.
4. See *A Criticism of Dr. Atkinson's Glossary to Vols I-V of the Ancient Laws of Ireland* by Whitley Stokes, D.C.L. London 1903. Dr. Atkinson seems to have decided many years earlier that the production of an Irish dictionary was beyond him. John T. Gilbert, writing to Kuno Meyer on 24 January 1888, from Villa Nova, Blackrock, states: 'At a recent meeting of the Council of the Academy Dr. Atkinson announced that he had decided to do nothing further in relation to an Irish Dictionary.' T.C.D. Ms No. 4222 (7).
5. Meyer to Best 26.6.1907 from Liverpool. NLI Ms No. 11002.
6. Meyer to Best 4.7.1907. NLI Ms No. 11002.
7. Meyer to Best 21.7.1907. NLI Ms No. 11002.
8. *Ibid.*
9. Meyer to Best 8.12.1907 from 41 Huskisson Street, Liverpool . NLI Ms No 11002.
10. Meyer to Best 21.7.1907. NLI Ms No. 11002.
11. Meyer to Best 28.7.1907. NLI Ms No. 11002.
12. Meyer to Best 7.8.1907 from Villa Hungaria, Pöstyén. NLI Ms No. 11002.
13. Meyer to Best 18.8.1907 from Pöstyén. NLI Ms No. 11002.

14. Meyer to Best 27.8.1907 from Villa Männer, Gossensass. NLI Ms No. 11002.
15. Meyer to Best 29.8.1907 from Gossensass. NLI Ms No. 11002.
16. Meyer to Best 3.9.1907 from Gossensass. NLI Ms No. 11002.
17. Meyer to Best 13.9.1907 from Gossensass. NLI Ms No. 11002.
18. *Ibid.*
19. Meyer to Best 22.9.1907 from Basel. NLI Ms No. 11002.
20. Osthoff to Meyer 29.9.1907 from Heidelberg. NLI Ms No. 11002.

Chapter 5

'**A** TRAGIC year for Celtic studies',[1] remarked Meyer as news arrived of the deaths of Sophus Bugge and Constantino Nigra, distinguished Celtists both, the former of Norway, the latter of Italy. Celtic studies had been impoverished earlier that year, through the death in January of another great scholar, Graziadio Ascoli, leaving his important work *Glossario dell' antico Irlandese* unfinished. There was a rumour in Paris, said D'Arbois, that Stern was dead, but happily this turned out to be groundless. Mediaeval scholarship suffered an immense loss in the death of Ludwig Traube of Munich, 'nach langen schweren Leiden', sad tidings for Meyer who heard of it in May. They had last been in correspondence about an edition of Esposito. Traube's work and interests covered the heritage and terrain of Irish scholars in Europe and his vital contributions in these realms were appreciated by specialists in the field, among whom was the distinguished mediaevalist of a later time, Ludwig Bieler. A year of sorrow indeed for Celtic scholarship.

At a lecture in Manchester on the last day of January Meyer wound up with an appeal for a Celtic chair for John Strachan. Wandering from place to place in Central Europe he had reached Basel in time for the philologists' congress when he was struck with dismay at the news from Best that Strachan was grievously ill with pneumonia. He wrote back at once on 25 September:

> This is indeed most alarming and dreadful news, and I am anxiously awaiting to hear more. If he has tided over the crisis yesterday, and as you say, his constitution is really strong, all may be well. I am afraid he had been working far too much having his Welsh grammar on his brains and hands ... and had no proper holiday which he needed so much ... Let me know what you hear ...

A brief and pathetic note of Mrs Strachan's written apparently to Best, gives a final record of imminent tragedy. 'My husband is dangerously ill with acute pneumonia ... His death is very close'.[2]

On the night of the 26th Meyer attended a recital at the Minster in Basel. The music was Berlioz' *Requiem*. Listening to it he could only think of Strachan, not knowing that the worst had already happened. At 7 a.m. the following morning he was awakened to receive a telegram from Best. John Strachan was dead. The cause pneumonia, contracted from sleeping in a damp room in a Penarth hotel. Meyer was numbed with the shock. He write in a shaky and agitated hand, so unlike his normally neat and regular script:

Your telegram woke me this morning at 7. I was quite stunned for a long time and cried like a child. Oh the senseless brutality of it. A damp room! But we will bring an action against the churlish scoundrel who put him into it. And his wife and children. And the loss to science. But more than all the dear gentle fellow with his kind blue eyes. His sufferings too, and all so unnecessary and so meaningless ... I heard Berlioz' 'Requiem' in the Minster here last night and thought but of him.[3]

In Basel he spoke of Strachan to the Indogermanic section and the Congress as good as commissioned him to investigate the tragedy. Next day Meyer left for Paris. He would not be in time for the funeral but his sister Toni attended. James G. O'Keeffe crossed from Dublin to represent the School. Grieved and much upset, Meyer wrote to the hotel-keeper of Penarth who had put Strachan in the fatal room, charging him with grave and culpable neglect and also to the *Manchester Guardian,* evidently in accusatory vein against the same man, but the *Guardian* refused to print, saying it was waiting for 'corroboration'.

Strachan's untimely death shocked his fellow-Celticists. Thurneysen, who had coached him at Jena in philology, felt his loss keenly, Stokes said it was the greatest blow to Celtic studies since the death of Ebel and that they must all work harder. Meyer got a touching note from Zimmer, whose own health was wavering. Kenneth Jackson in retrospect, groups Strachan with Loth, Meyer and John Rhys as one of the heroic age of Celtic scholars. Tadhg Ó Donnchadha (Tórna), a student of the School, mentions Strachan's manuals as books that opened for all the gateway to a knowledge of Old-Irish. 'Anois a bhraithimid an chreach do bhuail umainn nuair do cailleadh an Strachánach'.[4]

With Strachan's death the School suffered its first serious loss. So much had depended on him. Irish scholarship owes an immeasurable debt to this gentle and erudite Scotsman, born 1862 at Keith in Banffshire, whose career reads like a triumphal progress in learning, steps in which included the highest distinction in classics at Cambridge, the coveted Porson scholarship, a term of philological study at Jena, where he came under the influence of Rudolf Thurneysen, the Professorship of Greek in 1885, aged 23, at Owens College, later Manchester University, plus the chair of Comparative Philology in 1889. An authority on the dialect of Herodotus, with a brilliant career in the ancient classics in prospect, he turned to Celtic studies in which he became a master and in this field as co-author with Whitley Stokes of the massive *Thesaurus Palaeohibernicus* in two volumes, 1901 and 1903, supplied the indispensable source book for students of Old Irish up to the present day. It was reprinted in 1975 by the Dublin Institute of Advanced Studies.

Celtic languages, chiefly Irish and Welsh, became the great love of John Strachan's life. He would recommend a classical education as an important basis for the study of Celtic. He drew up two useful manuals for the students of the School of Irish Learning, *Selections from Old Irish Glosses* (1904) and *Old Irish Paradigms* (1905) These were followed, after his death, by *Stories from the Táin* (1908). One can still happen on these texts, relics of the School's early years, thumbed and annotated, textual witnesses to the intensive way in which they were studied, word, phrase and idiom, under the tuition of Strachan or his successor Bergin.

Of Strachan's classroom work his friend and colleague Professor T.F. Tout has written: 'His success was wonderful, and he showed in the teaching of Celtic a fire, an enthusiasm, and a power of stimulus which excited the unrestrained admiration of his pupils.' For administration and business he had little taste, and with few conspicuous public gifts he never became widely known in Manchester. For learning alone he carried the torch.

John Strachan left a widow and eight children. Meyer, who had reached Liverpool on 5 October, went next day with his sister Toni and Professor Tout of Manchester University to see Mrs Strachan at her home, Thorndale, Hilton Park, Prestwich. 'She still bears up wonderfully well, but we fear a reaction'. Strachan, who had been busy at a Welsh grammar when he died, had left a mass of material, which Meyer returned to examine on October 26, finding endless papers, transcripts, catalogues of Mss and other material, an enormous mass which it would take a long time to sift and arrange. Meyer undertook to publish Strachan's Welsh grammar and in doing so unwittingly ran into a sea of trouble, which he described to Mrs Hutton.

> My plans are all upset for the moment by an action brought against Professor Strachan's posthumous book for infringement of copyright. It proceeds from Mr. Gwenogfryn Evans who pretends that Strachan made unlawful use of texts published by him. As I saw the book through the Press and signed the Preface I must appear. Indeed I am one of the defendants. The action is to come on at the High Court of Chancery on Feb 1st.[5]

A settlement was reached, however, but the costs to both sides were enormous.[6] A fund was opened for Mrs Strachan and her family, but she refused to accept any aid. She went to see Meyer at Liverpool, indignant at the attempt, considering it a slight on her husband and Meyer had to rush off to Manchester to interview people there and try and rectify matters, all in vain. 'She refuses and will hear of nothing. Ways and means have to be devised to benefit her, or rather the children against her will.'[7] Mrs Strachan, formerly Mina Grant, was the daughter of Dr James Grant, Strachan's old schoolmaster at Keith, and a woman of spirit.

Meyer published in *Ériu* (III, 200) a notice and bibliography of Strachan which show his achievements as covering almost the whole field of Celtic philology while he was yet only beginning to plan great and comprehensive works that would have enhanced the perspective of Celtic learning. He had difficulty in writing it there were so many things interfering. He had an extremely busy interval in Liverpool. Rhys came from Oxford to visit him on 20 November. On the morrow they were to have a great meeting in Liverpool Town Hall to launch a scheme for excavating Wales and the marches, for which they needed £5,000. Meyer now had an assistant in Welsh, his old pupil Glyn Davies. News came that Douglas Hyde had pneumonia and Meyer had written to ask for information. Mary Hutton had sent him her book *The Táin,* a huge tome, 'quite indigestible', which she wished him to review and recommend.[8] He was not enthusiastic.

Wanting rest and recuperation, Meyer set out from Liverpool on 13 December for Amélie-les-Bains in the eastern Pyrénées where he arrived on 20 December and put up at the Hôtel des Bains Romains. Next day he sent Christmas and New Year greetings to the Bests. He had stayed a night en route at Lyon and another at Nîmes where he saw the marvellous antiquities in clear moonlight. 'I am greatly taken with this place and its people (Catalonians) a splendid race.' The hotel guests were less interesting. There was plenty of sunshine and the air was fine and pure. They were near the Spanish frontier, right up a splendid valley full of strange vegetation. He wanted *Ériu* sent to him when it came out.[9] Two days after Christmas he wrote again that he was leading a most monotonous and ennuyeux life and gradually losing the capacity for work. Lying lazily in the sun he thought of his lecture for the Royal Dublin Society which was to come off on 7 February but he had put nothing of it on paper as yet.

Meyer made many interesting friendships on his travels and his letter goes on to describe one of them.

> I am writing this in the café of my hotel where I mostly spend my evenings quite alone, for the rest of the company settle down to poker immediately after dinner in the drawing room where smoking in not allowed. My most interesting and pleasant acquaintance is Lord Walsingham, a splendid specimen of the English aristocracy, about 70 years old, but vigorous and active, a great entomologist (he has just brought out Vol 5 of his *Fauna Hawaiensis),* who spends every winter in some new corner of this planet, ranging from Samoa to Jamaica and Biskra. He has a lady with him who seems to fulfil all the duties and so enjoy all the privileges of a wife, though her name (she is entered as Mad. Guythern Williams) seems to contradict this; also there are two charming girls who again bear a different name, viz. Mademoiselles Williams de Grey. Could you enlighten me from the Peerage or *Who's Who?* One does not like to ask. We make little excursions together and play chess when it gets dark, which happens here about 3, when the sun sinks behind the enormous rocks against which we are built up. But from about 9.30 to 3 the whole valley is flooded with sunshine, which is so powerful that without a sunshade it gives you a headache. I am taking the sulphur baths which seem to do my feet good.
>
> Zimmer has written a most virulent onslaught on Stokes for hs treatment of the Würzburg Glosses in his separate edition (over 20 years ago!) and in the *Thesaurus.* Stern and I cut out the worst passages, but enough remains to make Stokes very angry. The position of an editor is occasionally most difficult and embarrassing.'[10]

Zimmer considered a glossary to the *Thesaurus* a frivolous waste of time and money, saying all that was needed was an index to Ascoli. That might be so, thought Meyer, but still a concise Old and Middle-Irish Dictionary would be a great boon. 'Has anything more been done or said in the matter?'[11] For a long time yet the problem of the Dictionary was to vex his mind. Meantime O'Malley was busy copying at the British Museum in continuation of the Catalogue of Irish Manuscripts of which Standish Hayes O'Grady had compiled his classic Volume One. Osthoff had discovered a new law in Celtic but did not say what it was; he was preparing a paper on it for a Festschrift for Karl Brugmann.[12]

It was almost prophetic that in life John Strachan had no difficulty about who should succeed him. His confidence in Osborn Bergin was complete. 'Bergin has a great chance, and seems to be using it. At last I feel easy about the future of our School, which you will be able to run without foreign aids.'[13] And again: 'It has struck me as absurd that *Ériu* should be edited by two foreigners. At one time there was some reason, but with Bergin running the School there is none now. So I would suggest that I should go off, and that he should take my place.'[14]

Bergin of Cork, his provenance being added to his name by colleagues as if by way of title, was appointed full time to the School, teaching regularly twice a week during 1908 and 1909,[15] besides holding Summer courses in 1907, and taking on as well the co-editorship of *Ériu* with Meyer. In scholarship his standards were impeccable. John MacNeill paid him the tribute that no one, in matters of learning, could get through his guard.[16] He was criticised at times by Meyer, *sotto voce* and confidentially, for being too slow in output or again being too tardy a correspondent, but no one was readier than Meyer to admit that he possessed an unrivalled knowledge of the Irish language, which he could weave into musical verse in praise of his favourite territory of Béarra or, good as any bard, fashion into technical metre to welcome to Ireland his fellow scholar Thurneysen.

This gifted man worked hard to serve his students. One who appreciated this was his pupil Tadhg Ó Donnchadha (Tórna), likewise of Cork, who has left this record:

> I should not finish without expressing thanks for myself and every student of the School to Dr. Bergin because of his dedication on our behalf. Hardly anyone living has greater authority than he in Irish language matters. Although he kept us hard at work he was sympathetic to our shortcomings and was always ready to clarify a problem for us. He never chose to be dry or grim; even when wrestling with the most intractable gloss he did not fail to draw a laugh. This used encourage us. All his students have a special affection for the Doctor because he does not spare himself when it comes to work. One would pity him there every sultry evening, in the stress of work, perspiration rolling off him, endeavouring to serve us. It would not matter if this were his only duty. But he had various examiner's tasks to perform. His students are exceedingly grateful to him because he served them nobly in spite of his immense pressures. Long may he live.[17]

'Consult Bergin on the gender of those words and on all other doubtful points.' So Meyer on one occasion, adding 'I am very pleased with his Keating',[18] a reference to Bergin's selection of stories from Keating's History of Ireland, first edition 1909, which became the classic handbook of 17th century literary Irish, studied by thousands. 'Consult Bergin' was advice he repeated time and again. In Irish language matters the final court of appeal was Bergin of Cork.

That the School came to form a close association with the Royal Irish Academy was natural. The Academy was a rich treasure house of the

Irish manuscript literature which it was the School's main object to edit and publish and to which the students of the School had frequent resort. Meyer had been appointed Todd Lecturer to the Academy in 1904 with the duty of reading and publishing a paper annually on a subject of Irish literature. The Dictionary of the Irish Language was another factor that brought the Academy and the School closer. The project of the Dictionary, which was planned to appear under the Academy's imprint, had lain dormant for decades until re-activated in 1907 under Meyer's direction. Meyer, based in Liverpool and charged with a variety of other duties, could only act in a supervisory way, so the task of excerpting was given to Bergin, under whom progress was slow for he too was overburdened and so the Dictionary problem became acute when he had to take up fresh duties on his appointment to the chair of Old Irish in the newly established National University. To Carl Marstrander, who succeeded Bergin as professor in the School, the duty fell of preparing the first fasciculus of the Dictionary for the press. He did a considerable amount of work in the Academy, where he had a workroom and a small staff of assistants, and formed many friendships with the Academy's personnel, before transferring his base to Norway. Although he carried out his task in time and successfully, the event was followed by a controversy that marred the significance of the event. The work was continued and completed by later scholars, who followed the principles laid down by Marstrander. The Dictionary controversy will be related in a later chapter.

NOTES

1. 'Une année funeste pour la Celtologie'. Meyer to Best 15.7.1907. NLI Ms No. 11002.
2. NLI Ms No. 13336.
3. Meyer to Best, p.c. postmarked Basel 27.9.1907. NLI Ms No. 11002.
4. 'Scoil na SeanGhaedhilge', *Gaelic Journal* (Lughnasa 1908) 365.
5. Meyer to Mary Hutton, Belfast 23.1.1909 on notepaper of Carlton Hotel Edinburgh. NLI Ms No. 8616 (4).
6. Meyer to Mary Hutton 7.3.1909. NLI Ms No. 8616 (4).
7. Meyer to Best 13.11.1907. NLI Ms No. 11002.
8. Meyer to Best 21.11.1907. NLI Ms No. 11002.
9. Meyer to Best p.c. 21.12.1907 from Hôtel des Bains Romains, Amélie-les-Bains. NLI Ms No. 11002.
10. Meyer to Best 27.12.1907 from Amélie-les-Bains. NLI Ms No. 11002.
11. *Ibid.*
12. Meyer to Best 30.12.1907 from Amélie. NLI Ms No. 11002.
13. John Strachan to R.I. Best 16.12.1906. NLI Ms No. 13336.
14. Strachan to Best 26.3.1907. NLI Ms No. 13336.
15. Advertisement in *Gaelic Journal* (Samhain 1908) 524:

School of Irish Learning
33 Dawson Street
Director: Kuno Meyer
Session 1908-9

Mr. Osborn J. Bergin, Ph.D. will hold the following courses during the terms October 20th to December 23rd; January 5th to April 7th; April 20th to June 16th:

1. Old Irish (a) Outlines of Old Irish Grammar; Strachan's *Old Irish Paradigms* (b) Strachan's *Selections from the Old Irish Glosses*. Mondays 7-9 p.m.
2. Old and Middle Irish texts. *Táin Bó Cuailgne* (Yellow Book of Lecan version). Tuesdays 8-9 p.m.
3. Celtic Philology. Tuesday 7-8 p.m. beginning January term.

16. '... Bergin seems to want some definite impulse, some well-defined and interesting line of work. Till now, he has kept too close to the English idea of philology, linguistic anatomy, and yet he has a great taste for literature, especially for poetry. Perhaps he is too cautious. He is always right. For my part, I find nothing so instructive or so stimulating as my own mistakes, when they are discovered. I shall probably be as proud of my scars as any duellist, and why not? I can always point to the marks where Stokes hit me, and Meyer and Thurneysen and Bergin himself, and sometimes the birds of the air might have flown through the holes made in me. But nobody can get through Bergin's guard ....' Eoin Mac Néill to Meyer 23 June 1913. Letter in Archives Department, University College Dublin.
17. 'Scoil na SeanGhaedhilge', *Gaelic Journal* (Lughnasa 1908) 365.
18. Meyer to Best 28.3.1909 from Amélie-les-Bains. NLI Ms No. 11002.

Chapter 6

RICHARD Irvine Best was a great letter writer. To him we owe a debt of gratitude for the way in which he has enriched our knowledge of Irish learning, its progress, rivalries, inner workings and personalities. One had a choice, he told Gogarty, between scholarship and religion. For himself, he decided on scholarship. In early life he had leanings towards Egyptology but in the end chose Celtic studies, thanks to the influence on him of Henri-Marie d'Arbois de Jubainville under whose inspiration he came during some years of residence in Paris and secondly of Kuno Meyer whose admirer and willing disciple he became.

The letter to Meyer printed below allows us the briefest glimpse into the arcana of the celebrated institution of which Best was a model and distinguished member, the Royal Irish Academy, founded 1783 for the advancement of science, literature and antiquities. The first part containing its date is missing, but its proximate dating can be ascertained from the reference to Joseph O'Neill. This is it:

> I see from your letter that the Irish advocates on the Commission of the Senate have no proper idea of what Scholarship is, and are unable to distinguish between individuals. Nor is it confined to them. I had quite a hot discussion with Praeger this afternoon on the respective merits of MacN. and Bergin. He surprised me by saying that *you* are now off the Council through non-attendance, and Fr. Hogan and Count Plunket by rotation. Gwynn then is the only Irish scholar on the Council. They propose to put MacN. on in place of you and Hogan. Scholarship being equal, a Catholic is to be preferred. I pointed out that scholarship is *not* equal, that Bergin should be on the Council – too young a man, MacN. the older member (he is not, both put up by me in the same year), that no one has ever heard of B. in the R.I.A. But surely it is their *business* to hear of him. They pay him £200 a year for his services. But all no good. MacN. talks. They want a talker who will persuade the Government to do great things for them. *Hyde* would be a better influence in this way. No! they had considered him. Can you believe it, some *Catholic* members have been seriously considering Bishop Donnelly as the next President!! I really think the R.I.A. is a hopeless body. They talk of doing *Irish* work, going to the Government etc. but who is to *do* the work, when they have got the money – the obscure Bergin! Just think of the quantity of good work published so unostentatiously by our School. It fills me with pride, and must you also, when I see seven numbers of *Ériu,* and our little handbooks, used now all over the world as the medium of instruction in Old Irish. And then to see the Proceedings of the R.I.A. produced during the same period at what enormous cost, and paraphernalia of officers, secretaries, mace-bearers, and sham state. And add to our publications the solid instruction given – the scholars created, u.a. the Assistant Editor of the Great R.I.A. Dictionary, which is to bring it renown.
>
> Joseph O'Neill tells me he has been appointed a Senior Inspector of Intermediate Schools, salary £500 rising by £20 annually to £700. Lucky man! I

hear that he refused a lectureship in Irish at Cork £500. Professing is not in his line! Had we not trained him for such a post, inspecting would not be in his line either. He has been a great disappointment. Cork will now be filled by an untrained man, no doubt. I suppose O'Malley will get Galway. I shouldn't advise him to go to Cork. *O'Neill's appointment is not public yet, so please do not mention it.* Keep the above details of R.I.A. maneouvers also to yourself. I write all this gossip for your own eyes. I cannot conceive how anyone can prefer a school inspectorship to the honourable post of Professor in a University. It makes me despair almost when I see men turning their backs on learning when they are among the very few who can advance it, and who have been actually trained for that end.

Now all this is most depressing, so I must not continue further. My *Suidiugad T.T.* is well advanced. ... My African brother who has been in Paris since November arrives here tomorrow. I have not seen him for 10 years.

Warmest greetings from us both.[1]

Joseph O'Neill became inspector in 1908. A native of Tuam, Co. Galway, his boyhood years in Aran gave him a natural command of Irish, in the study of which he became deeply interested. After graduating from Queen's College Galway he was appointed to a teaching post there but left to attend the School of Irish Learning for training in the skills and discipline of Celtic Studies. He gave great promise, contributed to *Ériu* and studied in Manchester under Strachan. His departure from the field of Celtic scholarship was looked on as a serious defection by Best and Meyer who expected their students to remain loyal to the discipline for which they had been trained. O'Neill in later years developed into a respected novelist and he had a distinguished career in the civil service. Following close on the departure of O'Neill came another piece of bad news as related by Meyer to Best; 'I have had a great disappointment. Lewis, following the example of O'Neill, has thrown up his Celtic studies! He pleads his health, his unfitness to do genuine work, etc. I must not attempt to dissuade him. He will probably go in for preaching now'.[2] This was Timothy Lewis who was later to compile a bibliography of Heinrich Zimmer.

Visiting Stokes in April Meyer found the veteran scholar wonderfully fresh and active and quite enchanted with some brilliant emendations by Bergin of obscure passages in the Würzburg Glosses. Throughout the course of eating two dinners together Stokes spoke not a word about Heinrich Zimmer, who in a large contribution to the recently printed *Zeitschrift* VI[II], editor Kuno Meyer, had taken Stokes flatly to task in retaliation for the latter's fierce attack of many years earlier on Zimmer's own edition of the Würzburg Glosses. Meyer discovered some lovely litle poems in the British Museum, late and difficult, one on a lady named Caitríona beginning 'Réalta na Cruinne Caitríona' – Star of the universe is Caitríona. To Oxford on 11 April, then Bath where he stayed in 4 Johnstone St., reporting bad weather, during which he worked a litle, not with zest, read Jane Austen 'for the xth time' and rejoiced in some old German books he had picked up. Bath was a wonderful place for books. He bought some very rare Welsh ones for little. There was a fine copy of the Book of Rights, large paper edition, to be had but at the

steep price of one pound he decided against purchase. The principal secondhand bookseller was Irish, Meehan by name. Communicating as
usual with Best, who was laid up with lumbago, he advised against
spending money on doctors or drugs.

O'Malley, better known as Tomás Ó Máille, was difficult to deal with.
He did not mix with English students nor did he read and study English.
He led a solitary life and Meyer supposed he did his thinking in Irish.
He had asked Maud Joynt to show Best her poem. She at any rate could
write English. He wondered if Thurneysen would be able to make much
of O'Malley. To 'the fortunate youth, O'Malley', Meyer's phrase, had
fallen the task of continuing the Catalogue of Irish Mss in the British
Museum begun by O'Grady, though Meyer was somewhat in doubt of
his capacity for it just yet. He was shocked to find that Dr. Warner of the
British Museum, under whom O'Malley would have to work, stam-
mered in the most painful way.

At the beginning of the year Sir John Brunner had given £500
towards providing a lectureship in Welsh in the University of Liverpool
and Glyn Davies was appointed to the post. Davies told Meyer that a
number of Welsh students would come to Dublin in the summer for Irish
if at the same time there were an advanced Welsh course available.
Meyer was already anxious to have the study of Welsh language and literature included in the School's curriculum.

Glyn Davies, formerly Meyer's student in Liverpool, had how come
back from Aberystwyth to take up his appointment. 'He has no degree.
You will like him greatly. Was there ever such an absurdity as to think of
making Galway a seat of learning, away from the great libraries and
every other resource! I do not think our School can do any good with
Birrell, who seems to take his advice from men like Dillon and other
parliamentarians rather than from scholars.'[3]

Meyer did not think much of MacNeill's introduction to the *Duanaire
Finn,* believing that MacNeill did not know the extent and age of the
Finn saga. Stokes was printing a most remarkable text in the *Revue
Celtique* on Cuchullin's sojourn with Scathach. He sent the School's
prospectus to Professors MacKinnon, Henderson, Robinson, Bugge,
Gaidoz, Loth, Zimmer, Windisch, Anwyl, Morris Jones and Rhys (who
was sending a student). Unfortunately no students from Continental
schools would be able to attend as the university courses in Europe went
on throughout July. Glyn Davies asked that a syllabus be sent to the
Welsh Methodist Chapel in Dublin, it being a little place of worship not
far from the General Post Office, where one or two of the members were
leading Welshmen.

The study of Welsh was introduced to the School and figured promi-
nently on the curriculum of the Summer sessions of 1908 and 1909,
under the instruction of Glyn Davies who in July 1908 taught a class
daily in Modern Welsh for beginners and lectured once a week on the
history of Welsh literature from the 14th to the 19th century. These were
in addition to Bergin's usual classes in Middle and Old Irish. A total of

twenty eight students attended the Summer School, of whom two came specially from Paris, one from Vienna, one from Amsterdam, one from Scotland, two from Wales and one from England. The work of the School was given publicity by Meyer's inaugural lecture on the well-chosen topic of Celtic Studies in a National University.

There was news from Germany that Thurneysen had accepted the vacant chair of Comparative Philology at Strassburg, but would not get there till the Wintersemester. In a busy week Meyer collected a lot of money for the new Welsh lectureship, to which Stokes had subscribed, and sent the preface for Strachan's book to the printer. He went for a few days to Bilsby House, near Alford, in Lincolnshire, but was unfortunate in the weather which made it so dark in the old and beautiful house that he could hardly see enough to write. From there the went to Lord Walsingham's place, Merton Hall, Thetford, in Norfolk, taking some work with him as usual. Strachan's *Stories from the Táin* was out and he sent copies to Mrs Strachan, now at 16 Brighton Grove, Rusholme, Manchester, to Professor Leahy and Alice Stopford Green while the Dublin University Press who printed it sent copies to D'Arbois, Stern, Stokes and Windisch.

Edith and Richard Best were holidaying in Derreen, near Kenmare in South Kerry. Meyer, relaxing in the luxury of Merton Hall, wrote:

My dear Best,

Kenmare has always sounded very enticing in my ears. I suppose it is an earthly paradise, in which I hope you will spend a happy time. Ever since I came here we have been having perfect weather and can be out of doors the whole day. There are 13,000 acres of woodland such as Marbhán would have loved, with lakes and ponds full of the rarest plants and birds. People come from all parts to see Lord Walsingham's gardens and collections. A Baron von Hugel, curator of the Archaeological Museum at Cambridge has been here for several days, excavating an old Roman site, but found nothing except a rusty sword and some broken pottery. He had just met Armstrong. Lord Walsingham has three men always working at his entomological collections, which occupy one wing of the house. I was never in such a big place before. It is like an hotel, only much more comfortable materially. I generally work undisturbed in the billiard room which opens into the flower-garden, in which peacocks walk about. The peace and quiet is most soothing. Lord Walsingham is in London today attending a meeting of the Trustees of the British Museum. After dinner we play whist (but not for money). As Mrs Williams is a great smoker of cigarettes, we may smoke all over the house, even in the drawing rooms. I shall stay here till August 3rd, then to Cambridge for a day or two (where I have not been since 1883) and then to meet my sister in London. On my way here I got photographed at Elliot and Fry's, but the proofs have not come yet. I sent Strachan's portrait to his widow .... Lloyd wrote to me what a capital teacher Glyn Davies is. We must have him again next year .... I am to give a course of 10 lectures at University College London next session on Celtic Studies. That and the Todd lectures which I must hold before Xmas will give me a pretty busy Autumn term.

Poor Bergin is still at his exam papers. I had no idea he would have to do so much. I hope he will give it up next year.[3a]

Meyer enjoyed himself in the aristocratic and castled milieu into which he fitted with ease and sympathy. He slept in the room on the first floor right over the entrance, while he generally worked in the billiard room on the ground floor which led out into the most perfect flower garden he had ever seen, it being one of Lord Walsingham's hobbies to acclimatise the rarest plants, both trees and flowers.

Two early August days in Cambridge were immensely enjoyable and interesting, so many people all known to him by name before did he meet at breakfasts, luncheons and dinners, George Leveson Gower, once Gladstone's secretary and Liberal Whip, a most charming man, Montague James, known to us for his powerful ghost stories but more seriously throughout academic Europe for his advanced mediaeval knowledge, who told him that only Irish scribes used *Finit,* all others *Explicit,* two sons of Darwin, Baron von Hugel, who showed him a fine collection of Irish antiquities in the Archaeological Museum, Lady Victoria Manners, P. Giles, Strachan's old fellow-pupil, to whom he asked the University Press to send the Táin Tales. Waldstein was his host and he was put in Austen Leigh's rooms. Cambridge he liked far better than Oxford as a town. The houses harmonized much better with the architecture of the colleges, and besides the general cleanliness and neatness was very pleasing, while in Oxford there was much decay and neglect. He asked Best to remind him when next they met of stories he heard from Leveson Gower.

At Fitzwilliam Museum Cambridge he examined a vellum Irish manuscript written in 1624 containing among other things several of the Death-Tales, a short and rare version of Táin Bó Cúalgne, some Ossianic poetry that was new to him and some new prose stories. It was beautifully and lavishly written and he suggested Quiggin should catalogue and edit it.

He hoped Best was happy at Ballyferriter, and sent his regards to Van Hamel who was holidaying there with him. Gallárus would now be a familiar object to Best and perhaps he had managed to read the alphabet and other stones at Kilmalkedar. He enclosed for Best part of an appreciative letter from Glyn Davies, which read:

> Yes I did enjoy the Irish work immensely – so much so that I preferred sticking indoors to prepare. It was pretty stiff work – but I feel certain that it has not been in vain. Tórna and Miss Byrne picked their way rapidly, and Lloyd, with his etymological nose, rapidly overhauled them.
>
> Cann er prys: nunc dimittis and I feel envious of the Irish Colleges with their magnificent raw material.
>
> At any rate my method has had a fair test, and I shall stick to it. I am afraid it is Bohemian – but it does the work.
>
> And what a lot I have learnt from Lloyd and Tórna!
>
> Irishmen I shall always hanker after – they are simply splendid. I felt I could let go entirely with them.
>
> I feel a bit tired and the Class Library (?) makes me shudder after Dublin. I wonder when I shall be definitely appointed.[4]

By 13 August, Meyer and Toni, ever on the move, were in Heidelberg enjoying the hospitality of the Osthoffs in their new house, 18 Blumenthalstrasse. They were lucky in arriving just in time for an illumination of the castle, a wonderful spectacle. They were to leave that night for Freiburg and should the prevailing cold continue would go to Italy. Osthoff, who sent his best regards, wanted some Irish books, and would Best procure for him Hogan's *Luibhleabhrán*, also O'Donovan's Four Masters, which Massey of Dublin was recently offering for £11, rather much, and could Best beat him down? Osthoff talked etymologies the whole day and had a big new book ready with many Celtic speculations.[5]

Meanwhile the Bests had moved from Derreen to Ballyferriter in West Kerry where they stayed in William Long's. Richard wrote on 11 August:

> My dear Professor,
>
> Your interesting letters reached me safely and relieved the monotony of my present Gaelic existence. This is a much better place than Derreen although we fare less well as regards our creature comforts.
>
> You seem to have made a host of friends at Cambridge. Their names are quite familiar to me. I shall not fail to remind you of the stories which you promise to regale me with. Gladstone's private secretary should I think be a most entertaining person. What was the occasion of your visit to Cambridge after so many years absence? I thought you had got rid of the Welsh grammar with the completion of the preface. It would be nice to have it out before the anniversary of Strachan's death has passed. You have had a lot of trouble with it.... Just fancy! I explored an old cist here yesterday, into which I crawled on hands and knees. It has three compartments, several feet underground. The horrified owner would not venture within 3 feet of the opening, dreading the wrath of the pouca which, they are all convinced, haunts these old burial grounds. He told me that some years ago, before he acquired the field, an old Manuscript was discovered in it which no one in the neighbourhood could read. He believed it was torn up, or that the parson, a Mr Moriarty, since dead, got possession of it. But what might it not have been! The people are all so ignorant that any relic of ancient civilization is either dreaded as an evil thing or allowed to perish.....
>
> Irish flourishes all around here. Nothing else is spoken. We (Van Hamel and I) have had many talks with the natives. I still find the same difficulty in understanding them: they all speak so terribly fast. For the most part they can't read, and so are unable to say where one word begins and another ends. Mr Long, who is the worst offender as to speed and indistinctness, reads with us in the evenings, and makes little excursions antiquity hunting with us. He is a very decent fellow, with a really wide knowledge of the spoken tongue. I have the postboy every forenoon reading to me. Although I carefully prepare the work beforehand, it is with difficulty I can follow him, without looking at the printed page. It is most disappointing. I never had such an experience before with language. I attribute it altogether to the absurd antiquated spelling. The spoken word and phrase has no identity with the written word. That is why so few native speakers can read Irish.... All the same I have learned something. I can now read fairly well, and have a better idea of the intonation of the language. Van Hamel, who feels pretty much as I do, sends his greetings. My wife sends her love to your sister, to whom please remember me. I hope you will enjoy your holiday.[6]

Cold weather persisting, the Meyers travelled south to Italy, resting at Hotel Eden in Sirmione. This was the peninsula of Sirmio celebrated by Catullus. On settling into their hotel a great laziness took hold of them which made letter-writing an effort. It was very hot but there was always a delicious breeze from the lake on which the hotel garden abutted. They had the whole place to themselves, since the travellers, who went in herds, shunned Italy in August. Meyer took a mild sulphur bath every day, as he had no doubt Catullus did when staying at his villa there, of which they still showed the ruins, mere walls and foundations. Like many a poet before and since, Meyer had done a translation of *Odi et amo,* the Latin poet's immortal couplet which has challenged, and baffled, translators throughout the centuries. Toni and himself often went on the lake and planned to visit Riva, four hours by steamer. They intended to stay at Sirmione until September 1st, then go to Venice, Hotel Victoria.

Meyer read Best's letter from Ballyferriter with interest, finding that Best's difficulties with spoken Irish were familiar to himself so much so that he thought the game not worth the candle. He wished Best were with him. Nothing was so refreshing as these beautiful surroundings with their different worlds. Meyer probably appreciated that Best's modest income did not enable him to take many foreign holidays. He hoped Bergin would take a good holiday. Toni was taking a siesta while he was writing this from the Caffé del Resorgimento.[7] Evidently delightful Sirmione was not overpraised by Catullus.

The School's Report from the hand of Richard Best, covering the years 1908-9, was succinct and encouraging, indicating the progress made and the pride in its achievement. In June 1909 Meyer gave a special course of five lectures on Old- and Middle-Irish Poetry which, though of a highly technical nature, drew an attendance of twenty-eight, many of whom had come considerable distances, including students from the United States, Edinburgh and the North of Ireland. At the Summer School of 1909 Osborn Bergin gave instruction in the palaeography of Middle-Irish manuscripts to hear which twenty-eight students again attended, of whom two came from Scotland, one from Wales, two from Harvard and two from England. Glyn Davies gave three courses in Modern and Mediaeval Welsh to a class of twelve, among whom were Tadhg O'Donoghue and J. H. Lloyd, both distinguished Irish scholars. Tomás Ó Máille, a leading alumnus, whose travelling studentship was provided by Alice Stopford Green, graduated as Doctor of Philosophy at Freiburg in Breisgau under Thurneysen.

Publications were an important function of the School. During 1908-9 there appeared John Strachan's *Stories from the Táin,* Meyer's *Primer of Irish Metrics,* with Glossary and Appendix containing a list of the poets of Ireland, Osborn Bergin's Stories from Keating's History of Ireland and two works of John Strachan's reprinted in one volume *Old Irish Paradigms* and *Selections from the Old-Irish Glosses.* In the main these have stood the test of time, with minor revision, as class books for university students to the present day, testifying to the durability of the work done by the School professors, and not least to the teaching genius of the all but forgotten John Strachan. Meyer's *Primer,* now out of print and out of date, largely owing to his own later researches, has been succeeded by H. Gerard Murphy's scholarly *Early Irish Metrics,* while E. G. Quin's *Old Irish Workbook* has since appeared to complement Strachan's texts.

Since its foundation in 1903 upwards of 180 students had received instruction in the School in Old and Middle Irish, Palaeography, Phonetics, Welsh and Celtic Philology and it had attained prestige on the Continent, Britain and the United States as a centre of learning.

Class attendance lists were not kept. A list specially compiled by Best for Meyer, undated but probably relating to 1910 or 1911, shows a talented gathering, comprising J. H. Lloyd (Seosamh Laoide), Owen Byrne, John Fraser, J. Pokorny (Póigín), R. Flower (Bláithín), E.B., Mrs. Eason, J. McM. Kavanagh native speaker!, J.W. Purcell, Wm. O'Brien, J.J. Doyle, ? Friend of Mrs. Eason, Liam Ua Rinn, Miss Hurley, C.M. (Ó Uaimhín), R.I.B., Miss Williams, Rev. Fr. Fitzgerald of Australia, Miss Ryan, ? Friend of Mrs E., O'Keeffe, J. Glyn Davies, and Miss Deane (Das Engelein!). Annotations by Best to individual students read: Owen Byrne, a veteran who attended J. Strachan's first class; J.W. Purcell, attended his second in 1904, and has never missed a class since; Kavanagh, a Dun Quin man who writes Irish column for *Sinn Féin,* and gives Irish lessons to the pupils is the description of the legendary Seán an Chóta who was to produce a massive Irish language Thesaurus of West Kerry vocabulary that would have delighted the heart of Kuno Meyer; William O'Brien is Liam Ó Briain, Dublin born, who was to become Professor of Romance Languages in University College Galway, and the author of one of the most candid and interesting contributions to the history of 1916, *Cuimhní Cinn,* for which he was awarded the Douglas Hyde literary prize; J.J. Doyle, under the pseudonym *Beirt Fhear,* produced many Irish language works; Liam Ua Rinn, one of five brothers who fought in the 1916 rising, was the friend and biographer of Stephen MacKenna, translator of Plotinus; Miss Hurley is identified signally as 'one of the best' and likewise Miss Deane, the 'Little Angel', as 'very good, said to know more than all the rest', great praise in the company of scholars like Flower, Fraser, Pokorny and others. C.M. was doubtless Carl Marstrander but how explain Ó Uaimhín in brackets after it? If it served as his Irish name, whence derived? Pokorny's bracketed appellation of 'Póigín' we may fairly construe as relating to his fondness for the company of young ladies and coaxing their osculatory blandishments. Father Fitzgerald, of Australia and Ireland, was the author of a series of books including *The Five of Trumps, A Good Third* and *Fits and Starts* which were popular in their day.

Altogether a company[8] of which the School might well be proud.

NOTES

1. Best to Meyer. First part of letter, including date, missing. NLI Ms No. 11002.
2. Meyer to Best, 3 April 1908, from University Club Liverpool. NLI Ms No. 11002.
3. Meyer to Best, 28 May 1908. NLI Ms No. 11002.
3a. Letter dated 27 July 1908. NLI Ms No. 11002.
4. Included with Meyer's letter to Best, 7 Aug. 1908. NLI Ms No 11002.
5. Meyer to Best, 13 Aug. 1908. NLI Ms No. 11002.

6. Best to Meyer, 11 Aug. 1908. NLI Ms No. 11002.
7. On 22 Aug. 1908. NLI Ms No. 11002.
8. The company is in fact composed of Carl Marstrander's class which attended Mrs. Eason's garden party in Rathgar, shown in the photograph in this book.

Chapter 7

'What will be the relation of the new University to our School?' was the question posed by Meyer at the end of a letter to Best on 3 April 1908[1], thereby raising a matter of the greatest importance and one which was to affect the whole future of the School. Obviously he gave the question some thought as we find him two months later considering a lecture on 'Celtic Studies and their place in a University' as a subject appropriate for the time.[2] He would like the chair to be taken by Father Delany but would greatly prefer not to have other speeches, 'by MacNeill or others', since it would be an academic lecture, but these things he left to Best's discretion.[3] By June he thought the best title would be 'The University and the teaching of Celtic'. He was going to speak a good deal about German universities as a model, and their experiences in Liverpool.[4]

Such was the theme of the lecture he delivered on Saturday 4 July 1908 in Leinster Lecture Hall, Molesworth Street, under the auspices of the School of Irish Learning. Amongst the large attendance were his sister Antonie, Osborn Bergin, Anton Gerard Van Hamel, Richard Best and his wife Edith, Glyn Davies, John MacNeill, R.A. Stewart Macalister, Norma Borthwick, Sarah Purser, Tadhg Ó Donnchadha and many others distinguished in the world of Irish learning.

In the course of his lecture Meyer recommended that Ireland should adopt the best features of the German university system, the methods of which differed from those of England, in that their object was to train and produce independent investigators and thinkers. 'All will agree that an Irish university should contain a school of Celtic studies, that it should, if possible, become the home and centre of these studies, and, though a great school cannot be founded all at once, the foundations should be laid on so broad and comprehensive a basis that a noble structure can be raised in time.' Such a special school of studies could only flourish within a great University that was well equipped for the pursuit of all kindred subjects; for the student who wished to make himself a good Celtic scholar had to go far afield, and should have the opportunity of training in many branches, such as phonetics, comparative philology, palaeography, not to mention history, literature and archaeology. His late colleague John Strachan had often pointed out the importance of a combined study of all the Celtic languages. It was absurd to learn any of them in isolation. The new University ought to have on its staff men capable of teaching the other Celtic tongues, ought to have a Professor of

Comparative Philology and Professors of the chief branches of the Indo-European family of languages. As to the scientific study of the spoken language and its dialects, a thorough phonetic training was absolutely indispensable and a good phonetician should be invited to fill an honourable post in the new University. In the important field of Irish palaeography next to nothing had been done, though it called loudly for workers. 'To determine the exact period of the origin of letters in Ireland, and with it the introduction of learning into Ireland, to determine the age and home of our oldest, and, indeed, various schools of writing MSS – these are tasks that can only be undertaken by a skilled palaeographer.' Who would not look forward with hope and confidence to the rise of a great and flourishing Irish University, in which the study of her ancient national language would assuredly occupy the place of honour?[5]

It was a blueprint for the ideal. The ideal did not happen, for many reasons, one of them being identified by Meyer as the total incapacity of those in authority to understand how Celtic studies should be developed and an adherence to the infallibility of the examination system. Many important fields could not be catered for due to lack of funds and qualified personnel. No great School of Celtic would arise from the University. So much became obvious to Meyer within a short time. He did not visualise the University as fulfilling the needs of Celtic studies to the standards which were being met by the School and he expressed his pleasure to O'Keeffe that the School was again being well-attended. 'I don't think we can afford to give it up. I have now little faith left in the University.'[6]

The School of Irish Learning was flourishing. This was the encouraging news Best had for Meyer early in February, in a letter the first part of which welcomed a favourable development in the case against Evans who had brought the action against Strachan's Welsh textbook and went on to notice an error of Zimmer's which, if committed by anyone else, would have been the subject of rebuke by Zimmer in at least fifty pages of his abominable German. The School's Celtic Philology class now numbered 17, unique in the history of Celtic studies. Several priests from Maynooth were attending the courses, Father Boylan whom Meyer had met and now Dr. Sheehan also. Had Meyer seen MacNeill's pamphlet, in which he dismissed the School in three lines and omitted all reference to *Ériu?* Dr. O'Hickey could not have said less. If Modern Irish was not to be taught, Best could not see how the University could advance on the School. His own impression was that the University would not achieve as much. Unless it had a School for postgraduates or outside students it would be merely an examination cramming institution of the Trinity type. If Bergin became Professor of Old and Middle Irish he supposed they need do no more than hold Summer courses as heretofore. 'The School is certainly flourishing'.[7]

Alice Stopford Green, who had been closely watching the course of events, and wished the University to take advantage of Meyer's unique abilities, sent a memorandum to Chief Baron Palles, Chairman of the Commission, along with a letter dated 10 February 1909. The document was marked 'Private and Confidential' and headed 'Memorandum as to the suggested Co-Ordination of the School of Irish Studies with the National University of Ireland'. Paragraph VII read:

> I attach the utmost importance to the connection of Dr. Meyer in some way with the School. If it was possible to secure his entire services, I should expect a very rapid and brilliant advance in every branch of the higher studies highly creditable to the University. With a more limited time he would give a personal influence and stimulus to students which no one else can supply .... I may say in fact that I think the University course I propose of Post-graduate Studies, would have a very stunted and struggling life without his help at the outset.[8]

Douglas Hyde told Best about Mrs Green's proposal, perhaps not in the most accurate detail. Best was upset. It looked like a recommendation that the School should be taken over by the University. His concern was allayed by a re-assurance from Meyer, who wrote him on the 5th of March:

> Set your mind at rest about the School. We will not give up anything. What Mrs. Green means is this: if the new University is going to have a *postgraduate* School of Celtic they should come to terms with our School so that the same work may not be done twice over in Dublin. That surely is reasonable. But we must have full guarantees, and there should be a body of governors consisting of our own and of members of the Senate in equal proportions. I should still be the Director, Bergin *the* Professor. Then, with the money of the University (which is all they have to give) we can develop the School further on the lines which we have laid down. The University must understand that we have everything to give except money, though we have assets there too. I for one would not hand anything over under other conditions.[9]

Meyer, taking a rest at Amélie-les-Bains, kept in touch with everybody, being the best of correspondents in following the golden rule of answering a card or letter without delay. He wrote voluminously. If ever a complete collection of his letters is made it will document to the smallest detail the progress and development of Celtic studies during the course of his career. His command of English was perfect and a large, perhaps a major part of his correspondence is in English, but since he naturally wrote in German to his fellow Celtologues in Germany, a full view of the actual extent, volume and range of his correspondence will have to await the results of future research, given that his German correspondence and diaries have survived.

From Amélie-les-Bains he kept Mary Hutton informed about the situation.

> ... The Commissioners and Senators, so far as I know, have not yet seriously approached the question of Irish teaching. Tot capita tot sensus. They will not be able to come to any decision for a long time. There should be a *postgraduate* school in Dublin which should be fed from Belfast, Cork and Galway. At present our School of Learning supplies the want to some extent. Dr. Bergin now lectures to 17 students on the Comparative Philology of the Celtic languages. Unless the new University will provide such instruction, and so far it does not seem likely, we shall continue the School.[10]

There was much speculation about who would be appointed to chairs and lectureships of the new University. Encouraged by his friends,

Osborn Bergin applied, tardily it must be said, for the chair of Old Irish, a post for which he was strongly recommended by Meyer. If successful he would have to make a choice between the School and the University, since Dr. Denis Coffey, the University President, envisaged that the University was to lead the world in Celtic studies and would hear of no connection with the School.

There was a prospect for a while of an arrangement by which Meyer's services might be available to the University arising from a move which had the active encouragement of Alice Stopford Green. It might have succeeded had enough money been available but funds ran out, which put an end to it. Whether it might have worked in any case was doubtful, since Meyer would want a free hand and this he was unlikely to get especially in the context which he outlined to the School's treasurer James G. O'Keeffe:

> As to the University and Irish, I have now very little hope of seeing a real school, a postgraduate school, established. My evidence before the Commissioners fell completely flat. *None* of them realise the requirements of Irish scholarship, and it is questionable, if they could be brought to realise them, whether they would be able to supply them. Talk about scholars and patriots! Where are the former? There is Bergin, and again Bergin. No, the only real interest in Irish studies is centred in our School and we must stick to that. If Bergin should be offered a post, we can still go on in many directions, and we might remodel the School a little. As for myself, I would only consent to such a post as director, or to any participation in the University work, if I am given a free hand, and that is not very likely. With Hyde and MacNeill you cannot found a real school. They are both amateurs, as Hyde will and Mac N. ought to admit.[11]

Turning to the prospects for the School, he looked forward with the utmost assurance to a good summer session. He would take a course himself, Glyn Davies must come again and Bergin would of course take beginners and advanced students. He already had applications from Paris and Wales for intending students. Pokorny talked of coming and no doubt there would be others. It was the outlook of an optimist who was in no way daunted at the university's rivalry. He was writing from Villa du Soleil, Amélie-les-Bains, where he would stay until about mid-April. The weather was wretched, everybody had a cold and 'so have I'.[12]

It is extraordinary how wrong Meyer was in his judgement of John MacNeill. He may have changed his opinion later, since we find them in correspondence on the level in which scholar writes to scholar, but at this time Meyer considered it absurd to give important university posts to Hyde and MacNeill.

The following letter tells of an overture made to Meyer and of his own strong conviction in favour of Bergin's appointment:

Villa du Soleil
Amélie
2 April 1909

My Dear Best,
    I had a most interesting letter from Rhys just returned from Dublin of which I must give you some account, though you will see that it is more or less confidential. Tell Bergin what you think right. He says that he has not been able to achieve

anything with regard to our School. They persist in the view that they can have no dealings with us. Next Rhys sounds me as to my accepting a chair of Old- and Middle-Irish with a salary of £800. This would be a good deal more than the ordinary salaries which are to range from £400-£600. Whether this is entirely his own idea, or comes as a feeler from the Commission I do not know. In any case I could not accept such a post and have already told the Chief Baron so. As Rhys makes no mention of Bergin at all, but speaks of Pedersen (incredible, but true) I wrote very strongly to him saying what whatever else is to be done, if there is to be any real School of Irish studies, Bergin must be not only in it, but hold the chief post as far as language is concerned. Fancy thinking of Pedersen, who might do as Professor of Comparative Philology, but who would of course never accept. The truth is, Rhys is as much out of it as the rest of the Commissioners and I now see perfectly clearly that with such a body of men to guide the destinies of the new University in Irish studies at any rate, no proper provision will be made. Hence the absolute necessity, if these studies are not to disappear from Ireland altogether for our School to go on. Mrs. Green, too is now fully persuaded of this .....

Kuno Meyer[13]

The wandering spirit of Meyer took him early in April 1909 to Barcelona, a place much to his pleasing, which instead of the vulgar modern city he had been led to expect he found to be a regional capital of splendid situation, with charming old quarters, a market place the like of which he had never seen, and a tram system unsurpassed anywhere. The peace of his stay was shattered by a bomb explosion which rattled his hotel windows. On 8 April he returned on a relaxing journey along the Mediterranean to Amélie. Here he got a postcard from Best on the 12th, so full of content that it remains a physical mystery how Best could get so much into a card, which told about events in Dublin, especially prospects for the new university.

Many thanks for your interesting letter. What you tell me about the new University in no way surprises me. I am beginning to lose interest in it. B[ergin] professes to be more interested in the School. He did not wish to hear anything of a confidential nature. Prefers to remain in a state of ignorance. The Dane [i..e. Holger Pedersen] would never do. There would be a hue and cry raised by the ultra-patriotic party. Ireland flouted again! Though I should like to see you settled here, I cannot but think that you are better off out of it. Your freedom would be curtailed. We must make the School the head centre of *Celtic* studies in Ireland. If only one could add historical research. I wonder would Z[immer] come over for a course of Lectures on Irish Literature, and its importance as supplementing what we know of the Celts from Roman sources, etc. You know what I mean. I am afraid B. is not ambitious. He does not say much. Of course from the point of view of scholarship, he should be preferred to another Irishman. But would not his usefulness be considerably curtailed in other and even more important directions:- Dictionary and our School. For your must know that this new University will folow the English models – the only ones they know anything about. German idals are to them up in the clouds, or only suited to a different order of beings. B. still has the paradigms. I wish he would mark his corrections ... It is clear to me that *Ériu*, and our little books must now pay their way. If only we could be assured of a habitation, all would be well. Once the University is started we must increase our fees. 5/- a term (1 hour per week) is about 6d a class. We lowered these because so few came. Now the classes average 15 and 16. Dont worry yourself and waste your time writing to these helpless people. They will do the wrong thing in the end. The question we have to decide is simply this. Would B. help and advance Irish studies better as a Professor in the new University than in his present position (School and R.I.A.). I am inclined to think in the latter. Of course, I influence him in no way. ... I got quite a start this morning seeing "Bomb outrage in Barcelona" placarded over the streets. ... We are delighted to hear of Osthoff's rally. I had begun to fear he was going to succumb.[14]

Meyer wrote back directly. He was anxious about Whitley Stokes, now in his 80th year and stricken with pneumonia, with two nurses in attendance. He went on to consider the case of Osborn Bergin:

Your card came this morning and I will answer it fully. The point which you omit to mention, but which is surely a weighty consideration, is that Bergin cannot afford to refuse a provision for life. He is a noble fellow and I am sure would always be guided more by ideal than practical considerations, but his friends must think and if necessary act for him. Even if Mrs Green carries out her intention of giving £300 annually to our School we shall never be rich enough to be able to pay Bergin a high salary. And there is always the precariousness of our existence at all. Since I wrote to you last, things have developed a little. I had a long letter from the Chief Baron in answer to mine of February 13th as well as to one written by me to Rhys, which contained my views on the whole subject. I have written very frankly and familiarly to Rhys, so the Chief Baron knows my mind.[15] He again urges me to accept a chair with £800 saying that all the Commissioners hope I will do so. It is to be the highest salary within the University. But I have once more and finally declined and submitted my counter proposals, which are mainly two: that Bergin should be *the* professor of Irish language and that in that case, but in that case only, I would gladly cooperate with him, supplement his teaching, direct and stimulate Irish studies in the University generally and reside in Dublin for one term. He will lay this before the Commission when they meet at the end of this month. I have informed Mrs Green of it all. I also said that I would not teach under any system of examinations, set books, prescribed periods or the like. Thus, you will see, I have given them a chance of my services to the best of my ability. This I think I was bound to do. If they do not meet me on these conditions, I can withdraw altogether with a clear conscience. If they accept we will then consider together what the future of our School is to be. There will be as much need of it in more than one direction as ever; for it will take many years before the proper spirit can be infused into the University.[16]

A few days earlier he had written to Mrs Green in similar terms, telling her he had let Chief Baron Palles know his mind on the absolute necessity of putting Bergin into *the* chair of Irish Language, their resolution to continue the School of Irish Learning and the absurdity of giving important posts to MacNeill and Hyde,[17] once more displaying the same puzzling blindness to MacNeill's merits.

At Perpignan on 14 April he had two telegrams, one from Best and one from Whitley Stokes' daughter, telling him the great Celtic scholar was dead. Though prepared for it Meyer found it hard to realise that his wonderfully active life was suddenly at an end. Two months earlier he had seen Stokes in his full mental health, hardly any the worse for the bronchitis that had been troubling him all winter. They had been friends since their first meeting in 1883, although Meyer seemed to regard Stokes, who was his senior by years, born 1830, more as a counsellor and fatherly guide. He asked could Best or O'Keeffe represent the School at his funeral. He would be late himself. Best was unable to go and in fact it was Bergin who represented the School, fittingly, as one of the younger scholars esteemed by Stokes, who had confided to him his regret that he had never learned modern Irish.

Best, unaware that he had been ill, and taken by complete surprise to see his death briefly announced in the morning paper, lamented that the narrow circle of Celticists which formed their audience was rapidly diminishing, having been not long since bereft of John Strachan and that there was no young man coming up, although Marstrander might ultimately take the place of Strachan as an etymologist. Stokes' death had not excited the interest it should have and some absurd things had been written about him such as the 'limited nature(!!) of his scholarship.'[18]

Meyer, having returned to London, paid a mournful visit to the Stokes family at Grenville Place, where he found Maive and Annie displeased with the silly articles in the papers. Stokes had been working up to practically the moment of his death on the text and translation of *In Cath Catharda*, an Irish version of Lucan's *Pharsalia*, the longest prose composition of the mediaeval Irish after *Táin Bó Cúalgne* and *Acallam na Senórach* and had begun the Preface, which breaks off in the middle of a sentence, *die Feder aus der Hand gefallen*, to be completed by his sorrowing colleague Windisch and published in Leipzig later that year. Stokes had 'made several attempts to work before he had to take to bed, and when he found he was too weak he cried. He did not suffer much; his death seemed to have resembled that of my good mother.' So wrote Meyer,[19] greatly bereft.

Though he had reached a fullness of years at 80, the loss of Stokes was irreplaceable. For more than five decades he had been one of the Olympeans of Celtic Studies. He is, no argument, the greatest of Irish scientific Celtic scholars. Learned and acerbic, he had brought a sharp critical acumen to his disputations which earned him few friends but made for higher standards of scholarship. Progress comes through contention, he would say, echoing Aristophanes. As Governor, the School of Irish Learning had been favoured with the prestige of his great name, he had been a valued contributor to its journal *Ériu* and had published an improved edition of his important *Félire Oengusso* for the School's benefit. Never unhappy in controversy, he fought great linguistic battles with Zimmer, Atkinson and Standish Hayes O'Grady. He was said by Meyer to be one of the only two men in Ireland who had mastered the difficult *Grammatica Celtica*, the other being his friend and teacher Rudolf Thomas Siegfried of Dessau who for a brief space held the chair of Sanskrit in Trinity College Dublin. Apart from his contributions to Celtic learning he completed the massive task of codifying the Anglo-Indian Laws which he himself regarded as his major achievement. No mean poet, he is represented in John Cooke's *Dublin Book of Irish Verse*. Despite Meyer's utmost persuasion to secure his valuable library of 3,000 volumes for Ireland, it went by the wishes of his daughters to the University of London. The reason may have been that they were displeased with some of the unappreciative things written in Irish papers about their father but even the lofty London *Athenaeum* carried, anonymously, a less than just obituary notice and the folklorist Alfred Nutt was obliged to write to it and correct the balance.[20]

Meyer had bad news of Hermann Osthoff, his doctors having now given up all hope. The university commissioners expected a deputation from the School of Irish Learning, to join which he left London for Dublin on 24 April, and the outcome of this he detailed to Best, briefly and in haste:

> Delany summed up everything in a perfectly masterly speech. I consented to become professor in the University, with one term's residence, and a seat on the Board of Studies and the Faculty. I am also to go to Galway and Cork occasionally to lecture. Jackson said that he was glad the School had been heard at last, and that it ought to have been consulted at the outset. All agreed that the School must be recognised by the University.[21]

The arrangement that Meyer should join the University fell through, however. In May he heard from Rhys that there would be no University chairs at all, the money being exhausted. 'So all our little schemes have come to an end. However, I do not regret what we have done. We have shown our readiness to serve the University'[22]

One feels that Best regarded the advent of the University with less than enthusiasm, coinciding as it did with the discontinuance of the £100 Treasury grant to the School. Speculating on what the School might do with a fraction of the £2,000 given to the University, he could not conceal his fears that both students and teachers would be drawn away from the School. Dr. Denis Coffey, the University's President, had expected Bergin on his appointment to the Chair of Old-Irish to sever his connection with the School, envisaging that the University would become the world centre for Irish studies. Best had strong doubts about that. The University had no chair of Sanskrit or Comparative Philology, and only a lectureship in Welsh, and was no better provided than the School, and in short the means were still wanting for forming the great School of Celtic that was Meyer's vision as expressed in his public lecture on 'The University and the teaching of Celtic'. While it might have given some satisfaction that the School was the agency through which the University was supplied with some of its most distinguished appointees, the University in effect became a rival. The notion of the Postgraduate School within the framework of the University was no doubt uppermost in his mind as he wrote to Meyer:

> Bergin and I have been discussing the future of our School daily. It is our sole topic of conversation almost. He thinks with me that with you, and himself, and possibly MacNeill as professors in the new University all that can be done for advanced Celtic will be done, especially also as there is likelihood of a Welsh lecturer being appointed. The University having taken over *our* professors, and added thereto, have virtually taken over the one half of our School.'[23]

Best had critical things to say about the interest of the Gaelic League in the University. The more he thought of it the more he was convinced that no School of Celtic or even Irish research would rise out of such a University, when even the desire for learning itself was absent. 'Irish Ireland as represented by the Gaelic League has never shown any interest in Irish learning as such .... Continental scholarship has been bringing all that they now crave for to their very doors for years, and they have not opened to take it in.' One would suppose, on reading the leading article in the *Claidheamh Soluis,* organ of the Gaelic League, last week, that nothing had been done hitherto, that all had yet to be done by the 'pioneers' who were to write their names in the history of this University. It was all very sad to see such an immense sum paid annually, over £2,000 for Celtic alone, and to feel it was all to no purpose. 'We have done in our School on a few hundred a year more than this University with its defective organisation will be able to do with its £2,000.'[24]

Best took his summer holidays in Tintagel, Cornwall, in August. There he was shocked to hear of the tragic drowning off the Blaskets of a very promising student of the School, Eveleen C. Nichols. He was reading slowly through Rudolf Thurneysen's recently published *Handbuch des Alt-Irischen,* which filled him with wonder. What, he mused, would be left now for the younger generation of grammarians to do, unless a Handbuch des Mittel-Irischen by Marstrander? The professors at the new University Colleges would have an easy time, when immense learning could be purchased for sixteen shillings, leaving further research unnecessary. He went on to speculate on the likely appointments in the new University:

> I suppose O'Malley is now pretty certain of Galway. Dr Henry may come in for the Lectureship in Celtic! Horrwitz has written to me to use any influence I have on his behalf for (1) the Lectureship in German and (2) Lectureship in Eastern Languages in Dublin. I told him I had none, and gave him to understand that a Fellow of the R.U.I. might succeed to the former, and a certain priest, skilled in Semitic languages to the latter. Horrwitz enclosed a circular announcing ten lectures which he is prepared to give on Hindu and Teutonic literature anywhere, adding testimonials from Mahaffy and others. I feel sorry for H. He is again bound to be disappointed. But he has no claims on a University appointment. He describes himself as sometime Lecturer in Sanskrit and German T.C.D. All the world is applying for berths in this curious University. Had W.S. [Whitley Stokes] lived he might have described it as a Narrenschiff.

All this, and much more, to the extent of 750 words in all, Best got into one of his wonderful minuscule postcards addressed to Meyer.[25]

Writing from Tintagel a week later he remarks that 'no doubt B. has by this time sent in his application'.[26] He had not. He left it until the very last minute and the agitation he caused Mrs Green is reflected in the following letter from Best written shortly after his return home.

35 Percy Place
1 September 1909

My Dear Professor

> We arrived home on Sunday morning after a tiring journey ...
>
> There is not much to relate. When I was up at O'Keeffe's on Sunday afternoon, Mrs. J.R.G. called here, distracted upon hearing officially that Bergin had not applied for the O.I. chair, and Tuesday was the last day. However he arrived on Monday evening (I had in the meantime written conjuring him in the name of the S.I.L. to apply, otherwise MacS. was to get it, *so* Mrs. G.!) having despatched the formidable application, with testimonials from Th[Thurneysen], Z.[Zimmer] and P. O'Leary, giving you as a Ref. Yes! I hear some of the aspirants for other chairs

are growing nervous. Things may after all not run so easily. There is a fluttering in the dovecots. Some say the Lord Chief B. may arise and let loose his thunderbolts. He has already written to the press, denying that any appointments have been made.

I had a long talk at the School with Mrs. G. the following day. She was greatly perturbed at the idea of B. not standing. She thinks it essential that some one 'friendly' to the School should occupy this particular chair. She thinks that if O'M. were appointed, good relations could not subsist. So O'M. is contesting the seat with B! Mod. Ir. in Galway or O. Ir. in Dublin, whichever offers. Mrs G. says he informed her that his qualifications for the latter were better than Bergin's. Optimistic youth! He ought to get his dissertations printed and fling them down at Bergin's feet – meantime the months are slipping by. I do hope he is not ungrateful to Mrs. G. and the School. He owes everything to her and you. She got him the British Museum job even, as she reminded me. It is too early a stage in his career to adopt such an attitude of independence. Probably however it is rivalry of Bergin rather than anything else which fills his mind. Mrs. G. hopes that the School will be 'recognised' in such a way that Bergin can give instruction in both institutions. That, in a word, recognition will be so complete, that we shall not be regarded as an outside institution. So I gathered from her. But of course this is impossible. She thinks it will be the 'postgraduate' school. How can an unendowed body, such as we shall then be, with no funds worth speaking of, do the work of the Celtic School in the University, while the actual School with professors drawing over £2,000 a year, does nothing but set examination papers, and grind pass candidates? The position would be absurd.

Mrs Green has been archaeologising with Macalister, and is greatly impressed by his good qualities. She is not absolutely without hope that he may win yet. ... We hope you are having a pleasing time at Weimar. How I should enjoy the Liszt relics, Goethe also, thanks to old Eckermann! By the way poor Miss Nicolls was at Weimar last August in a pension. She was not at the tea party, but at the Metrics. I introduced her. You used to call on her to translate, I remember. A tall fair girl – shy, with a low tremulous voice.

Our affectionate regards to you both.[27]

Meyer kept sending unpublished papers of Stokes to Best who, reading through them, had that curious feeling that Stokes, even in death, was having a fling at Robert Atkinson's Glossary to the ancient Irish laws, 'as if Stokes were alive in the grave'. But he hoped the ancient Irish brehons who had preceded them to the Elysian fields would make peace between them, giving just judgement. As for the University, Best was glad Meyer was out of it. If the same toleration for religious beliefs were only displayed in the election of professors all might yet be well. 'I fancy however it is the Catholic young man who is to be safeguarded and not the heretic. Under this declaration it should be impossible for a Catholic lecturer on Early Irish Church History to avoid offending a young Protestant (taught by Zimmer), as for a Protestant to avoid giving offence to Catholics'. And where did the Irish Jew come in? The Jews had a pretty bad time of it in Irish religious poetry. They also must be safeguarded.

Gertrude Schoepperle was back in Dublin. She was greatly impressed by Father Andrew Kelleher's ability and enthusiasm for Old Irish. They read all through Thurneysen's Grammar together. Kelleher had applied for the Lectureship in Modern Irish in the University and Best wondered if anything could be done for him should he fail to get it. He had a letter from Kelleher from which it was clear that the young man wished to devote himself to Irish. Best thought he had decided ability. In Maynooth, where he lectured in Modern Irish, his record was good, and he had just sent in a poem for *Ériu* which was well done. Miss Schoepperle, who knew him better than anyone, was loud in praise of him for his independent mind and marked ability. He could read off the texts in *Ériu* at sight. Could anything be done for him? In a fortnight's time he was due to go to Enniscorthy where he would be on a mission for six years, with no time for study or research and one could see that he did not relish the idea. He was not known in Gaelic League circles and had produced little except papers in Irish for the Maynooth journal. Best supposed that his chances of the Lectureship were slight though he would say Kelleher knew far more Irish, old and modern, than some in the running. He suggested to Kelleher that he come to Dublin to meet Meyer on his next visit. 'When are you coming? I hope you will stay with us.'[28]

Best had a visit from O'Malley, indignant that he had been rejected by the Galway people on a vote of 5 to 9 despite having some influential supporters.[29] O'Malley hoped the Commissioners would nevertheless use their own judgement and select him for the Celtic lectureship. He had withdrawn from the work of cataloguing the Irish manuscripts in the British Museum. The Museum wanted to put a time limit which he could not see his way to accept. The work remained to be taken on some years later by Robin Flower who completed it to establish his great name in Celtic scholarship. O'Malley had nothing to look forward to if the National University rejected him. Gwynn Jones had been recommended for the lectureship in Welsh. Was this Glyn Davies' friend, wondered Best. If so, a good man.

Douglas Hyde was in an odd position. Rumour had it that Sheehan was a favourite with the Governing Body. Andrew Kelleher and Agnes O'Farrelly were competing for the Modern Irish lectureship. Now, considered Best, if Douglas Hyde gets the chair, surely a native speaker should be appointed assistant, because Hyde and Miss O'Farrelly would never advance the scientific and historical study of Modern Irish since neither had the training nor native command of the language. Kelleher had come to the conclusion that Enniscorthy was not the place for him. He might, if not too late, get a post in a Liverpool mission. He was coming to Dublin at the weekend and would meet Meyer.

Best had a long talk with Gertrude Schoepperle, Bergin being present. She had great belief in Kelleher's ability and enthusiasm. In the end he was not appointed, the University thereby failing to secure the services of an excellent scholar. Nor did he go to Enniscorthy as he had feared but was by good fortune appointed to the Parish of SS. Peter and Paul at Great Cosby, Liverpool, and became temporarily, through the good offices of Kuno Meyer, lecturer in Celtic at the University there, commencing to teach on 10 November 'and capable he is of explaining with clarity every knotty problem and archaic expression'[30] as a news item put it in P.S. O'Hegarty's weekly.

In November 1916 he was offered and accepted an appointment as Research Fellow in the University of Illinois at Urbana, which was funded by the Irish Foundation of Chicago. In less than two years he produced, jointly with Gertrude Schoepperle, *Betha Colaim Chille*, the Life of Columcille, edited and translated from manuscript Rawlinson B. 514 in the Bodleian Library with all the furnishings of scholarship, making an imperial volume of some 600 pages, published by the University of Illinois in 1918. Written largely in popular sixteenth century Irish prose, it is a classic of its kind and much prized. Strange that thereafter Andrew Kelleher receded into the shadows, leaving us nothing else from his hand of major import.

When the appointments to the University were made known Best wrote to Meyer in the discursive manner which makes him the most readable of correspondents:

My dear Professor,

So all is at length settled. Macalister is most to be congratulated in having a special £600 chair created for him, but it has cost Fr. K. the Lectureship, or Miss O'F. The former tells me on the highest authority that there is to be no Lectureship, funds not permitting *now*. The German post has not been filled. It would have been much more to the point to have given Macal. £400, and added the remaining £200 to the German Lectureship, bringing it up to £500, for which sum a really good Teutonic scholar could have been obtained. General History and Eng Lit have been postponed. Many are of opinion that Dr. O'Sullivan, a brilliant young metaphysician, should have obtained the chair in that subject. It was given to Father Shine, a pupil of Bergin's at our School, and a pupil of Zimmer's I think also. At any rate he has studied in Germany where B. met him. There can be no doubt whatever of his competence. The priests are fairly well to the fore, and it is to their credit that they are *almost* all men of high ability and of German training.

I congratulated Miss Hayden yesterday in the Reading Room as she sat before B.B., her mind at peace with the world.

......P[raeger] was curious to know who Marstrander was. I praised him to the utmost, of course, and said were he to work on the Dictionary, things would begin to materialise wonderfully fast. He was greatly impressed, and hoped you would be able to carry the Council, who must now begin to grow anxious. Bergin he seemed to think would be able to continue. I pointed out, however, that you wanted a whole time man. B. could of course continue as an honorary assistant, making it his 'research'. Now however is the critical time. Something *must* appear - B. will have his hands full for many months to come, with meetings, etc. etc. and his own teaching in our School and the University. The Dictionary must accordingly suffer. I have no doubt whatever if a sure-footed rapid worker like M. were on the work, he would under your directions complete the whole work in 10 years, and then be able to return home, with a great reputation, to fill a chair in Norway. Nothing he could do in the meantime would be so likely to spread his name as the Dictionary and he is not the person to allow it to exclude him from throwing off many and varied studies, such as he has just done for ZCP. I only wish the excellent B. had the same desire to print. Of his ability to do so there can be no gainsaying.[31]

Early in November Bergin began his professorial duties in the University but was not obliged to drop his work at the School before December. The pressure of his new duties soon compelled him to withdraw from both the School and the Irish Dictionary, leaving Meyer and

Best with the duty of seeking a successor. Bergin retained his loyalties to the School nevertheless and returned to help out with lectures at periods of low ebb. His dear friend Best wished Bergin were not so constitutionally slow. Gertrude Schoepperle, a wonderfully bright creature, told Bergin with an engaging smile she would not care to be as slow as he was. Best feared there was no remedy for this, and forecast that 'He will never take that place in the National University which his learning and real scholarship entitles him to. I doubt' he went on, 'if he will on his own initiative publish anything on a big scale'.[32] Some one had said that science was advanced more by those who dared than those who feared and in this respect others might outdistance him whose mental equipment was inferior. Bergin was in much better spirits these days. The 'chair' might be responsible for this, or perhaps Miss Schoepperle. 'They lunch together every day at the Veg. She is brightening him up wonderfully, and seems to enjoy it'.[33]

The beginning of the National University coincided with the exit of the almost incorporeal institution known as the Royal University of Ireland, which was only an examining body. It came to an end 'yesterday, amid scenes of the wildest confusion and uproar. All the Senate had doctor's degrees conferred upon them, also Rev D'Alton, the "historian" whom Miss Hayden has triumphed over. I wonder will they now give him the chair of Modern History!'[34] For such exquisite items of academic lore we again thank Richard Best. Both he and Meyer, worried about the School's future, now that Bergin was leaving, looked to Norway and the rising star of Carl Marstrander.

NOTES

1. Meyer to Best from University Club, Liverpool. NLI Ms No. 11002.
2. Meyer to Best 10.6.1908. NLI Ms No. 11002.
3. Meyer to Best 17.6.1908. NLI Ms No. 11002.
4. Meyer to Best 30.6.1908. NLI Ms No. 11002.
5. *Freeman's Journal*, 6.7.1908.
6. Meyer to O'Keeffe 16.1.1909 from 41 Huskisson St. Liverpool. NLI Ms No. 2113.
7. Best to Meyer 3.2.1909 from National Library, Kildare Street, Dublin. NLI Ms No. 11002.
8. NLI Ms No. 11002.
9. Meyer to Best 5.3.1909 from Amélie-les-Bains. NLI Ms No. 11002.
10. Meyer to Mary Hutton 29.3.1909 from Villa du Soleil, Amélie-les-Bains. NLI Ms No 8616 (4).
11. Meyer to O'Keeffe 23.3.1909 from Amélie-les-Bains. NLI Ms No 2113.
12. *Ibid.*
13. NLI Ms No. 11002.
14. Best to Meyer, on postcard postmarked Dublin 9.4.1909 and Amélie 11.4.1909. NLI Ms No 11002.
15. Rhys had forwarded Meyer's letter to Chief Baron Palles.
16. Meyer to Best, 12 April 1909 from Amélie-les-Bains. NLI Ms No. 11002.
17. Meyer to Alice Stopford Green, 9 April 1909. NLI Ms No. 11002. *Scríobh 5* (Baile Átha Cliath) 263.

18. Best to Meyer at Thackeray Hotel, Great Russell Street, London 19 April 1909. NLI Ms No. 11002.
19. Meyer to Best, from Thackeray Hotel 21 April 1909. NLI Ms No. 11002.
20. *The Athenaeum*, 1 May 1909.
21. Meyer to Best, on Shelbourne Hotel notepaper, 26 April 1909. NLI Ms No. 11002.
22. Meyer to Best. Postcard postmarked Liverpool 25 May 1909. NLI Ms No. 11002.
23. Best to Meyer, 30 April 1909. NLI Ms No. 11002.
24. Best to Meyer 25 May 1909. NLI Ms No. 11002.
25. Best to Meyer at Mommsenstr. 7, Berlin 20 Aug. 1909. NLI Ms No 11002 (58).
26. Best to Meyer from Tintagel 27 August 1909 addressed to Oberhof, Thüringen, readdressed to Gross Lichterfelde, Berlin. NLI Ms No. 11002 (58).
27. Best to Meyer 1 Sept. 1909. NLI Ms No. 11002.
28. Best to Meyer 6 Oct. 1909. NLI Ms No 11002.
29. Best to Meyer 11 Oct. 1909. NLI Ms No. 11002 (58).
30. *The Irishman* (London) Samhain 1910.
31. Best to Meyer 26 Oct. 1909. NLI Ms No 11002.
32. Best to Meyer 2 Nov. 1909. NLI Ms No 11002 (58). Nobody could confirm this better than Bergin himself, when writing to Alice Stopford Green: '... my studies are tending more and more towards the elucidations of small points of detail and technicalities ...' 22 Sept. 1916 (A.S. Green papers) quoted in R.B. McDowell, *A passionate historian* (Dublin 1967) 80.
33. Best to Meyer, 30 Oct. 1909. NLI Ms No. 11002.
34. Best to Meyer 30 Oct. 1909. NLI Ms No. 11002.

Chapter 8

ARLY in 1910 eye trouble was making life difficult for Meyer, who blamed it largely on the University Press and the British Museum on both of which he heaped maledictions.[1] Best gave him good advice on foot of which he placed himself under the care of the best oculist available. The cheerful news was that Andrew Kelleher, lecturing in Liverpool University, had 59 students in his first class.

As far back as 1880 the Council of the Royal Irish Academy had invited Robert Atkinson to undertake the production of a comprehensive Irish Dictionary based on all phases and materials of the language. For various reasons he made no progress and in any case his capacity for the task might be doubted in the light of the severe criticism dealt his Glossary of the Ancient Irish Laws by Stokes, publicly, and by Meyer, in correspondence with Mary Hutton, privately, not to mention sundry other buffetings. Finally in 1907 he relinquished the project and Meyer, who was Todd Lecturer to the Academy, after much consideration, and even doubt as to the feasability of the project at all,[2] accepted the responsibility of editor, with Osborn Bergin as assistant. The projected Dictionary, a task of magnitude, began to occupy his thoughts and to cause him worry. The question might well be asked, was he wise to take it on at all? In his mind however was the constant awareness that a full and reliable Dictionary was a basic desideratum of Irish studies.

Preliminary model sheets were produced. Examining the first of these Meyer found it unsatisfactory.

> The meanings must be much better given. What troubles me most is that hardly anything has been properly excerpted. I relied on Bergin to see to that, sent him everything as soon as it was printed (*Anecdota III* for example) and find that the work has either not been done at all, or imperfectly. I am now asking Bergin to let me have a further instalment which I will go through. But dear me, it is slow work.[3]

The work was shown to Charles Plummer, who criticised the first sheet severely. 'He is particularly displeased with the way in which the meanings are given indiscriminately.'[4] These comments have an important significance for what happened later. They confirm in a striking way the views uttered by Marstrander when he was criticised for not producing from the chaos which he found a result which his critics themselves were not finding possible.

Nor did it improve things that Bergin did not answer letters. Although now installed in University College Dublin, he was still connected with

81

the Dictionary project and Meyer wished that Best or the Dictionary Committee would find out from him what work he would still do on it. '*I cannot*'.

Marstrander had promised to come and help with the Dictionary and Meyer hoped to coach him in Liverpool before setting him to the actual work. If only they could associate Plummer with the Dictionary, Meyer would be happy, since Plummer was compiling his own Thesaurus at Corpus Christi in Oxford and was the only scholar working at lexicography.

Early in February Meyer went for the good of his health to Brine Baths Hotel, Shrewbridge Hall, Nantwich, along with his eye doctor. The affected eye was still pretty bad and he was accustoming the other eye to work by itself. He blamed rheumatism which seemed to have accumulated in unusual quantities. The baths he took at the hotel seemed to do him no good. He had done no work for a long time and did not suppose he could do any before going abroad. Everything was at a standstill. To add to his difficulties, his fellow editor Stern, prematurely aged and now very feeble, had definitely retired from the *Zeitschrift*, leaving Meyer to manage it alone. Nantwich was a dull place, full of dull hunting people. It had a title to fame in being the birthplace of Milton's wife and there were still a lot of quakers in the village. [5]

Marstrander wrote saying he would shortly be in Liverpool. He was willing to bind himself for three years and might stay altogether.[6] Meyer was back briefly at Nantwich and the weather was at its worst. 'What an awful crossing Marstrander will have. But his Viking blood may not mind it.'[7] The Viking, *An Lochlannach*, as Marstrander came to be known in Ireland, arrived at Liverpool and Meyer took him through some Dictionary materials, including proofs of the specimen pages and Bergin's slips. Marstrander at once spotted every weak point and had the right thing ready. Meyer was delighted with this wonderfully keen and eager worker who would reform the Dictionary. Nothing escaped him. 'I feel that I can absolutely trust him and a great burden is off my mind.'[8]

Carl Johan Sverdrup Marstrander, born 1883, was a native of Kristiansand on the southern coast of Norway and a graduate of Kristiania (Oslo) University, where his gift for languages had impressed his professor, Sophus Bugge, on whose advice he had gone to the Blasket Island in 1907 to learn the modern Irish language. A personality of some splendour, he had forsaken athletics and the prospect of representing his country in the pole vault of the Olympic Games in Athens, preferring the disciplines of Celtic scholarship in which he progressed until his excellence came to be recognised far and wide. He knew more than Pedersen, said Meyer, that is Holger Pedersen of Denmark, author of the mighty *Vergleichende Grammatik der keltischen Sprachen*, 2 vols., and that was praise.[9]

In Dublin, Best looked after Marstrander, finding him suitable lodgings and initiating him into the Royal Irish Academy and the work of the School, where he was to be let down easy at first with whatever he liked and could best do until he got a better grip of English. Come July, he would have to step into Bergin's shoes and follow his old programme as best he could, the main essential being that he must give instruction in Old-Irish, especially for the foreigners.

Meyer was in negotiation with Fenwick of Cheltenham to buy his Irish MSS 'for our university',[10] meaning Liverpool, but it was difficult to price them. There was no conclusive result to this approach of Meyer's, but Richard Best, no mean diplomat, was successful to a remarkable degree in later negotiations with the Fenwick family in purchasing the rich Cheltenham collection of Irish manuscripts for a reasonable sum on behalf of the National Library of Ireland where they are now housed. Lever of Port Sunlight had just given a gift of £100,000 to the University, but it was all going to Architecture, Tropical Disease and Russian.[11]

Meyer left Liverpool on 12 March for a further round of travel which brought him to London where two days of rest, mainly in Kew Gardens in bright sunshine with lunch and tea in the open improved his vision wonderfully. While he kept away from the British Museum, he did go to University College to have a look at Whitley Stokes' library. 'It made me very sad to think that all that mass of learning is buried here'.[12] Miss Stokes had been refused permission to erect a monument to her father in Howth and suspected an intrigue of the Mahaffys.[13] Paris was Meyer's next stop, then Acqui, in Italy, a pretty place, old and new, surrounded in the distance by fine bold hills with castles and villages dotted about. The hotel, which was good, accommodated some twenty guests, English, American, German and Italian, who dined on Easter Sunday on an agnello pasquale of eggs painted in the Italian colours. He had a letter from Marstrander, now working hard at the letter D of the Dictionary, but very critical of what had been done hitherto. A thousand pities, thought Meyer, that they had to print. Still at Acqui a week later, he looked out on a landscape buried in snow. The guests sat around the great fireplace in the salon or tried to keep warm by playing billiards. Meyer, sitting in his top coat, read Zola's *Thérèse Raquin*, Dumas' *Madame de Volupté*, Napoleon's letters and whatever else he could find in the shops and when feeling particularly well, tried to translate some Irish poems for *Ériu*. He had a letter from Mrs Green, who was greatly pleased with Marstrander. 'The young man has the ball at his feet' wrote Meyer to Best. 'How things have changed from what they were 25 years ago! But there is still a good deal of apathy and sournoiserie to overcome.'[14]

A group of Scandinavians arrived, among them an interesting and fascinating Danish lady, in government employ, who was a professional designer and painter of porcelain, who was also, one thinks, good company and as such appreciated by Meyer. 'It is a great thing to have some one to talk to at meals.'[15] During a short stop at Genoa, on his way to San Remo, he found someone of note to talk to in the person of Theodore Roosevelt, a meeting he described to Best on a simple postcard:

You know my ancient habit of always coming across famous people on my wanderings. I have just had about 20 minutes with Roosevelt, who was lunching in an hotel just opposite mine. So I sent in my card and was asked to come in at once. I found him taking coffee. He received me very amiably, poured out a cup for me and began to talk at once on Irish matters, racial, linguistic, literary. A middle-aged, stout, shortnecked man, with an extraordinary mouth, from which one cannot keep one's eyes. His fleshy lips (almost like a negro's) are always in motion, he draws them back and shows his teeth which are very prominent. Strong American twang. He spoke of Gobineau's work and said it might have been done for the 17th century, but as for the 19th, it was like an albatross trying to learn from a dodo. He told me incidentally that the Nibelungen had accompanied him to Africa (as Napoleon took Ossian). I wanted to make him refer to Celtic studies in his lecture at Oxford, but he said, all his lectures (also at Berlin and Paris) were fully written out. Still, I think, I will write to him about it. He spoke with admiration of my brother and his conversation, when he entertained him at the White House. He asked all about my chair at Liverpool and the prospects of Celtic studies. Then his family came in and told him to get ready for starting. So I left, greatly pleased with my interview. ....I leave here on Monday for San Remo (Hotel de l'Europe et de la Paix) where the Walsinghams are.[16]

At San Remo, lovely spot, Meyer was warmly received by the Walsinghams and accompanied Lord Walsingham to the Casino where the noble man lost £15 before Meyer could stop him, that being money in those days. Meyer, who did not play, but acquired the bad habit later, watched the unlucky performers 'with interest mingled with pity',[17] all their schemes and systems coming to naught. Leaving San Remo on the 20th Meyer arrived in Paris on the 23rd, where he met Henri Gaidoz, Joseph Vendryes and the Rector of the Irish College to talk Celtica and learn that the chair of d'Arbois, which had been in danger of extinction, would be continued, and probably occupied by Joseph Loth. Vendryes was a very pleasant nice-looking young man, refined and easy to talk with, who invited Meyer to be his guest at déjeuner. The accounts of Zimmer were bad, and his case seemingly hopeless. 'To London tomorrow afternoon, home on Wednesday', home being Liverpool, from where he wrote to Best about a scheme of reform he proposed for the University, the exact details of which it would be interesting to discover.

We had a great meeting at my house last night. I had invited twelve of my most distinguished colleagues to put before them a scheme of complete reform of our University on real University lines. It was received, I may say, with enthusiasm, and we have at once decided on the next steps. It will take us three years to carry it through. We have to get a supplementary chapter etc. But the time is at last ripe for such a reform. The present conditions are insufferable.[18]

In July, Meyer, wandering again in Germany, visited Berlin to see his brother Eduard, whom he found in poor health and getting worse. Feeling himself in need of medical attention as well they both consulted the best physician in the city, who overhauled them thoroughly and gave them good advice. Kuno was to try the hot sand baths at a little place in Thüringen called Kostritz and he was going there shortly for a few weeks. First he went to Leipzig to see his old teacher Windisch. From there his letter to Best includes a paragraph unrelated to philology, except for the explanatory Irish glosses:

> My dear Best, I am sitting opposite the most beautiful woman that I have ever seen. She is American, of Irish-Spanish extraction, I should say, of the most perfect shape and hue (i.dénam i. cruth) and with a pair of eyes of such luminosity and expression that they fill the whole room with their radiance. I mention this to excuse myself if you notice any incoherence or distraction in my writing. Of course, she has a vile creature for a husband.[19]

Meyer's appreciation of feminine beauty was warm and unaffected. But there is no incoherence and his hand remains firm and regular. He was writing from the Grand Hotel de Rome, on 25 July 1910, having spent the afternoon of the previous day with Windisch and his family. Windisch had a small class of students for Irish with whom he read Thurneysen's selections, dry and uninteresting stuff. He wanted to know all about the school and Marstrander and Pokorny and *Ériu*.

Life in Germany was very pleasant. They made one very comfortable in hotels and restaurants and everything was reasonably cheap. He had been haunting the secondhand bookshops, not so much for himself as for his nephews and nieces who were all omnivorous readers. Such a different generation! One of his nieces had become an excellent pianist while another had ambitions to go on the stage, to her parents' horror. But this was an old occurrence in the family. His third niece, a girl of nineteen, wanted a complete set of Dostoyevsky! They had not yet made the acquaintance of George Moore, nor would Meyer introduce him. He was glad to hear from Best of Marstrander's popularity with his students.

Then came the news that changed the whole tenor of Kuno Meyer's life. This was the death on 29 July of Heinrich Zimmer, which left vacant the Chair of Celtic Philology in Berlin. In a postcard message to Best, Meyer said he had died of heart failure and confessed his own surprise as he had not thought Zimmer's disease fatal. He had just asked his brother Eduard to order a wreath on behalf of the School of Irish Learning with a suitable inscription. 'This sad event may change my whole life. For the choice of a successor will be between Thurneysen and myself. If they want a grammarian and philologist, they will of course elect Thurneysen who would, I fancy, accept, if the conditions are much better than those at Freiburg. For me, though I have no wife and children, the decision would also be very difficult. It may all come very suddenly'.[20] Although he did not hesitate for a moment in applying for the Berlin post the decision must have caused him some heart-searching and one thinks he primarily did it out of a sense of duty.

Three days later he wrote again from Schwartzburg that it now appeared poor Zimmer had taken his own life by drowning himself after repeated attempts, a deed which he had long contemplated and hinted at to one intimate friend. He believed his illness incurable and his sufferings must have been great. He was buried quietly in Hahnenklee in the Harz. It was impossible to send a wreath as intended. That same day Meyer left for Kostritz to take the course of baths he had been recommended.[21]

Arriving at Kostritz on 7 August, and looking at the way the baths had to be taken, he decided against them. He would be put up to the neck into artificially heated sand, a most disagreeable and distressing procedure, with the doctor standing by all the time, watch in hand and finger on pulse. It would be a very exhausting cure. So he proposed to leave on the morrow and go up into the hills instead for plenty of walks and climbs which always did him good. He had walked six hours the other day with his nephews, climbing a good deal. His brother Eduard had told him the Committee in charge of the appointment to the Berlin chair was not expected to report before Christmas and that the appointment if made would not take effect before Easter, perhaps not before October 1911. He was glad to hear from Best that the School meeting had been so satisfactory. 'Pokorny is a wonderful fellow'. [22]

Thurneysen and Pedersen had also applied for the Berlin chair but Meyer was the man chosen. He reported the news to Best in a letter marked 'Confidential'.

> My dear Best,
>   Jacta est alea! I heard from my brother this morning that I was unanimously proposed by the Faculty *primo loco*, Thurneysen *secundo*, Pedersen *tertio*. The matter will now go to the Ministry, and I shall probably have an interview next month. I wished to tell you at once, as it has such a bearing on the School, but please do not mention it to anyone else at present. It must not leak out or get into the papers. That would be most improper. ....The only one to whom I am also writing is Marstrander, as there has been a curious and unexpected development here lately. To him therefore you may talk about it; but please impress on him also that he must not mention the matter to anybody else.
>   The unanimity of the nomination has surprised me. I am very sorry for Thurneysen, who will feel this very much. I suppose that what decided most of the distinguished scholars who compose the Faculty is the fact that Thurneysen is already in Germany and students can go to him as they have always done. ....
>   One of my conditions will be that I do not enter on the Berlin post before October next.
>
> With kindest greetings
Yours always
Kuno Meyer. [23]

For Meyer it was a fateful decision. One speculates that he might have been happier had he remained in Liverpool where he had made many friends and found social life so pleasant. The fact that his brother Eduard was already in Berlin, in the chair of Ancient History, may very well have influenced him. So doubtless did his patriotism and the conviction that he must serve the Fatherland. That he admired the Emperor Wilhelm is clear from his youthful poems. Whether to remain in Liverpool was a decision he would have to face up to a few years later in any case, with the outbreak of war between England and Germany, and there seems little doubt what his choice would then be. So it happened, sooner rather than later, that he made a choice which was inevitable. On 19 December 1910 he wrote to Best: 'To-day I signed the contract which binds me to Berlin from October 1911 onward. The conditions are on the whole all very satisfactory, and the authorities have been most obliging...'[24]

Following the death of Heinrich Zimmer on 29 July 1910 there arose the question of what was to become of his valuable Celtic Library. Frau Martha Zimmer wrote to Meyer asking his advice. Meyer recommended a retail sale, which would mean preparing and printing a catalogue to be sent to various Celtic scholars and libraries. That was, however, before he had actually seen the library. Meyer hoped that Best would help him in fixing the prices. The library was the only thing Zimmer had left to his family and the sale would have to bring in as much money as possible, although his widow was getting a pension of some £150. There was a family of two boys, who by all accounts were gifted.[25] Mrs Zimmer asked Meyer to go through the library and manuscripts to see to what might best be done and Meyer accordingly planned to go to Berlin in September to visit the family. He hoped the library would be kept together and the thought occurred to him that it might go to the Celtic seminar in Berlin.[26]

Arriving in Berlin he stayed with his brother Eduard in Mommsenstrasse 8, and on 11 September, following lunch with Pokorny, 'restless as ever', he went to see Mrs Zimmer, a melancholy visit. She was resigned but still terribly sad. 'She looked beautiful in her grief'. The library was much finer than he had thought. It was worth about £750. It included all the *Zeitschriften*, Kuhn, BB., and *Revue Celtique*. It appears that Güterbock, known to Celtic students from his work on the Index to the *Grammatica Celtica,* made Zimmer a present of his entire library a few years since when he decided to give up Celtic studies for good. Meyer put a query to Best:

> Is there any chance of the Nat. Univ. buying it en bloc? Bergin is hardly the man to manage it. It will perhaps go to America. Both Washington and Philadelphia are bidding for it. I still advocate the retail sale.[27]

He spent some hours with Mrs Zimmer and her two boys, the younger of whom, Ernst, was studying philology, but at the request of his mother would not touch Celtic. It is probable that Frau Zimmer had felt the strain of the controversies in which her husband embroiled himself as well as the fierce dedication to his research that caused him to work late into the nights and shatter his health. Like John Strachan, he had over-taxed himself and might be said to have met his death from copying a St. Gall codex within a fortnight, sleeping only a few hours in the morning, merely to send it back in the stipulated time.[28]

Meyer came away with a large parcel of manuscript notes and other items of Zimmer's which contained the boldest and most ingenious ideas thrown out but not worked out from which Meyer thought he might be able to make a paper for the *Zeitschrift*. That evening he took his two nephews to hear Fidelio at the Royal Opera.[29]

In the enchanting autumn weather Meyer sat out mostly in the large garden of his brother's house in Mommsenstrasse, working at *Betha Colmáin* and going through Zimmer's manuscripts. These were of profound interest and he considered it imperative to publish them in some shape or form. The vastness of Zimmer's plans was astonishing. They included a history of Celtic speech from remotest times. His ingenuity, daring, vast knowledge and bitter invective, of which Rudolf Thurneysen was the main target, were all present in the manuscripts. On the afternoon of 15 September Meyer had another interview with Zimmer's widow. He put the value of the Library at between £750 and £1000. In the course of a conversation that morning with Ludwig Christian Stern, Librarian of the Berlin Royal Library, Stern told him his library would not be competing for it. 'I am sending a short note to the *Freeman* about the library. If Dublin is to have it, no time should be lost. I fear American interference.'[30] There was not much in the books in the way of manuscript notes but there was a full index verborum to the Würzburg Glosses. There was also a copy of LL., saved from the fire of 1903, charred all round but otherwise perfectly good, with a lot of entries. Meyer stressed the urgency of the matter to Best. 'Could not £1000 be raised if the University (Hyde, MacNeill, Bergin) appealed for funds. Would you see Hyde about it? Ireland might thus pay its debt to the dead scholar. But everything must be done in such a way as not to offend the feelings of Mrs Zimmer. I am thinking of Mrs Strachan. This is the third case of the kind with which I have to do and it is a delicate business always.'[31]

Meyer planned to stay in Berlin until the 21st September. He could not imagine his being happy there. The people were not pleasant, the rush was far worse than London and every scholar in the city was more or less a wreck. Mrs Zimmer told him that when she heard her husband speak to a friend about his plans last winter she was aghast. The friend said 'But, Zimmer, this needs ten lives', and Zimmer answered that he could do it if only he had his health back. 'His jottings give you the idea as if his brain had been on fire. He rushes on from one mighty problem to another.'[32]

Four days later he wrote urgently to Best and asked him to see Bergin and O'Donoghue the librarian of University College about the library. 'It should not go to America of which there is great danger. Start a subscription list. Write some letters to the papers on Z.'s claims to be commemorated. I have given Bergin details of the collection. If the money cannot be raised, Liverpool would buy the Welsh and Breton section, or Dublin and Liverpool might combine in some way'.[33]

He would be in Dublin himself in October, but it would be well to start a propaganda at once. He planned to publish all Zimmer's *Nachlass,* omitting his onslaughts on Thurneysen, Wilhelm Schulze, Harnack 'and yours always K.M.'[34] On the 20th he left Berlin, which he thought would kill him in a short while, and next day planned to go to Hamburg, intending to sail for England on the 24th. He had by now come firmly to the conclusion that Mrs Zimmer rnust dispose of the library *en bloc*, the trouble of a retail sale being too great, added to the fact that she would have to leave her present home. His great fear was that it would go to America unless he could raise the money in Liverpool. On his way to Hamburg he stopped at Braunschweig to see the library of Wolfenbüssel close by, where Lessing was librarian, in the hope of finding manuscripts of Irish origin. [35]

Having spent some time in London examining the Stokes Library at University College, Meyer returned to Liverpool, where term began on 4 October. It was his 26th session at the University and he wondered whether it might be the last. 'What a wrench it would be.' He did not consider £750 too much for Zimmer's library, seeing what prices were being asked in recent Dublin book catalogues. He had begun printing CZ.VIII[2] in which he was publishing a first instalment of Zimmer's *Nachlass* leaving out the combative scholar's worst passages of attack on Windisch and Thurneysen. Meyer thought he hated Thurneysen more than Windisch although he could not have his fling at him so easily.[36]

Meyer's exhortations that the National University should purchase the library were successful. Eoin MacNeill set out for Berlin with instructions on behalf of the University to negotiate with Mrs Zimmer and spent a night in Liverpool with the Meyers on his way. On viewing the library he considered Kuno Meyer's estimate of £750 very fair and recommended the purchase at that sum. 'All will probably *be settled* before he returns, whereat I am mighty pleased.'[37] He awaited confirmation of the purchase from MacNeill, who presently wrote him a letter, which Meyer forwarded to Best. Evidently it contained tidings that the bargain had been sealed, for Meyer commented 'I am very glad the business is now settled. It is a weight off my mind.'[38]

Never was £750, or 14,000 marks, better spent. Ireland can be grateful to Meyer for his part in securing for her Celtic language and literature students a collection that was virtually priceless. For the newly founded University, its Celtic shelves as yet unstocked, it was an acquisition of incalculable value. Zimmer had spent some thirty years collecting all the available books, pamphlets and journals relating to the Celtic languages. Part of this collection was destroyed in a disastrous fire at his house in 1903, the shock of which seriously impaired his health, about which time Meyer observed to Mrs Hutton, 'Poor Zimmer, I am afraid, will never lecture again. His health has completely broken down.'[39]

He rallied, however, and set about restoring the loss, aided in this object by scholars and institutions the world over who appreciated his great work for Celtic studies. The energy he expended in this task may be measured by the fact that only a small number of books was needed to bring the collection up to what it had been. The library acquired by University College Dublin was divided into seven sections, of which the largest, numbering 679 items, related to Irish language and literature, bearing in mind that a single item could be a slim pamphlet or a set of many volumes. Next came Breton with 591 items, followed by Welsh with 589, Scottish Gaelic with 242, saga literature and folklore 285, comparative philology as related to Celtic languages 157 and there were sections devoted to Cornish and Manx. There were in all about 7,000 items, between volumes, sets, pamphlets and fasciculi, in the calculation of the University librarian D.J. O'Donoghue (*Irish Independent* 19 December 1910), who commented that in this library were the materials in which generations of students might find sources of inspiration for their energy. 'What a calamity it would have been if such a library had been scattered in all directions.' [40]

Housed under the name of the Zimmer Library in University College, Earlsfort Terrace, the collection enabled successive ranks of the University's Celtic students to consult, in one library, all the material for the use of which they might otherwise have to visit many widely separated locations, even many lands.

The fault was not Meyer's that he was unsuccessful in acquiring for the nation another important library, that of Whitley Stokes. Although he brought all his influence and persuasion to bear on Maive and Annie Stokes to give their father's library to some Irish institution, they would not hear of it. He found it incredible that their 'animus', as he called it, could go so far. One wonders why 'animus'. Could it be related to some unappreciative notices of Stokes in Irish sources? The library went to University College, London, the formal presentation being made by Meyer and Sir Charles Lyall, on behalf of the donors, on 9 December 1910.

Meyer described the occasion briefly to Best. 'There was a very large gathering yesterday for the opening of the Stokes Library. Mrs Green was there looking wonderfully fresh and well. She told me that Bergin had given £100 towards the keep-up of the Stokes Library, to buy new books, etc. We were all delighted, doubly so as it came unsolicited and unexpected. I hope it will make London donors follow suit'.[41] But Meyer considered it a waste of a splendid resource to have it housed, in cold storage as it were, where the likelihood of it being used or consulted was remote.

At the presentation he made a short speech reviewing the achievements of Stokes in Irish scholarship and recalling how his thoughts wandered back to the time when his library 'was the workshop, the laboratory, of the great scholar whom for more than 25 years I was proud to be allowed to call my master and my friend.'

The library consisted of about 3500 volumes and pamphlets, the bulk of them relating to Celtic studies, philology and folklore, included among which were manuscript annotations, review cuttings, notes, letters and postcards from various scholars with whom Stokes had corresponded. There were early Irish printed books, collections of all the scholarly Celtic periodicals, several hundred volumes on mythology, folklore and folksong besides Celtic, numerous works on Indo-European philology as well as on early Indian, especially Sanskrit, philology, folklore and literature. One of Whitley Stokes' many pursuits was the folklore of all nations and it is of interest that his daughter Maive contributed an important volume to this field of study, in her *Indian Fairy Tales* (Calcutta 1879) to which her father added a valuable index of folklore themes.

90

Of all Irish philologists, Stokes was the one most respected and looked up to by Meyer. Writing to Mrs Hutton his regard is clear for the elder scholar who was in a sense both guide and counsellor to him:

> I managed to finish my London course just before the Xmas vacation. My last lecture was on Whitley Stokes and I was greatly pleased to see so many of his old freinds among the audience. Altogether I was astonished to have so many hearers – about 150 – for a second year's course. I have been asked to give a third course next year.

> I do indeed miss Dr. Strachan and Whitley Stokes every day. I have arranged the books and Mss left by the latter and am now seeing his 'Supplement to the Thesaurus' through the press. The books go to University College London; the daughters would unfortunately not hear of their going to Dublin, which would have been the proper place for them. But it is hoped that a permanent lectureship or chair for Celtic may be established in London.[43]

NOTES

1. Meyer to Best, 7 Jan. 1910, from Thackeray Hotel, opp. Brit. Museum. NLI Ms No. 11002.

2. The doubtings attached to the Dictionary project may be seen from the following extracts:

   > The R.I.A. seems to leave everything to Gwynn and he does not unfortunately realise the standard of work required both in the Dictionary and in the Catalogue. Atkinson now wishes me to be chief editor of the Dictionary but seems to make it a condition that Purton is to be my only assistant. No sane scholar would assent to such a programme.
   > Meyer to Best 8.11.1906. NLI MS No 11002 (11).

   > Strachan and I have come to the conclusion that the R.I.A. should drop the idea of a Dictionary for the present. It can simply not be done. They undertook it rashly and must pay the penalty for it.
   > Meyer to Best 6.12.1906. NLI Ms No. 11002 (11)

   > As to the Dictionary, I have now come to the conclusion that it is altogether premature and should be dropped for the present. What the Academy might do would be to get Strachan to bring out a Dictionary to the *Thesaurus Palaeohibernicus* and other undoubted Old-Irish texts.
   > Meyer to Best, 8.1.1907. NLI MS No 11002 (12)

3. Meyer to Best, 3 Feb. 1910. NLI Ms No 11002.
4. *Ibid.*
5. Meyer to Best, 13 Feb. 1910. NLI Ms No. 11002.
6. Meyer to Best, 17 Feb. 1910. NLI Ms No. 11002.
7. Meyer to Best, 19 Feb. 1910. NLI Ms No. 11002.
8. Meyer to Best, 25 Feb. 1910. NLI Ms No. 11002.
9. For a fuller account of Marstrander's career, see the present writer's *Carl Marstrander (1883-1965)* in Cork Hist. and Arch. Soc. *Journal* LXXXIX No 248 (Jan-Dec 1984) 108-124.
10. Meyer to Best, 7 March 1910. NLI Ms No 11002.
11. *Ibid.*
12. Meyer to Best, 15 March 1910. NLI Ms No 11002.
13. *Ibid.*
14. Meyer to Best, 4 April 1910. NLI Ms No. 11002.
15. *Ibid.*
16. Meyer to Best, 9 April 1910. NLI Ms No. 11002.
17. Meyer to Best, 12 April 1910. NLI Ms No. 11002.
18. Meyer to Best, 5 June 1910. NLI Ms No. 11002.

19. Meyer to Best, 25 July 1910. NLI Ms No 11002.
20. Meyer to Best, 31 July 1910. NLI Ms No. 11002.
21. Meyer to Best, 3 Aug. 1910, NLI Ms No. 11002.
22. Meyer to Best, 7 Aug. 1910. NLI Ms No 11002.
23. Meyer to Best, 21 November 1910, from Liverpool. NLI Ms No. 11002.
24. Meyer to Best, by postcard, 19 December 1910. NLI Ms No. 11002.
25. Meyer to Best, 27 Aug. 1910 from Tambach. NLI Ms No. 11002.
26. Meyer to Best, 22 Aug. 1910 from Tambach. NLI Ms No. 11002.
27. Meyer to Best, by postcard 12 Sept. 1910 from Gross-Lichterfelde, Mommsenstr. 8. NLI Ms No. 11002.
28. Meyer to Best, 11 Aug. 1910 from Tambach i Thür. NLI Ms No. 11002.
29. Meyer to Best, 12 Sept. 1910.
30. Meyer to Best, by postcard, 15 Sept. 1910.
31. *Ibid.*
32. *Ibid.*
33. Meyer to Best, by postcard 19 Sept. 1910 from Berlin. NLI Ms No. 11002.
34. *Ibid.*
35. Meyer to Best, by postcard 20 Sept. 1910 from Braunschweig. NLI Ms No. 11002.
36. Meyer to Best, by postcard 3 Oct. 1910 from Liverpool. NLI Ms No. 11002.
37. Meyer to Best, by p.c. postmarked Liverpool 19 Oct. 1910. NLI Ms No. 11002.
38. Meyer to Best, 31 Oct. 1910 from 41 Huskisson St. Liverpool. NLI Ms No. 11002.
39. Meyer to Mrs Hutton, 24 July (*recte* June) 1903. NLI Ms No. 8616 (3).
40. D.J. O'Donoghue, *Irish Independent* 19 Dec. 1910. O'Donoghue also contributed a notice of the library to the *Irish Book Lover,* Vol II., No. 7, 102-3, Feb. 1911, in the course of which he says: '... but above all Zimmer has abundantly annotated many of the volumes with his latest discoveries, and on margins and inter-leaves has written his accumulated stores of learning, which he never otherwise could have placed on permanent record. Many a lacuna in Celtic texts is effectively filled, or a learned explanation suggested. In short in this great collection are the materials in which generations of students will find sources of inspiration for their energies for all time. By this purchase, and the taking over of the libraries of the Royal and the old Catholic Universities, University College Dublin now possessed about 35,000 volumes. About 10,000 of the books and pamphlets had reference to Ireland and the Celtic peoples generally.'
41. Meyer to Best, 10 Dec. 1910 from Endsleigh Palace Hotel, London. NLI Ms No. 11002.
42. Booklet, 'Presentation of the Whitley Stokes Library.' p. 4.
43. Meyer to Mary Hutton, 27 Dec. 1909 from Imperial Hotel, Bournemouth. NLI Ms No. 8616 (4).

Chapter 9

MEYER, holidaying in Monte Carlo in January 1911, considered it might be useful to have a talk with David Lloyd George, who was relaxing in nearby Nice, about the School and other matters, mainly the modest sum of money which had been withdrawn. The Welsh-speaking Celt, now powerful in political life, should for all reasons be sympathetic, but was rather elusive, being out when Meyer called, so Meyer left his card and address, hoping the great man would send a message. At Monte Carlo Meyer remained out of doors all day in the sunshine, spending the evenings with the Walsinghams or Conybeares or in the International Sporting Club where the tables were not so crowded, since he had now become an addict and was, on this occasion at least, successful. With room and petit déjeuner at 4 francs Monte Carlo was not dear. Toni was in Berlin looking for houses or flats and finding them horribly dear and not to her taste.[1]

He hoped that in Berlin he would at last be able to work properly. Hitherto all he had done had been in a tearing hurry and never satisfactory. One could not serve two masters, much less half a dozen. He had heard from Heidelberg that Sütterliss, a pupil and friend of Osthoff's and a good Germanist, was inclined to accept his (Meyer's) German chair. So far Lloyd George had not replied. Was the Celt being wary or simply not interested? He was leaving Nice on the morrow, so Meyer supposed they would not meet.[2]

Meyer left Monte Carlo on the 10th, travelling via Paris, where he met Gaidoz[3] and 'the irrepressible Miss Schoepperle, with her everlasting Tristan and Iseult', to reach Liverpool on the 14th and find all in the University horribly disappointed that Postgate had not been elected to Cambridge. His London classes were beginning on January 20th and his lectures, which he had yet to write, in a fortnight. He had news from Constable that his little book on *Ancient Irish Poetry* would be out in ten days.[3]

In London a class of eleven and three lectures on Zimmer kept him busy. No biography of Zimmer had appeared up to now and since the scholar's career was lively with controversy, with personal attacks surging from every page he wrote, like Vendryes said, such a study would make absorbing reading and Celtic studies are the poorer for lack of it. Meyer, who would have been in a good position to write it, contributed just the three lectures on his life and work but regrettably did not publish them. But an essay on Zimmer by one of his students, Richard Henebry, published in the *Irish Educational Review*[4] was considered very unsatis-factory, and with reason, by Richard Best who sent a copy to Meyer along with a letter saying:

> I send you a copy of the *Irish Educational Review* containing the article on Zimmer by Henebry, which is deplorable. Though boasting of his friendship, love and intimacy he treats him as a vainglorious fool.... It is full of inaccuracies as you will see, and not free from malice. Bergin has read it. Marstrander to whom we spoke of it, said that Bergin as a pupil of Z. should reply to it.... Not a word of his great achievements.... I hear you have been lecturing in London on Zimmer. What would you say to publishing your lecture as a counterblast in the new 'Irish Review', which is shortly to appear. Moore, John Eglinton, Stephens, AE. etc., are all contributing. They asked me to send you a circular.... They would be delighted if you would contribute.[5]

Reacting with sharp disapproval, Meyer wrote Henebry in ironical terms a letter 'that will I hope put an end to any intercourse between us'[6] which reads:

> Dear Henebry,
>   Since I wrote to you I have read your article on Zimmer in the *Educational Review*. The lofty sentiment pervading it, the noble style and choice language, the deep and wide learning shown on every point, but above all the scrupulous impartiality reflect the greatest credit on the writer. But what will most appeal to every reader is the gentle and delicate manner in which you have dealt with Zimmer's failings, covering them up with the mantle of Christian charity. That was, of course, to be expected from your calling, and from the loyalty of an old pupil and friend who had been admitted to such intimacy with the dead scholar and his family. I hope you did not forget to send a copy to Mrs Zimmer. What a pity your old friends Strachan and Stokes are not alive to enjoy this masterly exposition of Zimmer's work, and to congratulate you on the success of your debut as the spokesman of Irish Scholarship, the cause of Ireland and your Church,
>
> Mise
Kuno Meyer[7]

Henebry wrote an answer which he never sent. It was dated at Sunday's Well, Cork, 28 February 1911, and has been published by his biographer Dr Stockley.[8] In the course of it Henebry wrote that 'Zimmer's works constitute a thesaurus of fable about the History of Religion in this country' and addressing himself to Meyer, says 'I have heard grave complaints about certain lectures of yours', meaning perhaps the lectures on Zimmer being given by Meyer in University College London.

Best in his critical letter of 9 February, acknowledged receipt of Meyer's *Selections from Ancient Irish Poetry* which Constable had sent him. 'It is an attractive little volume and will spread your name far and wide. You have skimmed off the cream of Irish literature. I only wish the printer and binder had shown as much taste in presenting it to the public. Many thanks for the gift of it.' The *Selections,* a volume of 114 pages including notes, consisted of poems already published by Meyer in various booklets and journals and now brought together in a collection which in its introduction and contents had a significant impact on students and readers of Irish literature in the English language. The dedication was 'To Edmund Knowles Muspratt, the enlightened and generous patron of Celtic studies in the University of Liverpool a small token of affectionate regard and gratitude'. Muspratt in his memoirs has only the briefest allusion to Meyer.

For such an important little volume, the work by which Meyer is best known, the production was dowdy. This was compensated for by its reception. Writing in words of high praise, Lascelles Abercrombie told Meyer that

> '.... in these translations of yours there is more than can be verbally appreciated. Please don't think I exaggerate their value to me: I wish I could. Without, I hope, impertinence, I want to tell you that your renderings strike me as most exquisite and genuine English poetry; for, unless I say that, I cannot indicate the extent of my gratitude. Only those to whom poetry is the main thing in this life can judge of the immoderate pleasure felt when their stores are increased as mine were today. Of one thing I am certain; I shall not learn Irish when I can get such versions as these.'[9]

The review in the *Times Literary Supplement* greatly pleased Meyer and he wondered who wrote it.[9a] A discerning and sympathetic piece of writing, it occupied pride of place in the first page of the TLS of 16 March under the heading of 'Celtic Origins', taking up a substantial two columns. The poetry in Professor Meyer's book, said the reviewer, had a style behind it 'and such a style as, perhaps, only a great literature can produce'. It was a representative anthology of exquisite lyrics.

> Nevertheless, exquisite in themselves though they are, these lyrics in Professor Meyer's 'Ancient Irish Poetry' are primarily interesting as authentic specimens of the metal which has so deeply alloyed European poetry .... When all is said, however, Professor Meyer's 'Ancient Irish Poetry' is much more a stimulus to critical speculation. It is a book of poetry, nothing less; and Professor Meyer makes it so as well as his nameless originals. His sense of the poetic value of English is admirable; and is at its best in the pieces where the material is best – the poems which read the earth. Let anyone who wants a book to companion him on a walking tour choose this one; he will assuredly not repent of putting it to that severe test.

There was academic strife in Liverpool University, where they were 'in a terrible state of things', according to Meyer 'and I am up to my neck in it'. It would soon, he thought, reach the public. At present he could say no more. He had cancelled all his engagements, including the London ones, until May. 'I doubt whether anything will be done here now for Celtic. Indeed even Glyn Davies may have to go. The Council are all in the hands of one man, an attorney without any ideas. He has stocked the whole Council with his creatures. However, we shall fight him to the knife.'[10]

Carl Marstrander, heavily overworked, was stricken with pleurisy in Dublin and Meyer, greatly disturbed, awaited definite news from Best. So much depended on the brilliant Norwegian. Meyer wrote to cheer him up and was ready to cross to Dublin at once should he be needed. Marstrander's recovery was now the question of first importance and Meyer was immensely relieved to hear that a lung operation had been successful. Better news followed and Meyer commented that with good care and a holiday Marstrander might not be any the worse for it. 'Like all of us he will have to buy his experience and wisdom. Give him my kind regards and tell him so from an old hand at making a mess of it',[11] a reference to the arthritis which had made his own life so difficult and which, with greater care in the beginning, might not have developed. Nobody could have shown more concern for Marstrander during his illness and convalescence than Meyer, who gave him good advice and stayed with him for company in Monte Carlo where he went for some weeks in April to recuperate, watching over him with something like paternal solicitude.

Early in May Meyer delivered a lecture in Oxford on the same day on which he received a Doctorate from the University which gave him the right to style himself D.Litt. Oxon. Writing from Magdalen College he described the proceedings to Best. Gilbert Murray made the introductory speech in traditional Latin and mentioned both the School and *Ériu*. Warren, with whom Meyer was staying in Oxford, admitted him.

> It was all very solemn and impressive…. The weather is perfectly lovely and Oxford looks its best. At 3 I had my lecture, which was well attended (Sweet was there and Plummer), and Warren once more spoke. Then a garden party in this fairy-like place, with the deer grazing around us. I met many old friends and made interesting new acquaintances. Now there is a short interval till dinner, which will be given to me by Raleigh and Gotch, two old Liverpool friends. I go back to London tomorrow to dine with Ker and Jeanroy, and again with Ker and Thurneysen on Thursday. You see it is an endless succession of pleasures.[12]

Presenting Meyer as an outstanding citizen of the republic of letters, Murray outlined his career, calling attention to two out of many examples from his incredible repertory of labours, firstly, the journals *Ériu* and *Zeitschrift für celtische Philologie,* Secundo, scholam criticam, quae doctrinam antiquam Hibernorum ex tenebris revocaret, inter Dublinienses fundavit, which had furnished a disciple of Meyer's as the first Irish language professor to the recently established National University of Ireland.

> It may be permitted to me, myself of Irish origin though unacquainted with the Irish tongue, at this time, when, with the revived study of the ancient Irish language, poetry, learning and civilisation, the Irish people itself has begun to hope for better things and to gird itself for loftier achievement, to offer gratitude to this regenerator of Irish scholarship and to commend him to you as one who by his genius and learning has earned the highest acclaim in Germany and England.[13]

It was a splendid oration, a model of classical composition, much appreciated by Meyer, who wrote to Murray from Endsleigh Palace Hotel, London on 11 May:

> Dear Professor Gilbert Murray,
>   I had no opportunity before leaving Oxford to tell you once more what pleasure it gave to be presented by you and to thank you for all the kind and generous things you said about me. I wish to do so now and to ask you for a loan of your speech so that I may copy it and keep it as a mnemosynon of one of the proudest days of my life. I regret very much that my hurried visit did not allow me to seek your further acquaintance. If ever you come to Berlin I hope you will let me

know. I am staying here till Saturday, after which my address is 41 Huskisson Street, Liverpool.

Yours faithfully,
Kuno Meyer

In London he gave his last lecture on Zimmer, after which he was able to breathe more freely. He thanked Best for his congratulations on his latest honour, paying Oxford the compliment that it was not as bad as painted, 'at least the men I met there are mostly good fellows and as a rule not without learning, though often in a curious, old fashioned way. But that too has its charm'. If he had to live there good cheer and good fellowship would soon put an end to all serious work. Walter Raleigh told him he had to live out of Oxford in order to escape its influence on that score. He had evidently nearly succumbed.[15]

In Liverpool they were in the midst of their meetings to appoint his successor. 41 candidates had applied, some of them very distinguished people from Germany.[16] Lehmann-Haupt had been elected to the Greek chair recently. Meyer was surprised to hear from Marstrander that he was on his way back to Dublin from Monte Carlo, and feared the change in climate would do him no good. He had urged Marstrander time and again to go to some sanatorium in Switzerland or Germany to learn how he should live and take care of himself. He had not the most elementary ideas of good air, in his bedroom for instance, exercise and the like, and these he would be taught in a few weeks in such a place. Meyer urged Best to try and arrange this. 'If he fell ill again now we would all blame ourselves very much.'[17] Meyer held his last class in London on 26 May and that evening gave a dinner at Pagani's to which he had invited the Clanna Stokes, the Thurneysens, Mrs Green, Norman Moore and the Priebsches, omitting George Moore from the list as he thought he would not fit well with the company.[18] Antonie, who had been stricken with peritonitis, was now making a rapid recovery and they were going to Berlin in July to look for a flat.[19] The dinner was a great success, with company well selected and congenial. Mrs Green told him that 10,000 copies of her little work *Irish Nationality* (1911) had been sold which was in contrast to the more modest sale of 900 of his own *Selections from Ancient Irish Poetry.*[30] The Thurneysens, who had been staying in Liverpool with Kuno and Toni, had left for Wales after Meyer had shown them around the docks to gratify Mrs Thurneysen's passion for the sea and ships. In the University they were suddenly plunged into a horrible mess over the appointment of Meyer's successor, 'so that all my plans are upset. I foresee weeks of strife and toil; and what with this and the impossibility to get to any settled work I am compelled to ask you to cancel my course in Dublin,' being six lectures on the history of the Irish language scheduled to begin on 19 June. On this subject he appears to have published nothing subsequently, which is a pity. But at present he never had his hands so full of business and his health was suffering under the continual strain and he would be glad when it was all over.[21]

At Meyer's request, Richard Best had been busy compiling a bibliography of Whitley Stokes which he finished early in June. It was a task thoroughly performed, a tribute both to the great Celtic scholar who was present at the birth of Celtic philology when the immortal *Grammatica Celtica* appeared, and to Best's own standing as a bibliographer and was acknowledged as 'a beautiful piece of work'[22] by Meyer, who added that if Zimmer had been done in the same way they would now have a more comprehensive bibliography of Celtic studies during their most important period. He was sending it off to Germany by Professor Petsch. It is printed, all fifty-five pages, in *Zeitschrift für celtische Philologie,* Vol. VIII, 351-406.

It seems that the choice of his successor was not easily arrived at. Writing to Best on June 9th, he said they had sat up the night before until 2 o'clock debating about the German candidates. 'The result I rejoice to say was a victory for my favourite, but there are still several stages to pass before that victory is assured'. His favourite then, obviously, was Robert Petsch, who was duly appointed his successor in the chair of German and held the post until 1914.

The time was now near when he had to bid goodbye to Liverpool, where he had been popular with all and had for twenty-seven years partaken with zest in the social and academic life of the University. It had been a good life amongst appreciative friends, two hundred[23] of whom subscribed to a portrait, to be painted by Augustus John and presented to him on the eve of his departure, as a mark of their esteem for a valued colleague. John and Meyer were old friends since 1901, when John had been appointed instructor in the art school affiliated to the University,[24] and they had together adventured along with Sampson into gypsy haunts of the Welsh highlands. The collection and disbursement of the money for the portrait was organised by Professor Alexander Mair.[25]

On a postcard of 15 June, Meyer related to Best the distractions that beset him at this time.

> All our plans are now upset as soon as we have made them, and to crown all I shall probably soon depend on the will or whim of one of the most eccentric and erratic of men, Augustus John, who is to paint my portrait. I half hope he will decline to do so, but he is an old friend and has been asked by friends.... At present I am going through my books and Mss to see what I can get rid of before I go. There is little leisure for work, and yet I ought to finish quite a number of things....'[26]

Farewells were said with ceremony. John Sampson, habitué of gypsy company, as well as artist in life and the lighter sorts of poesy, who had been instructed by Meyer in the prosody of Irish verse at which he proved an adept pupil, as in his poem in honour of Meyer's 40th birthday

Kuno Meyer
is a theme that might inspire
Balder bards than I to worse
verse

now again contributed a worthy recital, in the nature of the elegy, read at a supper party given by Edgar and Mrs Browne on 28 June on the occasion of 'Professor Meyer's departure from Liverpool', full of allusions to his fellow scholars and their jollities -

Kuno is going - hence these strains of woe!
These sad secretions of ophthalmic brine!
Kuno is going - All our great men go,
Rendall, Lodge, Aked, and De Beaumont Klein

....

Recall the Crocodile, that kindly spot,
When all were friends, and everywhere goodwill,
And Raleigh sang a song I've quite forgot,
And Strong, they tell me, dodged the waiter's bill.[27]

On the night of July 5th Meyer was guest of honour at a dinner in the University, which was attended by about 65 people, including some of his oldest friends from boyhood days in Edinburgh. Amongst those who spoke were Walter Raleigh, John MacDonald Mackay and Edmund Muspratt. At the dinner he was presented with a set of beautiful portraits, photographic probably, of all his arts colleagues.

John had begun his portrait in oils that afternoon, working with great rapidity, but discarded this first effort and began another in a different location, Gethin's studio in the Apothecaries Hall, Colquitt Street end of Bold Street, on which he made better progress, 'getting on *like a house on fire*', Meyer's words and emphasis. 'He is painting me without a waistcoat sitting in an armchair. I look like a sailor.'[28] Next day Meyer wrote: 'John hopes to finish today. It is a strange production, frightfully unconventional. Open shirt, one button of the trousers open (this I must really get him to change), a red tie which I never wear, no waistcoat &c.'[29] In such rapid time did John complete this remarkable portrait, the dimensions of which are 91 x 76 cm. While the finished work was probably a surprise to his sister Antonie, Meyer reports that she 'and all others like John's painting very much and all agree that it is a masterpiece.' In his own view it was meant for a large room or hall and had to be looked at from a great distance.[30]

The portrait, which on its presentation to Meyer became his property, was left by him in the custody of the University Club in Liverpool. It received the highest praise from critics like Sir Claude Phillipps and W.A. Sinclair who, after its exhibition at the Hibernian Academy in Dublin in 1912, applauded it in the *Irish Review* as a work 'justifying the whole art of painting .... the portrait of a strong sensitive man, painted with superb assurance and directness, forsaking old forms of expression ... startling in its simplicity and nervous characterisation.'[31] The portrait, which has a history, now hangs, fittingly, in the National Gallery of Ireland.[32]

'We are off tomorrow' wrote Antonie to Richard Best on 18 July from their Liverpool home, 41 Huskisson Street. She was going to Berlin in search of a suitable house or flat while Kuno proposed among other things to visit his old teacher Windisch and go for a rest cure to Pöstyén where, on medical advice, he might try radio emanations in conjunction with the baths. At Pöstyén he heard from Best that Marstrander had gone to Norway, taking all the dictionary slips with him, evidently intending to stay there a good while. Surprised, Meyer hoped he was not putting his health at risk and wrote to him at once, no doubt advising him to be prudent.

Meyer did not fail to thank Richard Best 'for all your kindness and hospitality which has made your house a second home to me',[33] in a note from Bryn Derwen, Denbighshire, where he was staying after a visit to Dublin in early October. He had been to see Augustine Birrell hoping his influence might obtain a modest grant for the School and found him most businesslike but hardly really interested, asking whether they were not a learned society reading papers to each other, which suggests that the admirably bookish Chief Secretary did not keep himself informed of the progress of Celtic studies. Everything now depended on Sir John Rhys and whether Lloyd George could see them soon, as Meyer had to return shortly to Berlin for his University duties.

There was genuine regret felt in Ireland at Meyer's departure from Liverpool amongst those, not many perhaps, who were informed and appreciative of the services he had performed for the nation's literature and learning. Liverpool was so near, with only the Irish Sea between, and Berlin so far, that it was feared his help and encouragement would be reduced or diminished. Their feelings were expressed and their apprehensions calmed by the influential *Freeman's Journal* (27 December 1910) when the news broke of his Berlin appointment, in the column headed 'By the way':

> Dr Kuno Meyer authorises us to announce that he has now definitely accepted the invitation to the Chair of Celtic in the University of Berlin, in succession to the great Zimmer. His acceptance means a great loss to Ireland, where his work at the School of Irish Learning has been an immense stimulus and the very best of practical aid to the establishment of the native School of Celticists of which Ireland may now legitimately boast ...
>
> This loss to Ireland will in some ways be tempered by the fact that Dr. Kuno Meyer will, beyond doubt, be instrumental in enforcing upon the numerous Celtic students of Germany that Ireland is the natural Mecca of the faithful. Here we have the historic places, the living language and folklore, and fervent and accomplished professors and students of the old literature. The Celticists of the past generation almost ignored the living Celtic people and the modern language which is still - whether in vocabulary, in phonetics, or in traditional literary and historic allusions - the key to the old treasury, and of all these Dr Meyer has firsthand and peculiarly sympathetic knowledge. Ireland itself, apart from a knot of poets and of linguistic students, has not fully appreciated the great work done by this eminent scholar.

Well said, and enlarged upon the following day by the same *Freeman's Journal* (28 December) in a striking tribute headed 'The new Celtic scholarship', an extract from which illuminates the regard felt for Kuno Meyer, the opening words being from his 1909 edition of *Tecosca Cormaic*, the Instructions of King Cormac mac Airt.

Firmness without anger, Patience without strife, Affability and no haughtiness, Taking care of ancient lore, Giving truth for truth, Hosting with reason, Truth without addition, Honouring Poets, Taking thought for every wretch' - these are some of the qualities which King Cormac Mac Airt, in the Teagasc traditionally ascribed to him, demanded of Kings. They are among the qualities of the great scholar also; and they are not inapplicable to the great scholar from whose work the English words are borrowed, from Dr Kuno Meyer in his edition of the noble tractate, the first complete publication of this valuable and beautiful ninth century document of social custom which gives unassailable proof of a luminous, instructed, courteous and merciful civilisation in the Ireland of a thousand years ago.

NOTES

1. Meyer to Best, postcard 3 Jan. 1911. NLI Ms No. 11002.
2. Meyer to Best, postcard 5 Jan. 1911 from Monte Carlo. NLI Ms No. 11002.
3. Meyer to Best, postcard 11 Jan. 1911 from Paris; letter 19 January 1911 from Liverpool. NLI Ms No. 11002.
4. Rev. Richard Henebry: 'Heinrich Zimmer' *Irish Educational Review* Vol 4 (1910-11) 257-72.
5. Best to Meyer, 9 Feb. 1911 from National Library of Ireland, Kildare Street. NLI Ms No. 11002.
6. Meyer to Best, 20 Feb. 1911 from 41 Huskisson Street, Liverpool. NLI Ms No. 11002.
7. Meyer to Henebry, 20 Feb. 1911 from Liverpool, in W.F.P. Stockley, *Essays in Irish Biography* (Cork U.P. 1933) 147.
8. *Ibid.* 148-9.
9. Lascelles Abercrombie to Kuno Meyer, 7 April (1911) from 47 Greenpark Road, Birkenhead. T.C.D. Ms No. 4224.
9a. Meyer to Best, 17 March 1911. NLI Ms No. 11002.
10. Meyer to Best, 20 Feb. 1911. NLI Ms No. 11002.
11. Meyer to Best, 23 Feb. 1911 from Liverpool. NLI Ms No. 11002.
12. Meyer to Best, 9 May 1911 from Magdalen College, Oxford. NLI Ms No 11002.
13. Bodleian Library Oxford. Ms Gilbert Murray 502 fol 57-8.
14. Bodleian Library Oxford. Ms Gilbert Murray 502 fol 296.
15. Meyer to Best, 13 May 1911 from Endsleigh Palace Hotel, London. NLI Ms No 11002.
16. Meyer to Best, 15 May 1911. NLI Ms No. 11002.
17. Meyer to Best, 20 May 1911 from Endsleigh Palace Hotel, London. NLI Ms No. 11002.
18. Meyer to Best, 26 May 1911 from Endsleigh Palace Hotel, London. NLI Ms No. 11002.
19. *Ibid.*
20. Meyer to Best, 28 May 1911 to Liverpool. NLI Ms No. 11002.
21. Meyer to Best, 31 May 1911 from Liverpool. NLI Ms No. 11002.
22. Meyer to Best, by postcard 7 June 1911 from Liverpool. NLI Ms No. 11002.
23. Michael Holroyd: *Augustus John, a biography,* 2 vols (London 1974) I, 309, footnote.
24. *Ibid,* 114.
25. Stanley Conway: *The University Club, Liverpool: its history from 1896-1956* (Liverpool 1969) 61.
26. NLI Ms No. 11002.
27. John Sampson: *In lighter moments.* University College Liverpool, Hodder and Stoughton, London 1934. 98 et seq.
28. Meyer to Best, 13 July 1911. NLI Ms No 11002.
29. Meyer to Best, 14 July 1911. NLI Ms No 11002.

30. Meyer to Best, 19 July 1911. NLI Ms No 11002.
31. *Irish Review,* April 1912, 97-8.
32. Seán O Lúing, 'Kuno Meyer by Augustus John; a brief history of a famous portrait' *Studies* (Winter 1982) 325-43.
33. Meyer to Best, 5 Oct. 1911. NLI Ms No. 11002.

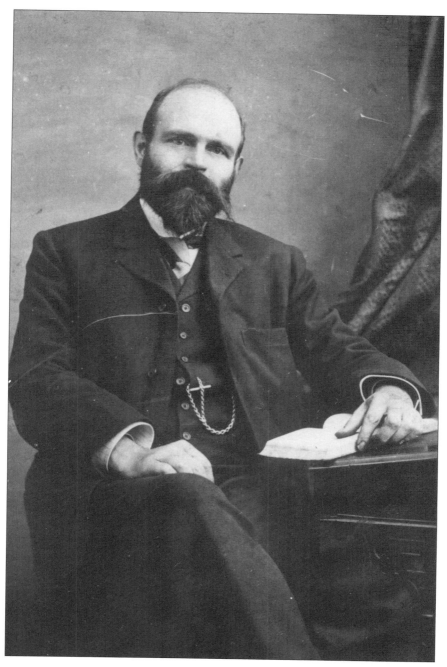

PLATE I:
Kuno Meyer (photograph by Messrs. Bassano, London). Copy courtesy of the
National Library of Ireland.

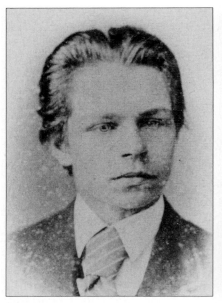

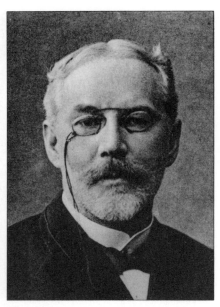

PLATE II:
Kuno Meyer at seventeen, Edinburgh,
1875 (by kind permission of the Royal
Irish Academy)

PLATE III:
Ludwig Christian Stern (courtesy of
the National Library of Ireland)

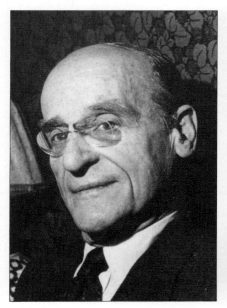

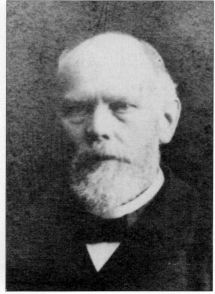

PLATE IV:
Carl Marstrander (courtesy of
Verdens Gang, Oslo)

PLATE V:
Ernst Windisch (courtesy of
Manuscript Department, Trinity
College Library, Dublin)

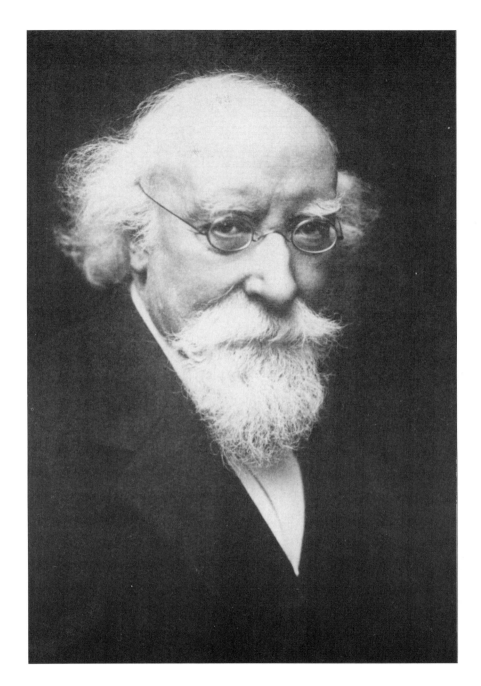

PLATE VI:
Whitley Stokes (courtesy of the National Library of Ireland)

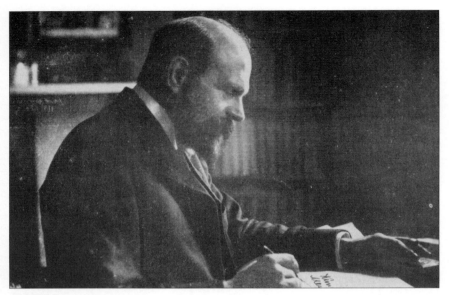

PLATE VII:
Kuno Meyer aged about fifty-four (reproduced from Irisleabhar Muighe Nuadhad, 1913, courtesy of the National Library of Ireland)

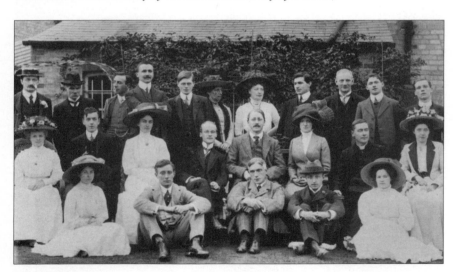

PLATE VIII:
School of Irish Learning, Summer 1910 (Carl Marstrander's class photographed at Mrs. Eason's Garden Party, Rathgar). Back row: J. H. Lloyd, Owen O'Byrne, J. Fraser, J. Pokorny, Robin Flower, Mrs. R. I. Best, Mrs. Eason, Seán Óg, — Purcell, Wm. O'Brien, J. J. Doyle. Second row: ——?, Liam Ó Rinn, Teresa Hurley, Carl Marstrander, R. I. Best, Miss Mary Rh. Williams, T. A. Fitzgerald, O.F.M., Miss Veronica Ryan. Front row: Miss Hurley (?), J. Aimers, J. G. O'Keeffe, Glyn Davies, Miss E. Deane.
(by kind permission of the Royal Irish Academy)

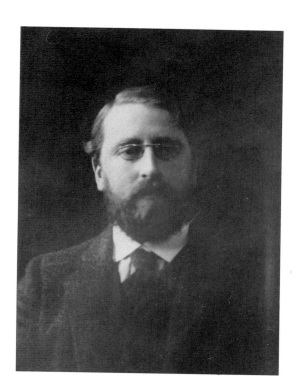

PLATE IX:
Richard Irvine Best,
November 1917 (courtesy
of the National Library of
Ireland)

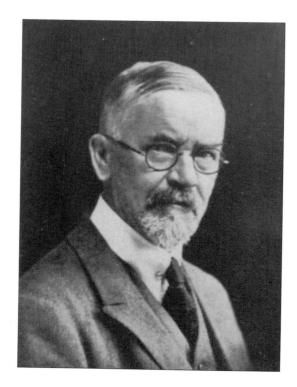

PLATE X:
Osborn Bergin (by kind
permission of Scoil an
Léinn Cheiltigh)

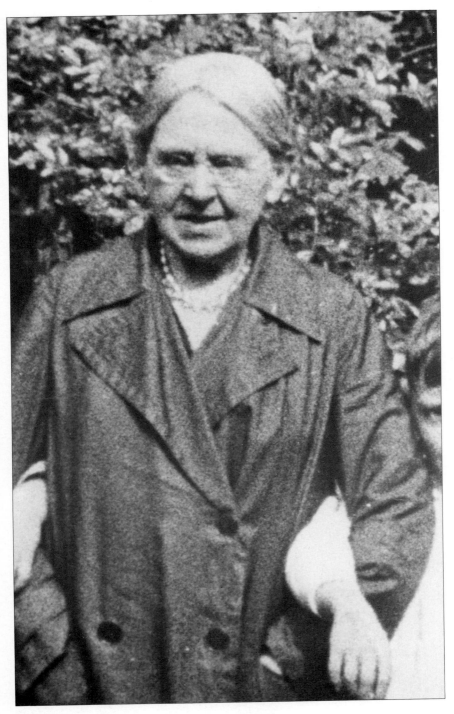

PLATE XI:
Antonie Meyer (probably taken in Templin, near Hamburg, in early 1920s)

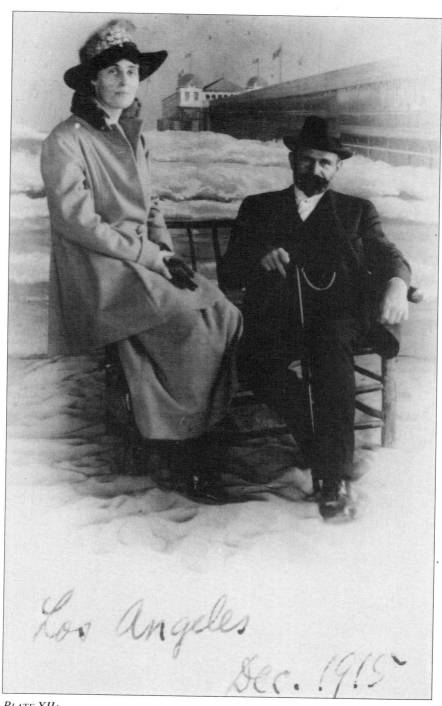

PLATE XII:
Kuno and Florence Meyer, Los Angeles, December 1915 (courtesy of the University of Liverpool, Central Photographic Service)

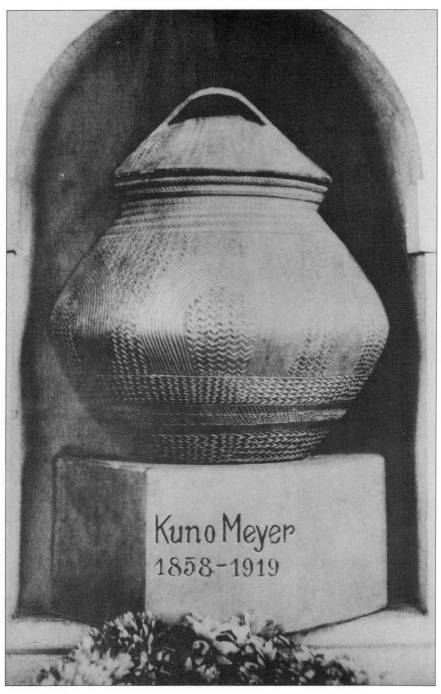

Plate XIII:
Burial urn of Kuno Meyer (courtesy of Manuscript Department, Trinity College Library, Dublin)

Chapter 10

BY early August Antonie found a suitable flat in Charlottenburg, Niebuhrstrasse llA, fairly central, not too far from the Tiergarten, at the top of the house, with good air, containing six rooms some of which were quite large, with electric light, automatic lift, gas-kitchen, bathroom, two toilets and all modern comforts, for £115, which was the yearly rental presumably. Flats in Berlin were dear, explained Meyer, but the landlord paid all taxes. What attracted him most was the free and open position of the house, at the corner of two streets, with a large clear space on one side, and the amenity of a balcony. They were not going into it before mid-October.[1]

When Kuno Meyer arrived at his new address late on the night of 14 October, his sister Antonie, already installed, met him with the news that Ludwig Christian Stern was dead. It was a shock. Meyer had been looking forward to his society and although he knew Stern's health was far from good he was not prepared for this.

No survey of Celtic studies can omit the name of Ludwig Christian Stern. Born 1846 in Hildesheim, he specialised in Egyptology during the earlier part of his career and after two years as director of Cairo Library became assistant in the Egyptian Museum of Berlin, contributing to the *Zeitschrift für Aegyptische Sprache und Altertumskunde* and publishing amongst other things *Hieroglyppisch-lateinisches Glossar*. At the age of thirty-nine he abandoned his distinguished career in Egyptology to devote himself entirely to Celtic studies and in this field he also became pre-eminent. In association with Meyer he founded the *Zeitschrift für celtische Philologie* and became joint editor with him of that celebrated journal which is still, happily, making a welcome appearance. On his appointment in 1886 as conservator to the manuscript department of the Royal Library of Berlin, a post he held till his death, he gave particular attention to Irish palaeography, published detailed descriptions of Irish manuscripts at Giessen, Stockholm, Copenhagen, Saint Paul in Carinthia, published a facsimile of an Old-Irish manuscript of Würzburg, besides enriching Old-Irish studies in many other directions. To readers of modern Irish he is best known for his excellent text with introduction, glossary and translation of the early l9th century *Cúirt an Mheádhoin Oidhche* (The Midnight Court), a long rabelaisian composition of exquisite Irish, the immense popularity of which has earned a distinction for Stern among Irish readers who are unaware of the significant body of scholarship he contributed to early Irish studies. A man of rich erudition, he was more littérateur than grammarian.

No one knew better than Meyer that his loss was considerable, aware from long acquaintance as he was that his richly endowed mind had acquired a large amount of rare knowledge possessed by no one else, nor likely to be soon acquired by anyone else. He wondered how Stern had disposed of his library and wrote to Mrs Stern offering his advice and help.[2] He was well pleased with his new quarters, but would not settle down to work there properly until he had arranged all his books. Besides he had to devote a few days to calling on his colleagues at the University where he was to be formally introduced on 24 October.

He went to see Mrs Stern, a long, sad visit. Her husband's death, from heart failure, was so sudden and unexpected that she would hardly trust her senses when she saw him dead. Like all other scholars he had made no arrangements about his books and manuscripts, and yet that had been uppermost in his mind during his last minutes. He kept on saying in an almost inaudible voice 'alles verbrennen', meaning no doubt his letters, sketches of work, etc. His widow had only too faithfully carried out his instruction and burnt all his correspondence with Lepsius, Brugsch, Ebers, etc., as well as all his other papers. Meyer asked her whether his MS Glossary to Dafyd ap Gwilym was amongst the material burned. She could not say. He was to go through the library with her in a fortnight's time. Although not a very large library it was well chosen and contained all necessary handbooks. He was going to divide it in 3 parts, one for his seminar, one for Best, Bergin, O'Keeffe and anyone else in Dublin, and one for himself. Would they all meet and draw up a list of the books they wanted, both Irish, Scotch, Welsh and Breton, and affix such prices as they were willing to pay. All his books were well bound, some beautifully so. He must find out who Stern's binder was.

On his formal introduction on the 24th Meyer became a full member of the Royal Prussian Academy of Sciences, a prodigiously learned assembly, but he found their proceedings dull and conventional, with none of the ceremony which marked Royal Irish Academy functions. He called on numerous colleagues, many of them high in the world of learning, such as Harnack, Wilamowitz and Waldeyer, by all of whom he was graciously received, though he felt he would become close to few of them, some being too old, others too busy.

Altogether Berlin was too huge a place. It took him two and a half hours to his brother's house, Mommsenstrasse 7/8, and back. Some of the younger men on the staff, like Schulze, Luders (Sanskrit) and Morf (French) he might perhaps get more intimate with but it would be a very long time, if ever, before there could be anything like the intimacy which bound him to his Liverpool colleagues. So far only two students had applied for his Old Irish course. They were both English, one a Northumbrian, the other from Cambridge.

Stern had a beautifully written original manuscript of his edition of the Midnight Court and Glossary which was to have been given to the flames by Mrs Stern but was rescued by Meyer who pointed out that they were already printed. Stern had the habit of writing all sorts of aperçus, quotations and observations in his books and there were some in this volume, all very apt. Meyer asked Mrs Stern to present it to the National Library of Ireland and hoped she would do so.[3]

There was a lull in Meyer's correspondence with Best. Meyer had been very busy with work, with his cure, which so far had no effect, and paying with an effort the last of his innumerable calls. It was time to break away from everything so he had come to his favourite Leipzig that morning to see friends. Noting from the English papers that his portrait by John had been exhibited at the New English Art Club and received a fine tribute from Sir Claude Phillipps as a work of tremendous power, he thought John was probably right in considering it one of his best works. He found his revered teacher Windisch in pretty good health and planning to begin the printing before the end of the year of his 'Celtic Britain' which would run to some 250 pages.

A curiously discordant note now intruded into Meyer's correspondence, far removed from the scholarly interests that were his normal preoccupation, and revealing a strong political feeling which, though probably always dormant, may have been influenced by his new environment. 'There is', he said, 'an extraordinary bitterness in Germany against England, which may well lead to war if it gets further nourishment. The fact that England grabbed Egypt and South Africa, let France grab Morocco, Italy Tripoli and now Russia Persia without any protest, but made difficulties when Germany sent a single cannon-boat to Agadir as a mild protest against the flagrant violation of a sworn treaty and grudges Germany a poor compensation in African territory will not easily be forgotten and as I read history will as certainly be avenged some day as England had to avenge Majuba Hill and Khartoum'.[4]

It may be explained as an utterance characteristic of the imperial age when the great nations of Europe competed in claiming arbitrary possession of distant regions, a state of affairs that seemed as natural and above question to Meyer as to fellow-scholars in England, Germany, France and other powerful countries. Ominous nevertheless and presaging naught for future comfort.

Feeling the better of his Leipzig visit Meyer returned to Berlin where he found a letter from Best awaiting him, giving him news of doings in Dublin, and other matters:

> Your card from Leipzig and my letter crossed. I hope you are not run down, but that you are beginning to feel the good effects which you expect from the radium treatment. McClelland was to have given a demonstration of radium emanations at the R.I.A. reception last night, but for some reason it did not come off.... on the whole the evening was more agreeable. The various Presidents of the Colleges of Surgeons etc. etc. were there in their robes, also the Provost, unrobed. J.P.M. [Mahaffy] wore his Presidential gown designed by himself Rossetti green with frontal stole of Buddhistic yellow. Bergin has managed to sprain his ankle again. I saw him hobbling up Dawson Street this afternoon leaning heavily on a stick. He showed me a long letter in Irish which he had from O'Brien, but no mention of his

escapade. Mrs Green has written that she saw Sir John Rhys who had not been able to see Ll. George. Lord MacD. has written 'I am not sanguine that you will extract anything from the Treasury. But why not ask Mr Binet to make you a grant from the Educational Funds placed at his disposal. He could surely spare a few hundred pounds from the Secondary Education grants. And possibly the Belfast and National University might make a subvention'. Indeed they would not! Bergin scouted the idea of Univ. Coll. helping us with money. The question is should you write to him now making the suggestion that if H.M. Treasury fails he could do this, pointing out the educational side of our School in teaching, and publication of manuals. Surely we might be eligible on that score. Kindest greetings to your sister and long life to her Bluthner! My wife has begun to talk of a Pleyel grand, but I fear these luxuries are beyond us. Our neighbour is bawling at the top of his voice, with the most horrid discords accompanying him from his organ. We shall have to leave. [5]

Meyer gave a survey of his first two months in Berlin to Alice Stopford Green:

Charlottenburg
Niebuhrstrasse llA
10/12.11

My dear Mrs Green,

I have been very remiss in not thanking you for your kind letter before this. But life in this huge place, where distances are even greater than in London, is such a rush that the day is gone before one realises it. I have had to pay about 80 visits to colleagues of the Faculty (60 of them) and fellow-Academicians. I have had to get my classes and lectures into shape, and as my students are all much older and riper than those I had in England (knowing what they want and seeing that they get it) my work is rather heavy and takes a good deal of preparing. I have altogether 8 students in Old-Irish, nearly all foreigners: one from the National University (O'Brien), a Scot, a Northumbrian (very good), a Cambridge graduate (Braunholtz), an American professor (the keenest of the lot), a Dutchman and only 2 Germans. This is not a bad beginning, considering that Thurneysen at Freiburg only has 3 students (Lucius Gwynn among them). I believe they will all of them do good work. I have also had much to do in selling the library of my old friend Stern, whose death was the first news that awaited me here. I have bought most of the books for my Seminar, the Government readily giving a large sum for the purpose. These things as you know are done much more easily here than in England. Shall we get our wretched pittance for the School? I am afraid not, after Mr. Birrell's letter. Who is there really to help us, or even take an interest? Not Mr. Birrell, nor Stephen Gwynn, I am afraid, nor anyone. I have written again to Sir John Rhys, but doubt whether he is well enough to tackle Lloyd George. And even if he does I am very doubtful of the result.

We have a very comfortable flat where if you ever come to Berlin I hope you will stay with us. But apart from my work life is very monotonous and lonely here. There can be no real intercourse. It takes us 2 ½ hours to my brother's and back.

I have been trying a new cure - radium inhalation, but so far without any success or the slightest effect, so that I shall soon give it up. The climate suits me well. We are having a wonderfully mild winter so far. We get a fortnight off at Xmas which my sister and I will spend at Monte Carlo, where we shall find the Walsinghams and the Conybeares from Oxford. At Easter on the other hand we have a very long vacation, nearly 2 months, which I hope to spend in England. I hear that they are getting up another course of lectures and classes at University College for me.

Like you I have not heard anything from Mr Marstrander for months. I hope he has had no relapse; but if he had I should no doubt have heard from Mr Best, my only faithful correspondent in Dublin. I have translated a fine old Irish poem on the Hill of Alenn (not Allen), now Knockawlin, or rather on the ancient hillfort there, which gives a vivid picture of the life and doings of such a royal seat. I will send you a copy when it comes out.

My sister joins me in very kind regards.

Always yours sincerely
Kuno Meyer[6]

Wishing to publish a volume of Zimmer's posthumous papers Meyer had gone to see the publisher Weidmann in Berlin but a long talk produced no results, Weidmann refusing point blank, saying that Zimmer's other publications, *Nennius Vindicatus* and *Pelagius in Irland*, had been ruinous with less than 200 sold out of 1000 printed. This showed again how minute was the interest in Celtic studies in Germany. Thurneysen also complained bitterly about the small sale of his Handbuch, which was the chief reason for not embarrassing his publisher further with another volume.[7]

It was time for Christmas holidays, and Meyer and Toni set out for Monte Carlo on 19 December. Within a few days Meyer was able to announce to Best that after several visits to the tables he was richer by 400 francs. 'Que ça dure!'[8]

Meyer wrote again to Marstrander, not the best of correspondents, asking him to break his silence and above all to write to Mrs Green. He had more luck at the tables, adding another 200 francs to his winnings, but Toni lacked the courage to try her luck. There was news from Berlin that the Academicians were to be received by the Emperor on the Centenary of Friedrich the Great's birthday, ladies not included in the invitation, unfortunately. He had just set a paper in Modern Irish for the Matriculation of London University for which there was only one candidate and he, if a good Gaelic Leaguer, would walk it.[9]

On the 31st Meyer and Toni moved to the magnificent Cap Martin Hotel near Mentone. A letter had arrived that morning from Best and Kuno, taking coffee on the terrace with his sister, sent his warmest greetings for the New Year to the Bests, wishing for their presence and described his surroundings, the Mediterranean all around them in its deepest blue, just slightly rippled, such a perfect summer sea. 'A bright Japanese parasol keeps off the brilliant sun over our table. There is not a soul here beside us; they are all taking their siesta after the huge table d'hôte lunch which we also had for 7 francs each - heavy American dishes, a hot lobster with an impossible sauce, nothing really enjoyable except the hors d'oeuvres and a meringue. No vegetables and very poor fruit. But the coffee is good, and if only I had a decent cigar or cigarette to smoke with it I should be quite happy'. But he found that maritime climates did not really agree with him. He felt rheumatism all over and even Toni had slight twitches. The contrast between the hot sun and the shade was too great. And then the cold floors! The view was splendid. Mentone and its bay stretched to the left, and Bordighera and its promontory against the horizon, and on the right the whole coast as far as Nice. They were expecting the Conybeares, father, mother and son to take tea with them later on. The family would soon separate, he going to Florence to work, she to Sicily and the boy back to Oxford. Their daughter was in Egypt! Such was modern life. Meyer and his sister were leaving for San Remo on the morrow, mainly because one was no longer admitted to the club at Monte Carlo without paying the entrance money to the private rooms in the Casino - 100 francs each, exorbitant, a German manager having been appointed who was trying a new system of levying money wherever he could. At San Remo there was a very comfortable club with winter-gardens which one could join for 10 francs. He could put his system to the test there. Although not so lucky lately he was still some hundreds to the good and felt the pleasurable sensation of making some surprising coups.

He promised Best to forward all the books of his (B's) third list when he returned to Berlin. He was glad the Zeuss had arrived for Christmas and hoped Best was pleased with it. Just as Meyer was writing, much to their annoyance, a wretched piano and fiddles had struck up some horribly vulgar music and the place was filling up with people of all nationalities. 'I dont suppose musical taste was ever so low as it is now amongst the bourgeois'.

Meyer wondered whether Celtic studies in Germany would have a future. It did not look like it. Thurneysen with his one student and Meyer himself with two, one of whom showed signs of giving up, was not a promising situation. 'There is hardly any interest and no knowledge among my colleagues, to whom everything Celtic is terra incognita.' Wilhelm Schulze was the only exception. Meyer could not understand Marstrander. Was he working at all? And what of his health? Meyer had no letters forwarded to him from Berlin and perhaps Marstrander had written to him there. As a duty of his new situation he was to read a paper to the Berlin Academy the following November..[10]

Kuno and Toni left San Remo on 6 January, fortunate in weather, if not in luck, having lost at the gaming tables all they had won, to be left without profit except the fun they had for their money.[11] The School of Irish Learning was at a low ebb. With Marstrander away in Norway and his intentions unclear there were no classes being held. To fill the gap Meyer thought of asking Holger Pedersen to come in the summer or autumn and give a course of lectures on comparative philology or the history of Irish.

The function in the Berlin Palace and Opera went well. Kuno's distinguished historian brother sat next to the Emperor Wilhelm who looked quite ill and hardly spoke to anyone. Still he addressed the Academy, granting them three new posts and various other things, in the presence of a magnificent gathering of princes, generals and marshals. Kuno's own health was improving[12] but he continued uneasy about the School's prospects. If Pedersen could not come and Marstrander failed them who would take the summer course? For reading he was engrossed in Gissing's *New Grub Street*.[13]

In February he was stricken for several days with a bad attack of rheumatism which left him exhausted and with the feeling that he would not have the strength to lecture as he had planned in London and Dublin or indeed go to England at all in March. The change to Germany had done him no good. 'Since last year my power of resistance is not what it was. How true it is that you should not transplant an old tree. It is not the climate or weather of Berlin, but the altered conditions of life, many of them very trying. Take my daily round. Waiting about on windswept platforms or street corners, then an overheated train, out again into the cold, then at the University horribly hot rooms so that after my lectures I am always bathed in perspiration, out again into the cold etc. ... at present I am fit for nothing'.[14]

Nor was he at all pleased with the way in which *Ériu* was progressing under Marstrander. Although joint editor himself he felt handicapped, for what, he asked, could one do with a fellow editor who never wrote nor acknowledged anything. Marstrander should retire from the task. Meyer hoped Best would look after the journal and save what could be saved. And in any case if he should have to give it up himself then Best would have to take his place. It was now clear that Meyer's departure from Liverpool was having serious consequences for the School. Berlin was a considerable distance from Dublin and the problems arising were proof of how much the School depended on his presence or proximity.

He had two long letters from Marstrander, with a lot of curious proposals and written in a dissatisfied spirit, which ruffled Meyer. Fancy Marstrander saying that '*many* of the younger Celtologists have got no fair chance of showing what they can do. At least I think I have not, and I doubt whether I shall ever get one.' This, from a young scholar for whom they had done so much, was extraordinary. 'I am afraid he is eaten up with conceit.'[15] Marstrander explained he could not carry on with both the Dictionary and teaching and proposed to retire from the School, a least for a year or so. He also proposed to retire from the editorship of *Ériu*, suggesting that it be handed over again to Bergin. Meyer recommended he talk matters over with Best and other good friends when next he came to Dublin. To Best he proposed that if Marstrander could not deliver any courses at Easter or in Summer, then they must either continue his leave or let him resign for a time.

So the School had to do without Marstrander for the present. Meyer was now doubly glad he had asked Pedersen. For what was to become of the School at this rate? As for *Ériu*, they might well agree to let Marstrander retire and would Best do the editing? He was on the spot, knew all the possible contributors personally and could deal with Mss and printing better than anyone. Meyer would continue with him as joint editor or not as Best might prefer. Think it over, urged Meyer, addressing his colleague as 'My dear friend' instead of in his usual formal manner.[15]

Later that month Meyer went to Amélie-les-Bains for a rest, arriving on the 11th to find a letter from Best which gave him great pleasure. His portrait by John had been exhibited in Dublin and called forth the highest praise from judges and critics, including Best himself whose comments would have pleased John. A great pity John did not make it a better likeness, said Meyer, but he blamed himself for not taking him more in hand.

Amélie had received him very well. He had found some old acquaintances and would no doubt make new ones. 'As for the editorship of *Ériu* I don't think B[ergin] would make a good editor with his dilatory habits and lack of enthusiasm. He does not produce much himself and would not stir others. No, do take it yourself.' It was a pity they did not know for certain that Pedersen could come.[16] As it turned out, he could not.

Meyer complained he was not lucky. On the morning of 20 March Amélie woke to a day of bitter winter weather. Many visitors, himself among them, fled for refuge to the old walled town of Carcasonne, a wise thing to do, for there in the lowlands it was much warmer. He went to bed early and read Balzac, *Une ténébreuse affaire*, most entrancing. What was that he heard from Gaidoz of a new periodical to be called *Gadelica?* Too much of a good thing. He should not be surprised if Marstrander were to start a journal of his own. 'The young man is morbidly ambitious. Bien à vous deux!'[17]

In a letter from Amélie-les-Bains he described to Mrs Green his reactions at leaving England and unburdened to her his concern for the School. Since their interests in Irish learning coincided he found in her a sympathetic listener with whom he could communicate on familiar terms. While there may have existed in Ireland a belief or impression, fostered perhaps by the predilections of Whitley Stokes, that Germany teemed with students and scholars with a devotion to Celtic studies, his correspondence on the subject discloses the cold reality.

My dear Mrs Green,

It was a great pleasure to receive your kind long letter which reached me in this forlorn corner of the Pyrenees, where I hope to recover from a really nasty attack of influenza. If all goes well I still hope to be in England about the middle of April and to spend at least some days in London, when perhaps we may meet again. In any case I will let you know my whereabouts. So far Berlin has not been able to lessen my regret at leaving England, where I have left too many good friends behind and most of the interests of my life. Berlin is so huge (14,000 students!) that one is lost in it. Intercourse is hardly possible, everybody busy with his own concerns, everything a rush. And as for Celtic, there is of course no interest whatever among the wider public, while my colleagues in the University and Academy - all dreadfully learned in their own subjects - are far more interested in Central Asiatic and Central American research. Did I tell you that Zimmer's old publisher would not take a volume of his posthumous works as he had lost too much money on his publications. Even *Nennius Vindicatus* and *Pelagius in Irland* have not paid their way. When I contrast this with Nutt's announcement the other day that new editions of the 'Celtic Church' and 'King and Hermit' are required I realised that there is no public for Celtic works in Germany while there undoubtedly is in Britain. I shall therefore continue to publish in English, with the exception of an annual contribution to the Berlin Academy's transactions which I as a full member, drawing an income of £120 from it, am obliged to hand in. But if Germany does not supply me with readers or a public, it is wonderful how every learned endeavour is encouraged and supported and organised by the Government. As to students, both Thurneysen and I have but one German among them, the rest are all English, Irish or American. I paid a visit to Freiburg on my way here and met Lucius Gwynn and Miss Power at Thurneysen's house, both very happy and getting on in their studies.

As for our School, it is at present in a perilous condition. Marstrander has written to say that his health will not allow him to carry on both the Dictionary and the School, so that he must, at least temporarily, resign from the latter. I am glad I asked Prof. Pedersen to hold a Summer course this year which he has promised to do if he can finish his great book before then. If he should not be able to come I don't know what to propose. We should then practically have had no teaching for a whole year. Bergin is going to hold a summer course in Ballingeary, or we might ask him. Let us hope that Pedersen will come either in August or September.

All your news has interested me very much. Best is indeed valuable and a mainstay of the School. As Marstrander also speaks of retiring from *Ériu*, I hope to induce Best to edit it with me. He takes more pains than anyone else. I am very glad to hear of your volume of essays. Though nothing will impress or shake Mr Mahaffy, I fancy his adherents are getting fewer every year, both within and outside Trinity, and your attack will open more eyes. I had already heard about young Martens from his professor in Berlin, Sering, and hope to see him next term.

Your generous offer of renewed support to the School comes at a critical time when all depends on carrying on the work over a difficult period. If the purely grammatical work must cease for a time, would it do to extend in other directions, historical, archaeological, or even palaeographical (diplomatics)? But there again unless we can get a first-rate scholar of undoubted reputation, such as the University cannot show, we will neither justify our existence nor draw students. Let us talk this over when I come to London. It is a pity that France has produced no great Celtic scholar. As for literature, say general mediaeval literature, there are many distinguished scholars but few of them even know the difference between Irish and Welsh! Entre nous, it took me years to prevent my friends Professors Priebsch, Bonnier, Friedel, etc., from saying 'Welsh' when they meant 'Irish'. The loose terminology (Celtic, Breton, British etc.) has caused all this mischief. But the chief reason is that for lack of textbooks and handbooks they cannot easily get oriented. Among the things that I should like to do would be a survey of the whole field of Celtic study, pointing out its relation to general philological and literary studies.

I must break off here and continue, I hope, some afternoon in your drawing room.

Yours always sincerely
Kuno Meyer[18]

NOTES

1. Meyer to Best, 4 Aug. 1911 from Gross Lichterfelde. NLI Ms No. 11002.
2. Meyer to Best, 15 Oct. 1911 from Charlottenburg, Niebuhrstrasse 11A. NLI Ms No. 11002.
3. Meyer to Best, by postcard 28 Oct. 1911. NLI Ms No. 11002.
4. Meyer to Best, by postcard from Leipzig, 1 Dec. 1911. NLI Ms No. 11002.
5. Meyer to Best, 8 December 1911. NLI Ms No. 11002 (59).
6. Meyer to A.S. Green, 10 Dec. 1911, from Niebuhrstrasse 11A. NLI Ms No 15091 (1).
7. Meyer to Best, by postcard 18 Dec. 1911. NLI Ms No. 11002.
8. Meyer to Best, by postcard 23 Dec. 1911 from Monte Carlo. NLI Ms No. 11002.

9. Meyer to Best by postcard 26 Dec. 1911 from Monte Carlo. NLI Ms No. 11002.
10. Meyer to Best, 31 Dec. 1911 from Cap Martin Hotel, près Mentone. NLI Ms No. 11002.
11. Meyer to Best, 6 Jan. 1912 from San Remo. NLI Ms No. 11002.
12. Meyer to Best, by postcard postmarked 29 Jan. 1912 from Charlottenburg. NLI Ms No. 11002.
13. Meyer to Best, postmark Charlottenburg 10 Feb. 1912. NLI Ms No. 11002.
14. Meyer to Best, 19 Feb. 1912 from Charlottenburg, Niebuhrstrasse 11A. NLI Ms No. 11002.
15. Meyer to Best, 2 March 1912 from Charlottenburg, Niebuhrstrasse 11A. NLI Ms No. 11002.
16. Meyer to Best, 11 March 1912 from Amélie-les-Bains. NLI Ms No. 11002.
17. Meyer to Best, 20 March 1912 from Carcasonne. NLI Ms No. 11002.
18. Meyer to Alice Stopford Green, 19 March 1912 from Thermes Romains, Amélie-les-Bains. NLI Ms No. 15091.

Chapter 11

O N 18 July 1911 the Corporation of Dublin formally resolved to confer the Freedom of the City on Kuno Meyer and Canon Peter O'Leary in tribute to their work for the Irish language. Time passed, as Canon O'Leary wrote in his ageless memoirs[1] and a date in April 1912 was set for the conferring, an honour which was proof, as he said, that the work done was well appreciated. Best, who had been negotiating a suitable date with the Corporation settled for Monday the 22nd and wrote 'So look out for festivities! I am delighted that matters have been so arranged. It will be a great pleasure to see you again... it will be a re-union of hearts, for if report be true, the young Norwegian gentleman will also re-visit these shores about the same time,' for so Macalister had told him, and so Purton was told by E.J. Gwynn of Trinity College, the young Norwegian being no other than Carl Marstrander, whose correspondence about his future intentions was reticent, except to say he would represent Norway at the T.C.D. Medical School Centenary.[2] Meyer, critical of Marstrander, wrote Best asking his help to make the coming number of *Ériu* passable, because good he feared it could not be, Marstrander having without his knowledge accepted and sent to the printers the most rubbishy stuff, including a contribution of Purton's which swarmed with absurdities.[3]

He would be delighted to let Augustus John have another trial at his portrait. As John painted so quickly it was no fatigue, the Liverpool portrait having been virtually finished in four hours. But the next time there must be somebody present who would talk and who better than George Moore. What was his address in Ebury Street? Meyer was afraid lack of time and health would prevent him from accepting all the proposed honours. He might have to go to Liverpool for a day or two where his good friends had collected enough money to found a Celtic chair, on condition that he would take it.[4] Best was greatly pleased at the prospect, stranger than fiction, which he hoped would come to pass, of Meyer being settled once more on Merseyside, where he would be able to advance his favourite study far better than on the continent. 'When you come over we shall talk about it, and the future of our School.' His Irish admirers would be greatly disappointed if he were to forego any of the festivities they had arranged, bands and torchlight processions and all. They were ready to receive him any day and hoped he would be able to stay more than a week. 'Goodness knows when we may meet again!'[5]

Monday the 22nd suited Meyer quite well for the ceremony and he was making arrangements not to return to Berlin until the beginning of May. He just had a letter from Marstrander from which he gathered that if the School had money enough to pay him a larger salary he would stay. Whether that would imply giving up the Dictionary he did not say. Meyer would wait until they met. Marstrander was returning to Dublin shortly.[6]

Having arrived in London Meyer visited the House of Commons on April 12th, where he had lunch with Stephen Gwynn and other Irish members and dinner later with the Liberal whip William Jones and Welsh members, while in between he heard Asquith, Carson and Redmond, thought he had never seen such a hideous face as that of Bonar Law, made him 'quite ill to look at him,' witnessed some regular schoolboy scenes at which Captain Craig excelled, the whole impression he received being that of 'a tricky, disingenuous and ignoble fight. But Asquith and Redmond too were at least dignified and never lost their balance or temper.'[7]

Best forwarded him an invitation from St. Patrick's College, Maynooth, which he accepted. The night of the 14th he had George Moore to dinner at Pagani's when there was a battle royal between the author and Creigenach, who took him seriously, on Shakespeare-Bacon. Moore was very witty and amusing.[8]

On Monday 22 April 1912 the Municipal Council of Dublin assembled in special meeting 'to witness the affixing to the Roll of Honorary Burgesses of the name of Dr Kuno Meyer ... and also the name of Very Rev. Peter Canon O'Leary' and to present to them the Certificates of Honorary Freedom of the City, conferred by Resolution of Council of the 18th day of July 1911.

In presence of a notable attendance the Lord Mayor, introducing both men, spoke of them in words of high praise. Meyer having signed the roll and acknowledged the honour as the greatest distinction that had ever fallen to his lot, said he was rewarded richly and beyond expectation by the recognition which his work in the cause of Irish letters and studies had thus obtained at the hands of a generous people, far beyond the small circle of scholars, fellow-workers and pupils. It was a new bond which tied him to a city and country, in which he had many dear friends – a country which by the nature of his studies was never out of his mind, and which a life-long occupation with its history and literature had taught him to love with an affection second only to that which he bore to his native land. His native city of Hamburg had in the past more than one link with Ireland, and one of these associations was brought home to him with a new significance when he remembered that his grandfather in that city of Hamburg did actually talk with Napper Tandy and did take him by the hand, as his father often told him as a boy long before he ever heard of the wearing of the green – he seemed to feel that his connection with Ireland extended even beyond his own life.[8A] Again his thoughts were carried back to a time, more than a generation ago, when he heard the first accents of Gaelic speech in the Highlands of Scotland; when at Leipzig he began his Irish studies with his revered master, Windisch, to the time of his first visit to Dublin and his first acquaintance with Whitley Stokes, Hennessy, John Fleming, and later on with Father O'Growney. It was a different Ireland to which he came now, and in nothing was the difference more marked than in the regard in which those men and the studies which they represent were now being held. It needed no prophet to foretell that their national literature would be a powerful factor in the unification of the country. The common possession of a rich heritage of memories would do more to bind a nation together than laws and enactments. They were the heirs of a great and unique literature dating from the fifth century, a national possession of which every Irishman should be proud, and which other less fortunate nations envied them. To resuscitate that ancient literature, to bring it before the Irish people, to win and train workers for that work had been a labour of love with him for more than thirty years. He would continue to devote the remainder of his life to that task, supported, he hoped, by an ever-increasing band of younger Irish scholars.

Canon Peter O'Leary followed, speaking first in Irish and going on to express his appreciation to Meyer and his own indebtedness to him for his translations from Old Irish in the *Gaelic Journal* which had unlocked for him the treasures of the early language. He expressed his faith in the future of the Irish language and thanked the Corporation for the honour conferred upon it through the persons of Dr Meyer and himself.

The vellums bearing the City Seal conferring the Freedom were richly coloured and ornamented in Celtic design and mounted on beautiful decorated white poplin, the whole wrought by the skilled hands of John F. Maxwell of Derrynane Parade.[9]

The ceremonies at the City Hall concluded, Meyer, Canon O'Leary and Osborn Bergin motored to St. Patrick's College, Maynooth, to spend the night there as guests of the President, Monsignor Mannix. That evening at a meeting in the MacMahon Hall chaired by Rev. Gerard O'Nolan and attended by the President and students, Canon O'Leary put forward reasons why Irish should be studied. He was followed by Meyer who said the Irish language was entitled to serious study because it enshrined a literature from the Bardic poetry of the seventh century to 'Séadna' and the other works of Canon O'Leary. It had been his good fortune to visit Maynooth in the early days of the language movement, and having returned now after twenty years he recalled a conversation he had then with Father O'Growney. They had been talking over the prospects of the revival of interest in the language, and they always came back to this – that if it was not a literary revival as well as a linguistic revival it would not be lasting. He had a sort of feeling that the Gaelic League setting up as it were, perhaps unintentionally, a contrast between the native speaker and the scholar had done harm to the movement. The two things were absolutely inseparable, so inseparable that the smaller nations of Eastern Europe, Bohemia and Hungary, when they started their revivals began by founding learned societies and academies to edit the national classics. Ireland had a unique literature, something to be proud of, something to make for the unification of the country, and surely that was more needed in Ireland at the present moment than in any other country. They had in this literature, with the thousands of associations of place and interest springing therefrom that which would unite the whole of Ireland. If a poet should arise as in Scotland Walter Scott had arisen and gathered the whole of the lore and traditions and associations of the country, he would do more to cement the different parts of Ireland together than any laws or enactments could do. That poet had yet to arise. Meanwhile it was for them who were in touch with this literature and language to make known to Irishmen and Irishwomen this glorious heritage of a great past. Father O'Growney had lamented to him the absence of a modern Irish literature. But Canon O'Leary had arisen since to enrich Irish literature and he must have younger men, trained for the task, to follow him.[10]

Canon O'Leary in the course of the evening had thoughts of his own. They related to the tomb in the college cemetery containing the relics of Father Eugene O'Growney whose body had been borne from Los Angeles over land and sea after a lifetime given to the Irish revival.[11]

Dublin's example was followed by Cork. On September 25, the feast of St. Finbarr, patron of the City, Meyer and Canon O'Leary were met at the railway station by the Lord Mayor and city dignitaries and escorted amid cheering thousands to the City Hall where the ceremony of signing the Roll of Freemen took place. After a brief speech of thanks by Canon O'Leary in Irish Meyer addressed the audience in a speech which was widely reported because of its allusions to contemporary politics.

He referred to the power of a national language and literature for bringing unity into nations and said that the young people of Ireland desired this common ground upon which all could meet. 'I believe that even in Ulster this feeling exists, and is so very widespread and strong that if the people there had been left to themselves better counsels would have prevailed. They would have chosen to cast in their lot with the rest of the motherland and to stand or fall with it. But an English party out of office, clinging to the one plank that is left to them, have once more interfered – let us hope for the last time – in the affairs of this country and are trying to fan ancient animosities into a flare. There might be some who would think it ill of him, a foreigner, to interfere in national politics, but the action of the Corporation had made him half an Irishman, and thus he might be allowed to give expression to feelings and convictions which he shared with all patriotic Irishmen.'[12]

It was a departure from matters of language and literature, but none the less applauded by his listeners, pointing as it did to problems of the hour. It received widespread attention in England and Meyer reported to Best that his Cork speech had got into all the English papers, *Morning Post, Manchester Guardian* and others.[13]

It is at this point that Canon O'Leary brings his memoirs to a close with an expression of wonder 'at how well the young boys spoke Irish to us,' in the crowded City Hall of Cork.[14]

NOTES

1. Peadar Ua Laoghaire, *Mo Sgéal Féin* (Baile Átha Cliath 1915), 215.
2. Best to Meyer, 22 March 1912 from 35 Percy Place, Dublin. NLI Ms No. 11002.
3. Meyer to Best, 25 March 1912. NLI Ms No. 11002.
4. Meyer to Best, by postcard 30 March 1912 from Amélie-les-Bains. NLI Ms No. 11002.
5. Best to Meyer, chez M. John Orr, Rue Amyot 8 bis Paris from Dublin, Good Friday 1912. NLI Ms No. 11002.
6. Meyer to Best, by postcard postmarked 9 April 1912 from Paris. NLI Ms No. 11002.
7. Meyer to Best, 13 April 1912 from Endsleigh Palace Hotel, London. NLI Ms No. 11002.
8. Meyer to Best, 15 April 1912 from Endsleigh Palace Hotel. NLI Ms No. 11002.
8a. At a later date, 3 Aug. 1912, Meyer wrote to Best from Charlottenburg - 'When you are back in Dublin I must ask you to have a bibliography of all that pertains to Napper Tandy. My old master Prof. Wohlwill in Hamburg is working at the subject and is sadly at a loss for material. He also asks me for an authorised version of the Wearing of the Green and the history of the song.'
9. *Freeman's Journal* (Dublin), Tuesday 23 April 1912. The *Irish Independent* of same date has a photograph which includes, besides Kuno Meyer and Canon O'Leary, Sir Joseph Downes, The Lord Mayor, Councillor Shortall, Miss Harrison, Mr. A. Byrne, Councillor Lennon, Councillor T. Rooney, Mr. M. J. Losty (Sword Bearer), Alderman J.T. Kelly, Councillor Crozier, Rev. Father Fitzgerald, Councillor Scully, Councillor P. O'Reilly, John Howard Parnell.
10. *Ibid.*
11. *Mo Sgéal Féin*, 217. Canon O'Leary gave the full text of his Irish address to *Irisleabhar Muighe Nuadhad*, Iml. II, Féile Pádraig, 1913.
12. From undated presscutting, source unidentified, in writer's possession.
13. Meyer to Best, 1 Oct. 1911 from University Club, Liverpool. NLI Ms No. 11002.
14. *Mo Sgéal Féin*, 219.

Chapter 12

IN the Report on the work of the School for the session 1910-1912[1] we are told that Professor Marstrander was obliged by pressure of other work to resign his post 'early in the present year' of 1912, and that 'the Governors take this opportunity of recording their warm appreciation of the services he rendered to the School'. The uncertainty which had attended Marstrander's intentions was now brought to an end by an agreement he came to with Meyer in Liverpool in the last week of April 1912, on his arrival fresh from Norway. Meyer was delighted to find him in such good spirits, better than he ever seemed before. They had spent a morning and afternoon together, talking matters over. They agreed on his temporary resignation from the School and *Ériu* until he had brought out the letter D of the Dictionary. Even a Summer course at the School was reckoned impossible as he would lose a month for the Dictionary. He was at last going to devote all his time to this one object and Meyer concluded that this was no doubt a correct decision.[2]

Meyer's friends in Liverpool wished to make him an honorary professor, that is without salary, so that he might have a seat on the Faculty and Senate, where his absence was much regretted. He could then, from Liverpool, lecture both in London and Dublin in the Summer term. He would try to arrange matters in Berlin to accord with this proposal. Pedersen had finally declined both for August and September and the unhappy prospect was that the School must close down for the Summer. What did Best think?[3] He was going to Weimar to the annual meeting of the Goethegesellschaft to which he had belonged almost from its foundation in 1880. Cycling, he told Best, would do him good. 'I was a good cyclist once! Now I could only manage a tricycle and have sometimes thought of getting one. But the motor cars frighten me, especially here in Berlin where they are allowed to go at a tremendous pace.' He now had seven students in Welsh. What child's play it was after Irish!

Toni and Kuno had lately taken to accepting invitations and were socially busy but his health was standing up to it. 'While I am writing three young artists are playing a heavenly Beethoven trio (op. 72) in the next room. I can always work much better with music and if I were a rich man would keep a little orchestra.' He had a letter from Marstrander, who had returned to Norway to work, saying that he felt particularly well and could do more work there in an hour than he could do in Dublin in a day. Marstrander, however, was not making a success of *Ériu*, which had got into bad ways and must be taken out of his hands.[4]

In July Meyer went on a week's tramp through Thüringen along with Toni, Eduard his brother and four nieces and nephews, 'quite a merry company', until the rains came and compelled them to postpone the ascent of the Inselberg. He wrote to Mrs Green and Best from Friedrichroda, an awfully pretty place embowered in wooded hills, with such quaint architecture, and a very pleasant people, a mixture of Angles, Franks and Saxons. The contents of his two letters largely correspond, though he gives more detail in that to Mrs Green which reads:

Friedrichroda
Thüringen
19/8.12

My dear Mrs Green,

On a rainy day in the heart of these hills and woods (where I came to join my brother and sister in a walking tour for a few days) I get some leisure at last to write to you. I have just been reading your last book again, of which I am to write a review for the Berlin 'Deutsche Literaturzeitung.' My last weeks were spent in writing out all that is of any value or interest in the mass of notes, sketches and excerpts among the posthumous papers of Zimmer, which his widow has confided to me. To the last he was a pioneer who kept his eyes open in all directions. Thus he has unearthed a wonderful document of the utmost importance for early Irish history, literature and what not. It is shortly this:

A Gaulish writer of the 6th century deploring the devastation of Gaul since the beginning of the 5th, through Alani, Huns, Goths and Vandals, says that 'then learned men began to leave these shores for Ireland, carrying their learning with them to the great advancement of wisdom and learning in that country.'

Here we have for the first time an authentic and almost contemporary statement as to the source of the great development in Irish learning during the 5th and following centuries. Now many things become clear at last, e.g. the 'rhetoricians' of whom Patrick complains in his 'Confession' – they were Gaulish professors and rhetors, Christians of course, but contemptuous of poor Patrick's lack of learning. The influence of Virgil the Grammarian on Irish philology, metrics, etc. now also receives a new light. We now have firm ground under our feet and can proceed much more confidently in our studies of those early centuries. I shall publish all this in my *Zeitschrift,* but hope to develop it much further later on. What interests me especially is the influence of Gaulish-Latin literature, both prose and poetry, on Gaelic literature, which is now assured. You know that one kind of rhythmical prose – most difficult to understand – was called *retoric* in Old-Irish. It is based upon the sort of rhythmical prose and which the Gaulish rhetors and rhetoricians spoke and wrote, of which we have many examples. It must not be forgotten that Latin literature in the 5th century meant almost exclusively Gaulish literature. Every famous writer of that age is of Gaulish origin.

I have my head full of these things at present and so I write of them, knowing well how interested you will be. I hear from Professor Fitzmaurice-Kelly that my engagement to lecture in London during January-March 1913 is a *fait accompli.* I am very glad. I shall hold regular classes for Old-Irish and give a set of new lectures on various recent discoveries and developments. Meanwhile I am to lecture in Dublin during the latter half of September. Marstrander has left us for good, Pedersen cannot come, and the School must not let a whole session pass without some activity. If only Bergin would work more! He is most disappointing. On the other hand Irish studies have got a capital recruit in Mr Robin Flower of the British Museum. Do you know him? He has made some fine discoveries amongst the Mss.

We wind up in Berlin at the end of this month. I may go to Aix-la-Chapelle for August. It will depend on the weather. The heat has been very great lately, but today a change has set in.

With kind regards
Always yours sincerely
Kuno Meyer[5]

Writing to Best from Göttingen, Meyer enclosed for him a letter from Stephen Gwynn which contained uncheerful news about the grant for the School. Such a quiet pretty place, Göttingen, where one might work much better, with the big library practically as good as one's own, and how much more, thought Meyer, one would enjoy life there than in Berlin. It was pleasant as well to share the society of Wilhelm Meyer the mediaeval Latinist, Morsbach the Anglist and his old friend Rietschmann the head Librarian. Meyer was journeying towards Aachen and would probably stay the night at Wetzlar for the sake of Goethe, Charlotte and Werther.[6]

The Festschrift[7] in his honour which had been organised and edited by Marstrander and Bergin had reached him on August 7, possibly an advance copy. This very fine volume, of all but 500 pages, entitled *Miscellany presented to Kuno Meyer*, was published in Halle a S. by Max Niemeyer and contained contributions from Meyer's friends and colleagues, the number and variety of which impressed him and gave promise of several days interesting reading. His portrait by Elliot and Fry he did not think a good reproduction and he noted it was mistakenly attributed to Augustus John in the index. And what on earth made Marstrander write in French or rather, he supposed, get his Norse translated, because when they were together in Monte Carlo he could not as much as order his lunch or coffee in French. But it was a volume to be proud of, which he hoped would sell a little, to libraries at any rate, and he ordered six to give away, proposing as well to thank all contributors in due course.[8] The review in the *Times Literary Supplement* of August 7 referred to the copious body of Irish literature now made accessible, for which thanks were due 'in a very special measure, to Dr Kuno Meyer, who has shown an extraordinary flair for good things, and a rare gift for rendering them, not alone with scholarly accuracy, but with a just equivalence of poetic effect. No one in our day has done more for the human and literary side of Celtic studies, and the Miscellany before us is a well-deserved tribute.' Mrs Green had heard of it, but not yet seen it, when she wrote:

Queens Park House,
Seaford, Sussex

Mr dear Dr Meyer
......I must see the Miscellany as soon as I can .... Who can tell what you have done for Ireland, or how deep is the gratitude of all of us who know - May much work still lie before you to help and cheer us all. No one, I am sure, has more devoted friends than you, and more persistent ones. But in this respect a man gets what he earns and deserves - and you have deserved well of your friends.

A.S. Green[9]

'Now I must pack at once', the oft repeated phrase, and Best was to write him at Aachen, *postlagernd*, where on arrival he settled in at the Union Hotel, most comfortable, and such a dear old-fashioned place, just what he liked, and so reasonable he would not have to move into lodgings as he had intended. On the morrow he was to take the cure, the baths being close at hand. His throat had felt better immediately he left Berlin. He had given up cigarettes and taken to cigars. Curious how little Berlin agreed with people. His new colleague, de Groot, professor of Chinese, was quite unhappy about it and another colleague said he could not sleep in the place. Reading through his Festschrift, he wondered why could not all folktales be published in such original form as that of Sampson's and the gorgeous first taking down by Peter O'Leary on p. 389.[10]

By August 20 Meyer was back in London, wishing Best were with him as he was going to see George Moore and W.K. Magee for company. Robin Flower, whom he met for lunch, was full of his last Blasket experiences and was doing excellent work on the Irish manuscripts in the British Museum. Best was laid up with lumbago, 'Now', advised Meyer, 'see that you get better soon. Hot flannels are the thing or rubbing if you can stand it or the old fashioned cupping which I had often to apply to my old Edinburgh tyrant whose amanuensis I was.'[11]

Meyer spent a pleasant evening with Moore, whom he found aged and in need of a holiday, having worked too strenuously on his Trilogy, Volume 2 of which, now finished, would contain a portrait of Meyer for which Moore begged pardon in advance. Flower, with whom he dined, talked mainly about his favourite Blasket Islands, the subject of a book he was going to write from which he read the introduction to Meyer, 'very good'.[12]

After a brief stay in Eastbourne Meyer went to Bath where he stayed at his former address, 4 Johnstone Street, sitting at a roaring fire for the days were cold and the nights frosty, working on the index to *Cormac*[13] and reading Moore who was making them all look ridiculous. He felt very stiff and his neck seemed to be getting worse, a condition he thought was caused by the baths at Aachen, and not knowing what to do he felt annoyed.[14]

He read Meredith, *The Egoist* and *The Amazing Marriage*, 'but one gets tired of his mannerisms'. Visits to Salisbury and Wells were enchanting. 'What a beautiful country with pretty villages and what splendid buildings everywhere. I am ashamed of having lived 30 years in England without knowing it. How my good old mother would have enjoyed these rides.' They were made possible by the motor car and so cheaply, a whole day's ride for 4/6 and so comfortable. Glastonbury was exactly as he imagined it, a 'quiet watered', meadowy place with orchards (Avalon). How one could work in these old retired places, at least one imagined so. In Wells he visited an old friend, Dean Armitage Robinson, now very feeble and almost blind, which was why he gave up the Deanship of Westminster. To Oxford next, then Waterford which he wanted to see, then Dublin.[15]

For Dublin he had arranged an important programme. Part of this was the course of lectures on Old and Middle Irish Poetry and Metrics which he was to deliver in the latter half of September, in the absence of Marstrander and Pedersen, to the School of Irish Learning which, had he not come to its rescue, would have been moribund for 1912. Students from England and Scotland attended. To inaugurate the course he delivered on Wednesday 18 September in the Hall, 35 Dawson Street, one of his most celebrated lectures, open to the public, on 'Irish Learning in the 5th Century A.D.' He had it published with a rich furniture of notes by the School in the following year under the title 'Learning in Ireland in the Fifth Century and the Transmission of Letters'. In it Meyer drew heavily on the unpublished writings of Zimmer. Zimmer had focussed attention on a scribal reference of early origin, found in a Leyden manuscript, to an exodus of Gaulish scholars to Ireland who had fled from the demon-begotten Huns, Vandals and Goths and having settled in Ireland brought about a great increase in learning therein and laid the foundations for the cultivation of classical scholarship. Mainly on this premise, but reinforced by his own learning, Meyer built up a brilliant and elaborate argument for the existence of a high standard of civilisation and letters in 5th century Ireland. As a stimulus to national pride and morale on the intellectual level its effects might be seen as significant. Meyer brought his lecture to a close with the words: 'A field of study is opened up which needs skilled workers to explore it. I have endeavoured to point out the various directions in which further research will, I think, have to proceed; and I hope that the students of this School will continue to contribute to the solution of these as of many other problems connected with ancient Ireland'.[16] Although the premises on which Meyer built up this thesis might appear tenuous or disputable nevertheless the general tenor of his argument appears to have the support of so distinguished a scholar as Nora K. Chadwick, writing in 1960.[17]

Having received the honours from Cork City described earlier, Meyer spent a few days amid old scenes in Liverpool, arriving there on 30 September and staying with Percy Newberry, Professor of Egyptology, who lived in The Grange, a beautiful house with garden in St. Michael's Hamlet on the Mersey. Most of his old colleagues had returned and he stayed up late hours in their company, his health bearing up well and things being 'as if I had returned to my native heath'. It was lovely autumn weather.[18]

The publishers, Constable, sent him their statement on his *Ancient Irish Poetry*, which was poor enough news, with only 75 copies sold for the half-year January-July.[19] Getting fatigued with the social diversions of Liverpool, Meyer left on October 6 for London where he lunched with Flower and heard from him about his work on the Irish manuscripts and marvellous discoveries of literary sources. He wrote to Best about recording the speech and sounds of modern Irish. 'Now that the spoken language is disappearing the School should do everything in its power to take down what is left, or future generations will justly blame us.'[20] There was a pleasant evening with W.P. Ker as host at the gorgeous Prince's Restaurant in Piccadilly, where he had never been before, the company including Professor Constantia Maxwell of Trinity College Dublin and other friends.

He was captivated by Miss Maxwell, a very charming girl and in spite of her position very simple and modest and no blue-stocking. He was due to dine with Stephen Gwynn and William Jones, the Liberal whip, that night (10 October) when the Home Rule battle would be in full swing.[21] It is not hard to guess that their talk would be about the pittance of £100 withdrawn from the School in 1910 and the hopes of its recovery. Much careful diplomacy on this quest by Meyer went unhappily for nothing. His university duties now called him back to Berlin, where he went to see Hermann Ebel's widow on 22 October. Ebel, who died young, is one of the great names in the succession of German Celtic scholarship. His widow was now nearly eighty. It was most pathetic. She had actually tried to keep herself informed of the progress of Celtic studies since her husband's death in 1875. She quoted to Meyer Whitley Stokes' application of Schiller's distich to Ebel's discovery of the origin of *maicc*, when it was confirmed by ogam *maqi*:

Mit dem genius steht die Natur in eifrigem Bunde,
Was der eine verspricht, leistet die andre gewiss,

tears running down her cheeks. She said that was the proudest moment of their lives. She was going to let Meyer have her husband's Ms. Dictionary of Old Irish. He was very curious to know what it was like.[22]

His class at the University had got larger and now numbered 8 students. But adapting to his new environment was not easy.

It will take a long time before I feel at home in Berlin. It has many drawbacks and even some of the attractions turn out to be a delusion. It is e.g. almost impossible to go to a theatre. The prices are simply forbidding. Nothing under 7 or 8 marks and as soon as there is some special attraction as e.g. Strauss' new opera (Der Rosenkavalier) they rise to 30 or 40 marks! And yet hardly a seat to be had! Life is indeed very expensive here. My sister says that everything is *twice* as dear as in England. What a change from my younger days. I am going to have some new invention called *fibrolysin* injected into me. It is said to loosen the fibres. Nous verrons. I manage to do some work every day and have sent off a big instalment of *Cormac* to Karras. .... I hear nothing from Marstrander. The weather is still fine. Plenty of sunshine and bright air. But I cannot say that I feel as yet any good effect of the climate. On the contrary when I have finished this card I am going to take a Turkish bath - price 5/-![23]

To provide a forum for social life in Berlin such as he had enjoyed in Liverpool, Meyer planned to form a University Club, a new thing in Germany, and in this he was very successful. His colleague Harnack was so enthusiastic about it that he proposed to lecture in order to collect funds and as a lecture of his would bring in £100 it was a noble offer. They had got the site of a house which would be built according to their plans and would be ready in the spring of 1914. At a rent of £300 this was £100 less than they paid in Liverpool.[24]

The School, which had been lapsing, would require an outstanding scholar to lecture in the Summer session of 1913 in order to keep alive its prestige and the thoughts of Best and Meyer ran on Holger Pedersen of Copenhagen. It would be a great thing to have him, said Meyer. 'He is of all Celtists the most scientific, I think. It is wonderful what philological genius these Scandinavians have.' Thurneysen might have rueful thoughts about that. Pedersen had recently written a long review on Thurneysen's *Handbuch des Alt-Irischen* in the *Göttingische Gelehrte Anzeigen* 1912, No. 1 and Meyer thought it must be horribly unpleasant for Thurneysen to be criticised so severely and taken to task like a schoolboy. He could well understand why some people would never publish. And yet Pedersen's criticism was quite *sachlich*, without any animus.[25]

Pedersen agreed to come to Dublin and the School Report for 1910-1912 ends with the announcement that the Governors were happy to state he would lecture in July next.[26]

By mid-December Meyer was 'horribly busy'. In addition to all his other work the foundation of the university club which he had taken on himself gave extra to do though it looked a going concern. He had printed and distributed a leaflet dated 7 December 1912 headed *Hochverehter Herr Kollege!* announcing a meeting in aid of the project for the 14th. Some of the great names of German scholarship were appended, including besides Meyer himself, Harnack and Wilamowitz-Moellendorff. Money was needed and he expected about 400 colleagues at the meeting, which took place before the rectorial dinner and was a good opportunity for getting people to subscribe.[27]

Van Hamel was coming to Berlin next semester to take up some Irish work. With regard to School matters, 'Bergin is not a good man to consult about the affairs of the School or indeed any other project.'[28] With regard to recording the Irish language Meyer was thinking of a much bigger thing than mere lectures on phonetics. He would like to have the English scholar Wyld associated with the project, which needed organisation and Wyld was the man for that. Perhaps the School might combine with the Berlin Academy and the Royal Irish Academy to take down the language. The money question was secondary and should not stand in the way. He would talk it over with Mrs Green. For the present he must hurry.[29]

On the 20th Meyer celebrated his 54th birthday, 'six years removed from old age.' He had a long letter from Vendryes, who complained of overwork, and was sending his best pupil to Meyer to work at the Finn legend.[30] Meyer's full year in Berlin had not been easy and needing a rest he planned to go with Toni to Monte Carlo for Christmas. Before setting out Toni sent Edith Best some Strauss music, 'which you are not to play till Christmas Day'. She hoped Edith and her husband would like the pieces, which she herself thought perfectly charming, especially No

1 and 2. She had heard a new quartet by Beethoven the other day, that is, recently discovered, on the theme of his E Major Sonata. He had followed the Sonata closely and it made a most beautiful quartet. That night she was going to hear Elena Gerhardt with Nikesch' accompaniment, which would be a treat in itself. She was glad for Kuno's sake that they were getting away soon, as he needed a change badly after that lowering cure. She hoped the good effects might still appear, otherwise it was most disappointing.[31]

Whether or not it was the Berlin air, Meyer was cross and irritable in the early days of 1913, 'in a demon of a temper' with Tempest of Dundalk who had shelved his lecture on Irish Learning, and displeased with Robert Lloyd Praeger, the publications officer of the Royal Irish Academy who 'as usual' was ignoring his requests.[32] Tactfully as he could, Best softened him. Praeger, he explained, was laid up and could not write. Meyer felt contrite but was still out of humour with Dublin University Press whose ways were intolerable. Meyer was in fact feeling isolated and depressed, for who was there now, he asked, to take much interest? 'I still feel the loss of Stokes, Strachan and Z[immer], and Stern too,' a circumstance that placed him typically in the context of the old Irish saying *Is maol guala gan bráthair,* 'bereft is the shoulder that has no brother'. *The Zeitschrift* was out and he would send Best a copy. Printer Karras was already far advanced with the second heft. Would Bergin not contribute to *Ériu*? The old restless urge was on him. 'We are packing up. I start on Sunday. My London address is University College, Gower Street, W.C.' Tempest had not yet sent him the end of his lecture and notes,[33] and he was vexed with the man's slowness.

Nor was he one bit pleased with Mario Esposito, the Italo-Irish scholar who was investigating classical learning in early Ireland. Part of Meyer's lecture was printed in the *Irish Review*[34] and Esposito contributed a well-reasoned essay to *Studies*[35] rejecting his arguments about the existence of Greek in Ireland. Esposito, said Meyer, was not adequately qualified to pronounce on the question and would never do the 'work he might do and ought to do until he learns Irish.' The question of Greek in Ireland could not be decided until all the Old-Irish and Middle-Irish grammatical and glossarial treatises had been minutely examined. 'It is a pity that Esposito is so inaccurate in his achievements. He trusts Manitius, a most laborious compiler, but a man of little judgment, who often goes astray. In his whole paper there is no word about the Irish *provenance* of classical MSS, the Irish commentary on Vergil (the so-called enlarged Servius), the Liber Fabularum Robartaig, the Greek school grammar and all the other evidence produced by Zimmer; nor any mention of the all-important passage in Aldhelm, where the superior Greek learning of Ireland is so clearly stated'.[36]

In less than a week of writing the above Meyer was in London, where he stayed at Endsleigh Palace Hotel. A social and business round included lunch at University College with Provost Gregory Fisher and Karl Pearson, a flying visit to W.P. Ker in Gower Street and an arrangement to dine with him at the Savile. On Wednesday he was off to Oxford where he would stay with Rhys till Friday, when he was going to propose a great project for Wales at Carmarthen, where the Antiquaries had made him their Vice-President. A card awaited him from Marstrander, who was much interested in the Irish Dictionary being compiled in Germany by Hans Hessen. Marstrander had asked the Council of the Royal Irish Academy for three more assistants. He thought the letter D would run to 300 pages. Meyer referred again to Esposito's paper, which he had only glanced at the previous week, but had since read carefully and considered such a wretched performance that it would be best to take no notice of it. Esposito merely copied Roger[37] and Manitius[38], and when having to stand on his own legs, as in the case of Cormac's Glossary, he was quite incapable of stating the facts. His summing up was ridiculous and his appeal to Truth (with a capital) no less than childish 'He will, if he goes on like that, become the most conceited pedant in Ireland. For God's sake get him away from Dublin. Has he no imagination at all? Surely our business is to endeavour to explain how Ireland came to be the high-school of classical learning and continued to be so for so long a time, and not to pick out a number of chance instances, in which no great learning is shown.' And surely no Irish chauvinist could be so committed as Meyer to glorifying Ireland's past.

He wrote to Esposito, in Latin, saying he would answer him presently. On second thoughts however, he decided to do so without referring to his paper at all, facts being best left to speak for themselves.[39] This was no doubt prudent, as a printed challenge to Esposito's paper would embroil him in controversy with a formidable opponent.

His letter to Esposito reads, in translation:

> Greetings from K.M. to colleague Mario. You sent me your investigations into Greek learning in ancient Ireland, which I have gone through very carefully. I must say I am in total disagreement with you. Not only do you ignore the unanimous testimony of the times, of Aldhelm, Bede, Alcuin and all the others, but you pass over in silence the evidence which actually appears in Irish sources from the close of the sixth century. However on this subject I intend to reply to you in more composed and detailed terms. I have noted these few points as proof that I have read your essay with close attention.
>
> Leipzig 10 January 1913[40]

Latin is more diplomatic than plain English. The question of Greek in early mediaeval Ireland has been much debated, with its existence supported and doubted. Meyer gives details on the transcription of Greek as practised by the Irish in a note at page 27 of his printed lecture. Given all Meyer's erudition in its favour, however, it would seem that the claim for a serious knowledge of Greek existing in early Ireland still awaits definitive study.

NOTES

1. *Ériu* VI (1912) 175-6.
2. Meyer to Best, 27 April 1912 from University Club Liverpool. NLI Ms No. 11002.

3. Meyer to Best, 6 May 1912 from Berlin. NLI Ms No. 11002.
4. Meyer to Best, 10 June 1912 from Charlottenburg, Nieburhrstrasse 11A. NLI Ms No. 11002.
5. Meyer to Alice Stopford Green, 19 July 1912, from Friedrichroda, Thüringen. NLI Ms No. 15091(1).
6. Meyer to Best, 8 Aug. 1912. NLI Ms No. 11002.
7. A circular inviting contributions to a Festschrift, signed by Bergin and Marstrander, was sent to Celtic scholars in Ireland, Great Britain and Europe. It reads, in part:

Confidential

Dublin, 28th January, 1911

Dear Sir,

The appointment of Kuno Meyer to the Chair of Celtic Philology in the University of Berlin seems to several of his friends to be a fitting occasion to offer him some mark of their appreciation of his great services to Celtic Studies, and of their personal regard. They think that the tribute should take the form of a *Miscellany* or *Festschrift*, to which his fellow-workers and some of his pupils would contribute. Mr. Max Niemeyer of Halle, the well-known publisher, has shown his interest and sympathy by generously undertaking the publication of such a volume.

It would greatly increase the value and interest of the *Festchrift* if Continental scholars were to add their tribute. Invitations are accordingly being sent to the following:-

[List follows]

We venture to hope that this project will meet with your approval and sympathy, and that we may count upon your cordial co-operation.

(Copy of circular in RIA MS 12 0 23)

8. Meyer to Best, 8 Aug. 1912. NLI Ms No. 11002.
9. A.S. Green to Meyer, 30 Aug. [1912]. NLI Ms No 11001(2).
10. Meyer to Best, 10 Aug. 1912 from Union Hotel, Aachen. NLI Ms No. 11002.
11. Meyer to Best, 20 Aug. 1912 from Endsleigh Palace Hotel, Endsleigh Gardens, London. NLI Ms No. 11002.
12. Meyer to Best, 23 Aug. 1912 from Beachy Head Hotel, Eastbourne. NLI Ms No. 11002.
13. *Sanas Cormaic.* An Old-Irish Glossary compiled by Cormac Úa Cuilennáin, King-Bishop of Cashel in the 10th Century. Edited from the copy in the Yellow Book of Lecan by Kuno Meyer, Professor of Celtic in the University of Berlin, Halle 1912. This text was Vol IV of Anecdota from Irish MSS. In the introduction, p. xvii, Meyer explains that a handy and cheap edition of Cormac's Glossary had long been a want felt by students of Irish. It had first been edited from the Lebor Brecc in 1862 by Whitley Stokes who considered the time had not arrived for a critical edition, on which Meyer observed that 'So slow has been the progress of Irish studies that fifty years later we still have to be content with mere *ekdoseis*' (texts only).
14. Meyer to Best, 28 and 29 Aug. 1912 from 4 Johnstone Street, Bath. NLI Ms No. 11002.
15. Meyer to Best, 1 and 5 Sept. 1912 from 4 Johnstone Street, Bath. NLI Ms No. 11002.
16. *Learning in Ireland in the Fifth Century* (Dublin 1913) 20.
17. *The age of the saints in the early Celtic church* (London 1961) 52-6.
18. Meyer to Best, 3 Oct. 1912 from The Grange, St. Michael's Hamlet, Liverpool. NLI Ms No. 11002.
19. Meyer to Best, 5 Oct. 1912. NLI Ms No. 11002.
20. Meyer to Best 10 Oct. 1912. NLI Ms No. 11002.
21. Meyer to Best, 10 Oct. 1912 from Endsleigh Palace Hotel, London. NLI Ms No. 11002.
22. Meyer to Best, 23 Oct. 1912 from Charlottenburg, Niebuhrstrasse 11A, Berlin. NLI Ms No. 11002.

23. Meyer to Best, postcard postmarked Berlin 9 Nov. 1912. NLI Ms No. 11002.
24. Meyer to Best, 2 Dec. 1912 from Charlottenburg, Niebuhrstrasse 11A. NLI Ms No. 11002.
25. Meyer to Best, postcard postmarked Charlottenburg, 3 Dec. 1912. NLI Ms No. 11002.
26. Report, *Ériu* VI (1912) 176.
27. Meyer to Best, 14 Dec. 1912. NLI Ms No. 11002.
28. *Ibid.*
29. *Ibid.*
30. Meyer to Best, 19 Dec. 1912. NLI Ms No. 11002.
31. Toni Meyer to Edith Best, postcard 15 Dec. 1912 addressed to Royal Irish Academy of Music, 36 Westland Row, Dublin. NLI Ms No. 11002.
32. Meyer to Best, by postcard postmarked Charlottenburg 2 Jan. 1913. NLI Ms No. 11002 (39).
33. Meyer to Best, by postcard postmarked Charlottenburg, 9 Jan. 1913. NLI Ms No. 11002 (39).
34. Vol II [1912] 449-459.
35. Vol I [1912] 665-683.
36. Meyer to Best, 9 Jan. 1913 from Charlottenburg, Niebuhrstrasse 11A. NLI Ms No. 11002.
37. M. Roger, *L'enseignement des lettres classiques d'Ausone à Alcuin*. Paris 1905.
38. Max Manitius, *Geschichte der lateinischen Literatur des Mittelalters*. Munich 1911-23.
39. Meyer to Best, 13 Jan. 1913. NLI Ms No. 11002.
40. Meyer to Mario Esposito, in Esposito letters, NLI 425 A fol 56. Meyer's Latin reads:

    K.M. Mario suo salutem. Misisti mihi elucubrationes tuas de Argiva apud veteres Hibernos scientia, quas studiosissime perlustravi. Confiteor quod tota mente a te dissentiam. Non solum unanimum saeculorum testimonium, Aldhelmi, Baedae, Alcuini ceterorumque omnium negleges, sed etiam quae in libris Hibernicis iam ab exeunte saeculo sexto inveniuntur silentio praetermittis. Sed de hac re diligentius et pleniore sermone sibi respondere in animo est. Haec pauca exaravi ne dubites quin opusculum tuum diligenter legerim.
    Datum Lipsiae, 10mo Ian. mens. die 1913.

Chapter 13

AN expression that occurs ever more frequently in Meyer's correspondence from Germany was 'horribly busy'. The more he
became involved in the social and academic life of Berlin the
more was Dublin becoming difficult to reach. With so much to do until
the middle of March he feared a visit to Dublin was out of the question
and unless there was a heavenly spring he would go south to a sunnier
clime, possibly Amélie-les-Bains. There are times when one gets the
impression that overwork was affecting him. He was worried about his
former Liverpool colleague Robert Priebsch, now Professor of German
at University College London, who had a nervous breakdown and was
spending his leave in Amélie. Meyer thought he would get sick of lecturing this term and give it up for life.

In the course of a visit to London he went to see Mrs Green to talk
about the future of the School of Irish Learning which he considered the
responsibility of his life. Mrs Green, helpful as ever, suggested they ask
Paul Vinogradoff to give three or four lectures on the tribal system. To
get him to come would be a notable advertisement for the School. Paul
Gavrilovitch Vinogradoff (1854-1925) had a world-wide reputation.
Born in Russia, he studied in Berlin under Mommsen, who influenced
him greatly, and Brunner. In 1901 he resigned his professorship of history in Moscow university, where his liberal mind found the environment oppressive, arrived in England and in 1903 was elected to the chair
of jurisprudence in Corpus Christi College Oxford, a post he held for
life. There he introduced a new method of seminar teaching which gathered round him a group of enthusiastic students of history and law.
Author of many books, a gifted linguist and teacher, he became an
authority on the feudal land system in England and a master of the social
and legal institutions both of the ancient and modern world.

In addition Meyer proposed to get Henry Cecil Wyld, an old
Liverpool colleague and authority on the English language, to lecture on
phonetics. Mrs Green offered to finance both courses, which were to be
widely advertised, with students brought to Dublin by paying their
expenses. Meyer was finding it hard to get suitable accommodation in
London. 'All the private hotels and lodging houses in this neighbourhood are no better than brothels or maisons d'assignation.' He would
have to try in the suburbs.[1] He found a suitable place at 36 Howitt Road,
N.W. and notified Best. A large audience attended his first lecture in
London. Flower was a most assiduous student and so was W.P. Ker 'of

whom I hope to make an Irish scholar yet'.[2] But he must have been feeling hard pressed, as he complained that the London classes were hanging like a millstone round his neck.

Mrs Green had spoken to Vinogradoff. He was willing and eager to hold a seminar at the School any time that Summer to set some people working at the Irish land and tribal system. He would explain the method of work, give some notion of the better known Welsh system on which he had written and set them work which he would return afterwards to examine. A good programme, thought Meyer, and if he could get Wyld as well this Summer session would be one of the most important yet. 'Mrs Green will finance everything.' The three important names of Pedersen, Vinogradoff and Wyld would look well together. They must advertise as soon as possible, and if any distant students applied and were in need of funds Mrs Green would also pay their expenses. How one must admire Mrs Green, whose support was so important to the School. Would it be possible, asked Meyer, to have all three together in July? They would find each other's society pleasant. Would Best be there to start them off ?[3] In the event Vinogradoff, busy with examinations and accumulated work, was unable to come, to his regret,[4] and his course was deferred until as far as 1915. By then the dogs of war were in action and a unique prospect of learning and interpretation which would have brought enhancement to the School was left unrealised.

Nothing if not frank, Meyer had told George Calder he did not think it fair of him to bring out another 'Old Gaelic Grammar' pilfered from Thurneysen. He had spent a pleasant evening with George Moore and was to dine with him that night with an American called Bergen. He had also made the acquaintance of Tonks, a most charming fellow, at D.S. McColl's, who lived close to him. Moore was in low spirits. He was suffering from a bad cold and talked about his age and 'the days of his potency' gone by! Meyer managed to cheer him up. He found Moore reading Petronius. That afternoon he was having tea with Mrs Boothby at the Carlton Hotel. She had now made the discovery that her husband had married her with all his debts unpaid. She was paying them off gradually and retrenchments were necessary.[5]

Meyer had an enormous amount of work to do in London but so far he was equal to it. He was campaigning for the establishment of Celtic chairs, or at least lectureships, in London and Liverpool. Ridgeway also wished him to plead before the University of Cambridge for a chair there and he could not well refuse. Meyer was sorry to say that Marstrander on the occasion of his two visits to Liverpool did not impress the people there favourably. Meyer hoped they would take him in London if anything substantial were done there. Calder had written him a letter which Meyer forwarded to Best. Meyer did not warm to Calder, disliking 'the man and his ways'. On an article about Ancient Rome in Ireland written by Haverfield for the *English Historical Review* he commented that the first seven pages contained a lot of questionable reasoning, much like Esposito's. He had signed his lecture on *Irish*

130

Learning for press and ordered 500 copies. The Plautine scholar W.M. Lindsay was going to write on the Gaulish exodus from the palaeographical side. Perhaps it would be better to reserve Wyld till the next year, suggested Meyer. He had a very pleasant time at Carmarthen.[6]

Tempest sent him 30 copies of his lecture on Fifth Century Ireland. Nothing but illness everywhere. Mrs Green had a low fever and had to cancel all engagements for weeks. Windisch had an ulcerated leg and would have to undergo an operation.[7] Flower was back from Oxford. He had got a fine job, on which Meyer congratulated him. 'Voynich has asked him to catalogue for him 300 Mss, mostly gorgeously illuminated missals, for which he will pay him at the rate of £5 each, in summa £1500'.[8] James George O'Keeffe was coming to London next week, leaving his family in Greystones and hoping to rent an apartment. Meyer had lost two students, Eleanor Hull who was ill and Miss MacNaughton whose father Lord MacNaughton had just died. 'She was most promising and read the Táin as well as Flower'.[9] Meyer was to be the guest of the London Irish on St Patrick's Day at the Hotel Cecil, John Redmond in the chair. By February 25th Meyer had got his last lecture off his mind and could breathe more freely. It was a great success, subject Arthurian Legend. He pleaded once more for a permanent Celtic chair in London. He confided to Best 'I have to write to the Norse *Storthing* to recommend a chair for C.M. - but this *entre nous*'.

At Cambridge he lectured to 'a capital audience' at which J.E. Sandys, E.C. Quiggin and William Ridgeway spoke. All were much interested and there was a great demand for the printed lecture. He stayed with Waldstein, the noted authority on Greek sculpture, who lived in great state with two motors and three manservants, a rich American widow, three stepdaughters and two children of his own.

Meyer wished Eoin MacNeill would publish more. He had a letter of twelve quarto pages from him full of the most interesting matter. Was Meyer by now coming to appreciate MacNeill's excellence? Best was planning to leave 35 Percy Place, so pleasantly situated on the south bank of the Grand Canal. His neighbour who aspired to be a musician and singer was making the most horribly discordant noises which Best could not stand. But he was staying on until October. Meyer asked him would he not write down some reminiscences of Synge. 'Lady Gregory managed to write more about herself than him in her paper on him'.[10]

Meyer asked Best to send a prospectus of Pedersen's lectures to Miss MacNaughton, Runkerry, Bushmills, Co. Antrim, who wanted to attend the course. Baudis was also coming. 'I am packing up. Had my last dinner with Ker and Flower last night at Pagani's. ... Moore asked me to remember him to you and your wife. He misses your society very much. Altogether he is pretty lonely here, I think.' On Monday night at the Hotel Cecil Meyer sat between Swift MacNeill, a fine old fellow, and a pretty Papist named Miss O'Malley, a great friend of the Redmonds. He was introduced to a lot of people. There were fine speeches. 'But among all their enthusiasm I thought of Parnell and how they chucked him.'

Miss Hull was to edit for Dent all translations of Irish texts the copyright of which had expired.[12]

With his cacophonous neighbour making life impossible, Best moved from 35 Percy Place earlier than planned, going to live not so far away at 57 Upper Leeson Street in a solid double-fronted residence with good gardens front and rear, one of a group of three similar houses cosily recessed off the main thoroughfare at the junction of Leeson Street and Appian Way. Happily it stands yet, with its companions, but one trembles for their future. There Edith and he spent the rest of their days and made it a truly hospitable salon for native and visiting scholars, writers and artists. Meyer was surprised. 'You have been quick about it and it meant some days hard work and discomfort. May you enjoy the house and garden for many years in happiness and comfort.' Meyer recalled that he and his sister had lodged in Upper Leeson Street about 1888. Best's home being detached he would have peace from his neighbours and yet, said Meyer, 'I am sorry I shall not find you again in your old surroundings, which had their own charm. Perhaps after all you will miss the gentle susurrus of the harmonium next door on Sundays.'[12]

In April Meyer was back in old haunts of Leipzig, places he hoped to show the Bests when they came to Germany, as they hoped, in July or August. He saw the important library of D'Arbois de Jubainville at Fock's, the booksellers, who was asking £375 for the lot which Meyer was greatly tempted to buy. He was sure Bergin, Marstrander, Vendryes, Quiggin and others would like to purchase many items and he would let them have them at reasonable prices, although it would give him much trouble. What did Best think and would he care to see the catalogue? The School, the National Library and other institutions might buy too. All Celtic scholars should avail of this unique opportunity. The Berlin Seminar might buy some books and so might Thurneysen. 'The danger is that the whole library is sold to America'. He asked Best to write him at Leipzig for he would not be back in Berlin before the 22nd of April.[14]

Macalister was planning to edit the *Lebor Gabála* or Book of Invasions of Ireland, a lengthy and curious assembly of pseudo-history and mythology, with help from Eoin MacNeill. Robert Alexander Stewart Macalister, whose name splendidly echoed his Scottish ancestry, nevertheless Dublin born, and intensely patriotic, was a man of much learning and many interests, whose metier was archaeology, on which he had written volumes, but his talents included skills in music, a contribution to Dickensian literature by providing an ending to *The mystery of Edwin Drood* and a creditable competence in writing modern Irish as his correspondence with Eoin MacNeill shows. But of his capacity to edit the *Lebor Gabála* Meyer had grave doubts, which he expressed to Eoin MacNeill who had evidently apprised him of the project:

> My dear MacNeill
> I got yr letter before I left London, and only find the time now to answer it. Macalister is one of those unfortunate people who will always attempt things which he cannot do, and not stick to what he can do. Instead of archaeological

work which tout le monde is expecting of him he is going to bring out a difficult Irish text with which he could not possibly deal alone. You are going to help him, but I ask you is that right?[15]

To Best he put an equally adamant view. 'Why will Macalister try to do things that are beyond him.'[16] His opinion was to be confirmed by future judgement. Macalister went on to edit the text in which the participation of MacNeill was minimal, only to have the result reviewed in terms of such severity that one is left in no doubt as to the correctness of Meyer's judgement.[17] Meyer dined with Windisch who was very poorly and had not been out of doors since Christmas, stricken with asthma, bronchitis and now blood poisoning.[18]

Best was faced with increased expenses because of his change of house and had to forego his projected visit to Germany. He wrote:

My dear Professor,
    Not until now have I had time to reply to your Leipzig letter. Every moment of my time has been occupied feeding the printer with proofs of my Bibliography, and ordering things in our new abode. At last we have got settled down. It was only yesterday that I managed to see Bergin and have a talk about D'Arbois' library. He is willing to purchase to the extent of £50 or so. To buy the library en bloc is out of the question, he says. He would have arranged matters otherwise had the notion occurred to him earlier. I unfortunately must forswear book-buying for many months to come. So do not count on me in any way, except to help you to dispose of them or estimate their value, which I shall be glad to do. I must now retrench in order to meet the increased rent and expenses of moving. You speak of my looking at the books in July. I am afraid my German trip is also knocked on the head. Six months ago I swore to my wife that she would be listening to Wagner in Munich this summer. But I cannot do it, and the good soul is quite reconciled to a humdrum holiday in Wales .... Pedersen's course would in any case prevent our going to you in Berlin. You know he lectures from July 14 to August 9. It is essential for me to be here, even if I were not keen about following his course. The School is now reduced to Miss Knott and myself as local representatives. It would never do for me to absent myself, while Pedersen, Loth, not to speak of the minor lights, were in Dublin. Someone must look after them'.[19]

Best's letter obviously crossed with one from Meyer dated 23 April which contained news of Marstrander's Norwegian appointment. 'You will have heard from C.M. that the Storthing has voted the Celtic Chair for him with ninety against twenty-nine votes – not bad for an assembly of peasants as he called it scornfully some time ago'.[20] Flower was going to continue Meyer's Irish classes at University College London on his return from the Blaskets at the end of May. Mrs Green was giving some travelling scholarships to members of the class for the purpose of attending Pedersen's lectures. Van Hamel also turned up in Berlin, very eager and much improved both in health (he had been quite stout) and in his knowledge of Irish and Welsh. Meyer's university classes were beginning the following Monday. He had asked Fock to send Best the catalogue of D'Arbois' library. Could Best give him an idea of when he was coming to Berlin? Any time before the second week in August would suit fine.

Meantime Best's letter arrived. Kuno replied at once. It would be well, he agreed, if Best remained in Dublin during Pedersen's course, but after such devotion a proper long holiday was absolutely necessary and Best must really keep his promise to visit them. 'Do not procrastinate, it is a bad habit, life is short and uncertain' and he quoted Goethe as saying that two things were the curse of life, Übereilung und Verabsäumung.[21]

Toni and Kuno were sorry that the Bests had to forego their visit. In Germany they were mourning the loss of Erich Schmidt, foremost among the country's modern literary historians. Meyer's classes had begun with a very good attendance, eight in Irish and ten in Welsh. He was also holding a course of popular lectures, 'Einleitung in die Keltologie', attended by about seventy students.[22] Pokorny had nineteen students, 'Flower is happy in his beloved Blasket Island, Marstrander envies him, Esposito writes to say that he is going to give up Hiberno-Latin studies and I am just beginning them.'[23]

Meyer was doubtful whether he could visit Dublin in October. Many duties kept him busy. 'The longer I stay in Germany the more I am getting tied up here'. Meanwhile Van Hamel was coming that evening to play sonatas with Toni, and Priebsch and Kuno would be the audience, though Priebsch usually used the opportunity to read Casanova and Kuno to correct proofs to the accompaniment of Mozart or Beethoven. Kuno advised the Bests not to think of visiting Germany at Easter with its cold weather. He expected Best's Bibliography of Irish Philology and of Printed Irish Literature to be out soon. It must have cost him a lot of trouble. 'Marstrander remains the same queer fish he always was.'[24]

Marstrander, occupied with multiple duties and a desperate race against time to complete his Dictionary work, found opportunity to let Best know Pedersen's requirements:

> I am writing to ask you whether you could get Dr. Pedersen 2 rooms in Kingstown or Howth with 4 beds. He will keep the rooms from July 12 to August 12.
>
> Pedersen will bring his wife, his son (aged 12) and his daughter (aged 7). I gather from his letter that he is anxious to obtain cheap lodgings; breakfast to be included in the terms, if possible (I presume his wife will do the rest of the housekeeping). He also seems anxious to be left with himself. I have told him, of course, that you and Bergin are 'unavoidable'. Please correspond with Dr. Pedersen about the matter. (Adr. Eleanorsvej 8, Charlottenland ved Köbenhavn).
>
> I know no one in Dublin who can settle this better than you and I trust you do not mind my troubling you with it.

Nor did Best mind preparing for the comforts of Pedersen and others, apprehensive though he was about the prospects of the course. Things looked far from good. He was greatly disappointed at the fewness of the entries. Although he advertised the lectures twice in the *Athenaeum*, and in weekly and daily papers and in the *Revue Celtique* not a single person had been attracted by these announcements. He had sent around a whip and a fresh circular, to which there were only two responses. Miss Byrne, Tadhg O'Donoghue and others were occupied with Intermediate examination papers. The Summer colleges attracted others as did the Oireachtas, the annual congress of the Gaelic League. Bergin, teaching in University College, had apparently no pupils to send. 'Things look pretty bad here. We shall have only twelve students, and some may drop out.' Had Best foreseen this he would have put Pedersen off. In fact Pedersen had written twice to say he should never have consented to come and Best believed he was coming only to keep his promise. Rev. Gerard O'Nolan, who was going to Germany for a month, was particularly disappointing when so great a scholar as Pedersen was brought over to Dublin expressly to cater for him and his like. Tomás Ó Máille had entered his name but would probably only remain a week, since he was expected in Galway for the Oireachtas. Eleanor Hull could not come as she was attending Robin Flower's classes in London University nor could Flower himself. James George O'Keeffe was holidaying in Dublin and would not come. Father Paul Walsh had taken no notice of Best's circular but was thought to be teaching in Ring. How glad Best was that they did not get Wyld to come as well.[26]

Best did not have time to worry when Pedersen arrived, for he did not have a moment's leisure after that, especially with the sudden appearance of Baudis and his wife, both of whom happily left soon for Galway, proposing to return in September for a longer stay. Joseph Loth arrived and John Fraser brought him around to meet Best at the National Library. Bergin and Fraser were devoted to Loth, whom they had met in Ballingeary at the Irish College. Loth was 'an exceedingly nice fellow, with a complete absence of side and self-importance', who worked most of the day in the Library at the archaeological reviews, and attended Pedersen's classes, but took no notes. He was looking out for new lodgings and in this wanted Best's assistance.

The classes were in full swing from July 14, with an attendance of sixteen, the list of whom Best forwarded to Meyer, along with an account of his distinguished visitors:

> Pedersen's lectures are of the greatest interest, Miss Knott says the best we have ever had. He writes them out in perfect English, and delivers them in a low monotonous tone – somewhat jaded, and in strong contrast to his powerful appearance. His accent is scarcely noticeable. He generally stops at 11.30. He is a short thick-set man, with fair hair brushed back from his forehead, beard beginning to fade, chubby hands, powerful shoulders, and large head. He is very quiet and reserved. Has no nerves, I should say; does not smoke. He says very little, rarely ventures on a remark, but answers questions.
>
> I called upon him on Sunday morning, and we had the family here in the afternoon. Mrs Pedersen does not know English, or I think German either. She has a perturbed, anxious look. There is a dear little girl of six, and a nice intelligent boy of 15. My wife played with them in the garden, giving them runs on the bicycle, which the little one enjoyed hugely. The Baudis's also came. Pedersen spoke a few words to Mrs. B. in Bohemian, but she sat silent beside him, most of the time. As you may imagine, entertaining them was something of an effort. I had out the phonograph, which interested Baudis more than Pedersen. The latter appeared to be most interested in the portrait groups containing Thurneysen and yourself. Fancy he had never seen either your photograph or Thurneysen's. When I described Thurneysen and his nervous manner, he exclaimed with surprise 'I should never have thought him nervous from his writings.' And Baudis remarked of Pedersen when he had gone that he would never have imagined him so impassive and reserved from his reviews of Thurneysen's grammar.

He has been lecturing on the pre-verbal particles up to the present, discussing their etymology and above all the origin and development of their meanings. Today he was on *ro*, which was almost a revelation. Yesterday he treated *air*. Everyone is delighted. He showed me the complete proofs of the concluding part of his grammar to be published in October. He treats the irregular verbs very fully, giving all their inflections with copious citations from the Glosses. The index is practically an Old-Irish vocabulary......

We were all photographed in the Green today. I'll send you a copy. I suggested to Pedersen that we should print these groups with the Annual Report in *Ériu*. They might tend to create a better understanding among scholars!! We could print Thurneysen's of two years ago at the same time. It would give a human interest to our proceedings, and would be welcome to everybody.[27]

The Bests were ideal hosts. They entertained the Pedersens with lunch followed by a visit to the Zoo which, one surmises, was enjoyed as much by the grown-ups as by the children. 'I like Pedersen. He is a thorough good fellow. When you meet him and hear his generous praise of other scholars, and his gratitude for work that is sincere and helpful, all the preconceived notion of bumptiousness which his review of Thurneysen's Handbuch gives me, disappears. It is merely his quiet outspoken way of comparing dissimilar methods'.[28] Such was Best's impression of the Danish linguist. Loth, whom he had at dinner to meet Van Hamel, seemed depressed and ill, the cause being an inflamed foot.

Meyer was delighted to hear of Pedersen's success. He had a fine class such as he could get nowhere else and would enjoy it as much as his audience. Writing while Toni, a cousin and Van Hamel were playing Mozart trios, he was sorry he could not say much on his postcard because he was 'horribly busy' trying to finish a book for the Berlin Academy on the oldest Irish poetry which he had to hand in by Thursday. F.N. Robinson from Harvard was coming to Europe next year and would no doubt appear in Dublin. Loth, whom Best liked so much, was a very unassuming bonhomme and pleasant company, though why Gaidoz bore him such a grudge Meyer could not fathom. Pokorny was happy in the Baltic, looking about for a wife. Thurneysen in the new number of the *Celtische Zeitschrift* was full of praise for Best's work on *Lebor na Huidre*.

On his return to Denmark, Pedersen wrote to thank Best and his wife 'for the help you have given us and the care you have taken of us from the first day to the last'.[29] They did not know it, but it was the last great flourish of the School. The ominous year of 1914 was approaching and events were to happen elsewhere which would affect the destinies of Celtic and other scholarship. Later in 1913 the more or less tranquil tenor of progress was gravely disturbed by the great Dictionary controversy which is related in the next chapter and had damaging results.

NOTES

1. Meyer to Best, 22 Jan. 1913 from Endsleigh Palace Hotel, London. NLI Ms No. 11002.
2. Meyer to Best, 1 Feb. 1913 from 36 Howitt Road, London NW. NLI Ms No. 11002 (4).

3. Meyer to Best, 5 Feb. 1913. NLI Ms No. 11002.
4. Vinogradoff to Meyer, 18 Oct. 1913 from Corpus Christi College Oxford. NLI Ms No. 11002.
5. Meyer to Best, 5 Feb. 1913. NLI Ms No. 11002.
6. Meyer to Best, 8 Feb. 1913. NLI Ms No. 11002.
7. Meyer to Best, 21 Feb. 1913. NLI Ms No. 11002.
8. Meyer to Best, postmarked Hampstead, 22 Feb. 1913. NLI Ms No. 11002 (41).
9. Meyer to Best, 22 Feb. 1913.
10. Meyer to Best, 25 Feb. 1913 from 36 Howitt Road, Haverstock Hill, NW. NLI Ms No. 11002 (40).
11. Meyer to Best, Féil Pátraic 1913 from 36 Howitt Road, NW. NLI Ms No. 11002 (39).
12. Meyer to Best, 18 March 1913. NLI Ms No. 11002 (39).
13. Meyer to Best, 7 April 1913 from Hotel Corneille, 5 Rue Corneille, Paris. NLI Ms No. 11002 (39).
14. Meyer to Best, 15 April 1913 from Central-Hotel de Pologne, Leipzig. NLI Ms No 11002.
15. Meyer to MacNeill, 30 March 1913, from Hotel Moderne, Amélie-les-Bains. NLI Ms No. 10882.
16. Meyer to Best, 15 April 1913, from Leipzig. NLI Ms No. 11002.
17. Cf *Irish Historical Studies* II, 88-91, 330-3; *Celtica* II Pt 1, 195-209.
18. Meyer to Best, 15 April 1913 from Central-Hotel de Pologne, Leipzig. NLI Ms No. 11002.
19. Best to Meyer, 22 April 1913, from 57 Upper Leeson Street, Dublin. NLI Ms No. 11002.
20. Meyer to Best, postcard 23 April 1913. NLI Ms No. 11002.
21. Meyer to Best, p.c. postmarked Berlin 24 April 1913. NLI Ms No. 11002 (39).
22. Meyer to Best, p.c. postmarked Charlottenburg 2 May 1913. NLI Ms No. 11002 (39).
23. Meyer to Best, postcard 7 May 1913 from Charlottenburg. NLI Ms No. 11002 (37).
24. Meyer to Best, postcard 26 May 1913 from Charlottenburg. NLI Ms No. 11002 (40).
25. Marstrander to Best, 12 June 1913. NLI Ms No. 11001 (28).
26. Best to Meyer, 9 July 1913. NLI Ms No. 11002.
27. Best to Meyer, 16 July 1913 from 57 Upper Leeson Street, Dublin. NLI Ms No. 11002.
28. Best to Meyer, 1 Aug. 1913. NLI Ms No. 11002.
29. Pedersen to Best, 18 Aug. 1913. NLI Ms No. 11002.

Chapter 14

What Whitley Stokes wrote in 1858 might serve as prolegomenon to the task undertaken by Carl Marstrander in 1912, which was to produce the first fasciculus of a full-scale Dictionary of the Irish Language, long considered as an essential basis to any progress in Irish studies.

> Some persons may ask, (he remarked), why should the Irish Archaeological Society expend its funds in publishing a document which merely illustrates the Irish language? Let such persons try to understand that every contribution to a more accurate knowledge of this Irish language is ultimately a contribution to Irish history. For this can never be written until trustworthy versions are produced of all the surviving chronicles, laws, romances, and poetry of ancient Celtic Ireland. Moreover, immediate results of high historical importance may be obtained by comparison of the words and forms of the Irish with those of the other Indo-European languages. Chronicles may, and often do, lie; laws may have been the work of a despot, and fail to correspond with the ethical ideas of the people for whom they were made ... But the evidence given by words and forms is conclusive ....[1]

About the same time his friend and mentor, Rudolf Thomas Siegfried, who held the Chair of Sanskrit in Trinity College Dublin, in a memorandum proposing the preparation of a complete Dictionary of the Irish Language under the superintendence of the Royal Irish Academy and the Irish Archaeological and Celtic Societies, envisaged such a Dictionary as a 'full interpretation, critical and historical, of every word of the language in which the past of the country speaks to us, in which the annals, the laws, the poetry, the records of religion and family life are present and the echo of which will sound for ages to come in the names of places and of persons.'[2] On the twenty-seven year old Norwegian scholar fell the responsibility of producing this Dictionary, in its first part, after an interval of some fifty years.

In taking on the work he found himself facing a handicap which in ordinary circumstances should never be imposed on a project of scholarship, namely, a time limit, of short duration, expiring in his case on a date before September 1913. This unusual circumstance had originated from the will of a great and generous supporter of the Irish language, the Rev. Maxwell Henry Close, who left a bequest of £1,000 to the Royal Irish Academy on his death in September 1903 towards the expenses of an Irish Dictionary, on condition that portion of the Dictionary had to be in print within ten years of his death. If not, the money was to be withdrawn. The condition, when made, was not arbitrary, for ten years was a generous term. But nothing had been done until the performance of the task was placed in Meyer's hands in 1907 and delegated by him to Bergin, who was too slow and inexperienced and, early in 1910, to Marstrander, by whose abilities Meyer was greatly impressed.

> I am delighted with him. He is wonderfully keen and eager and looks forward to his work with zest. He will reform the Dictionary. Nothing escapes him. He went through the proof and Bergin's slips and he at once spotted every weak point and had the right thing ready. I feel that I can absolutely trust him and a great burden is off my mind.[3]

The fiercely dedicated Marstrander was presently stricken with pleurisy brought on by overwork and carelessness and following his recovery left Dublin to continue his Dictionary work in Norway where he found he could make better progress. He was faced with a mammoth task, and the question occurs more than once, was it fair to burden him with it, given that the time for its completion was so short, and considering how many years had been let lapse before serious work was commenced.

Throughout the late Autumn of 1912 and the early winter months of 1913 he laboured ceaselessly in Kristiania, racing against the clock, with the defective and heterogeneous materials out of which he was expected to fashion the first instalment of the projected Dictionary. He was unable to take a holiday. 'I would love to go to the mountains for a week but cannot'. The more he worked the more it became clear to him that the raw material given him was useless for all scholarly purposes, gathered as it was from east to west without any general plan, and to some extent by people who even lacked the most elementary knowledge of older Irish. He made this clear to the Royal Irish Academy by letter late in 1912. To help him at his task he was given three women assistants in Dublin, Maud Joynt and Mary Byrne, both appointed in 1909, and Eleanor Knott, appointed in 1911, all of whom produced excellent work. Marstrander could point to the literal truth that never before had editor faced single-handed such a gigantic task. The high speed he worked at left him no time even to check proofs.

Within the Royal Irish Academy a Dictionary Committee functioned, but how real or relevant was its connection with the actual work remains unclear. Edward Gwynn seems to have been closest to what went on. Best was on the Committee and described how Maud Joynt was receiving batches of proofs of the Dictionary, 'enormous rolls. No eyes save hers and Gwynn's are permitted to behold them.'[4] Best was piqued, and told Meyer that as a member of the Committee he would demand that, before printing off, each member have submitted to him a set of the proofs.

Meyer reported from Berlin that Marstrander had 'at last' sent him a batch of proofs. He was critical of Marstrander's English which he thought should be altered by a competent person, Gwynn perhaps. As to the Irish the first thing that struck him was that it was a motley mixture from all periods of the language down to Peter O'Leary. Proper names were included in all sorts of spellings. There were doubtful etymologies.

'Of course he has amassed a lot of information and nothing comes amiss; but it comes in very questionable form. However, all that is now too late to mend. The great thing is to bring it out. I suppose it will remain a torso'.[5]

Richard Best was greatly agitated when Maud Joynt showed him, by 'an act of high treason or lèse majesté', the wrapper of the Dictionary with Marstrander's preface on the inner cover. Best was so disgusted that he took it to show to Macalister and Praeger. Fancy, (one can imagine the dear man choking), he set out by gravely stating that the aims of the R.I.A. Dictionary of the Irish Language was to introduce order into the chaos of Irish lexicography, and to mark his astonishment he put down a treble exclamation mark at this statement, which seems no more than a plain recital of fact.

> Then he proceeds to define the scope of the Dictionary which, beginning with the dawn of the Irish Language, traces the shape, meaning, and grammatical inflection etc. of all words in use among the *Celts* of *Ireland*. He stated that his predecessors had your Contribb. as a model. *He* however thought that the time had come for a bigger thing. He winds up by thanking his 3 assistants in alphabetical order, and Miss Joynt for indefatigable help in proof reading, and then couples *you* and Gwynn together for reading the proofs of *several* slips and supplying many illustrations, which called for the most grateful recognition. Fancy not a word about Bergin, not a mention of Purton. Your published D – Dno not mentioned. I was so disgusted that I expressed my mind to Miss Joynt. She poor girl was greatly worried over this preface, and felt something was wrong, but her [task?] was merely to correct English. When Praeger saw it he agreed it could not be published. So we have called the Dictionary Committee for Friday. We shall print instead a bald business-like statement, explaining why this Fasciculus 1 (not Part 1) begins with D rather than A, and what its price will be, and how it will be sold. The Introduction should come at the end of Volume 1 and Praeger and I think there should be a sort of historical or official preface stating how the Dictionary arose, and who worked upon it. But fancy ignoring Bergin and his work upon it, and bracketing you with Gwynn. He had sent me two paragraphs for insertion, explaining his use of etymology, and referring to the dawn, the broad daylight of Old and Middle Irish and the gloomy eve of Modern Irish!!! all of which are represented in the Dictionary. He writes like a school-boy. All of this *entre nous*.[6]

His confidant to this breathless communication was Meyer. Best wondered how Marstrander, by now 'incorrigible', would take the brief announcement which was put in place of his Preliminary Notice. My dear Best, C.M. is a great sinner, rejoined Meyer, who had half a mind to let all his frightful blunders stand, which would teach him a lesson. Not to acknowledge what he must owe to Bergin and Purton, not to speak of his, Meyer's, work was absurd. 'He wrote me a most offensive post card the other day after all the trouble I had taken with his damned sheets. He meant to be ironical, but it did not come off in his English, which as you say is often that of a schoolboy. I cannot understand why the Dictionary Committee has not had proofs all along. You should look into the Dictionary itself...'[7]

Meyer sent Best a revised proof of the Dictionary, to show him how much it stood in need of correction and claiming to mean the best for the Academy, Marstrander, the magnum opus itself, and all and everything concerned. Best was to see for himself that the task had been in many ways beyond C.M. especially in the proper names. Of course it was too late now to do anything to alter C.M.'s methods and Meyer seemed to regret that Gwynn did not exert some influence over him or correct certain things. Was anything printed off? Couldn't the whole thing be stopped for a month or two at any rate? Could Best not move on the Committee that the final proofs be submitted to it before final printing? All of which suggestions came from Meyer on 29 July, so close to the dateline that to have carried them out was impossible. Meyer wanted the proof back by return of post so that he could forward it to Marstrander.[7]

Meyer must have made numerous changes in the proof, to judge from Best's reaction. But how utterly changed a view Best presents about Marstrander whom he had seen some short years previously as too brilliant for words. His long and agitated reply reveals as well what he thought about the interior politics of the Academy.

1 August 1913
57 Upr. Leeson St.

My dear Professor,

The proof is indeed awful! I hope this headstrong youth will have the sense to adopt your corrections. We can do nothing here. It is ludicrous that the members of the Dictionary Committee are not to be permitted to see the proofs of the Dictionary. The great mistake was for the Academy to regard M. as master of the situation, and pander to his petty vanity. It is all due to this miserable £1,000 - the fear of losing it. When you reflect that this sum, if it will ever be paid, will not go into the coffers of the Academy, but to the printer, one might well pause and ask *a quoi bon*. Why spend money printing such a pretentious and untrustworthy work. It has all the appearance of profound learning without the reality. It looks more like a hotch-potch .... M. has no sense of what is fitting. He must be swollen with vanity, and a belief in the importance of his method and his analyses. The remarks you have made in the margins are not a whit too severe ... If this sheet is a fair specimen, I tremble for M's reputation. He should be eternally grateful to you. But this would be too much to expect. It is not a Dictionary, but often rather a series of discussions. ... There is far too much that is problematical and hypothetical. And to think of the labour he has expended on this inflated work! It will take a generation of scholars to purge it of its grosser errors, if you do not succeed in bringing him to reason. It will be known as Marstrander's Folly. If it were critically reviewed by you or Bergin his budding reputation would be blasted.

I talked to Praeger about it to-day, without showing him the proof. But I got no satisfaction. He merely said the Irish scholars should fall on it and tear it to pieces. That from an officer of the Academy! I complained of the supineness of the Academy in acquiescing with his orders that no one was to see the proofs but Gwynn and Miss Joynt. And also that the Dictionary Committee was so seldom summoned. I renewed my protest against the order of the Council referring your resignation to the Dictionary Committee and that Committee never having been summoned to consider it, and the matter allowed to drop. It was only a few weeks ago when a new Committee was summoned to consider a wild proposal of Marstrander to increase the staff and widen the scope of the Dictionary that I learned of this. When I raised the whole question at the next meeting I was ruled out of order and told that it was too late, that the business of the meeting was merely to consider the draft of a reply to C.M. Technically that may have been so. Praeger argued contemptibly that the Dictionary Committee was summoned. Yes, I said, but over a year later than the Order of Council, and your resignation was not on the Agenda, merely M.'s proposal. He quibbled at my protest, and I threatened to resign the Committee which I will do when the Academy meets again. He cast the blame on 'us Irish Scholars'. I retorted that it was the organisation of the Academy and he walked off. I have gone to some trouble drafting announcements and correcting *surreptitiously* the errors in his list of abbreviations. Now I shall trouble no further. I cannot forget his omission to mention Bergin and Purton, and his coupling you with Gwynn, who seems to have done nothing. Miss Joynt told me he had made very few corrections in the English. The MS came to her from Gwynn. Your corrections condemn Gwynn as a reviser. The only suggestion I can make is that you write to the Council, suggesting that after the First Fasciculus appears on August 10th - (It is being printed off now - it cannot be delayed any longer) that 2nd proofs be sent out to the Academy, to you, Bergin, Thurneysen, Pedersen, MacNeill and such scholars and members of the Committee as may desire them. That there would be no wish to over-ride Marstrander or interfere with his editing but only the general interest of Irish Scholarship would be considered, and care taken to remove obvious blemishes - that care which all scholars are grateful for when seeing complex and difficult works through the press. Marstrander should be made to realise that this is not *his* concern, his private work, but that of an institution, of a *nation*. His position in the whole matter is petty and vain to a degree. 'Alone I did it' will not avail him, when his work has to submit to the criticism of his fellow-workers, who may be misled by his wanton refusal to accept assistance. You are the only one who can do this. Bergin won't move. I should not be listened to. Gwynn has the ear of the Council and is regarded as an authority. Failing this, in the interest of scholarship the work when it appears should be subjected to a drastic criticism, as Praeger suggests. This might damage the Academy considerably. But what of that. Suppose it led to questions in Parliament, and the Academy grant was jeopardised, it might not in the end be an evil. The R.I.A. is run by a clique of scientists. Irish is a necessary evil. Irish studies which involve so great an expenditure of funds are not properly represented. The officers with the exception of Purser, who is not interested, are scientists. I have scruples as a member of the Academy from accepting the Close bequest for such a work, which I am convinced will remain a mere fragment. I ask myself is it bona fide. Marstrander is incapable of taking a lesson. Witness *Ériu* V, the Miscellany. Only an exposure will bring his limitations home to him. His vanity would then be hurt.[9]

Best returned the proof to Meyer, who sent it back to Marstrander. Without question he had put a lot of work into the proofs and was disenchanted with Marstrander, with the Dictionary Committee and with the Royal Irish Academy in general, contrasting it unfavourably with the Royal Prussian Academy. With growing impatience, he told Best that 'from now on I do not wish to hear or see anything more of this Dictionary. "He that will to Coupar, maun to Coupar". When I think of the difference between the proceedings of the Academy here and the R.I.A. I realise the whole thing. But I think the Dictionary Committee should wash their hands of the concern, or the scandal will fall on their heads. Praeger's attitude is absurd.'[10] He wrote at the same time to Edward Gwynn, no doubt in the same terms, and Gwynn, holidaying in West Cork, made as diplomatic an answer as he could, realising the pressures on Marstrander, his independent ways, the looming dateline and the necessity of soothing relations between himself and Meyer so that the latter's help might continue to be available.

Derrincorrin, Adrigole
8 Aug 1913

Dear Dr Meyer,

Your letter has reached me down here, where I am taking a holiday and trying to pick up some Irish. I am sorry you think so badly of the Dictionary. It is too late I am afraid to get any further corrections made in the first fasciculus, as it is due to appear on Aug. 10th: as you know, we cannot afford to hold it back. Let us hope that people will make charitable allowances for its imperfections: Marstrander has been working under severe pressure. It is a thousand pities that he will not make better use of the help that is to be had. You must have given a great deal of minute pains to examining his proofs, and I hope most sincerely that you will not give him up, trying as he undoubtedly is to work with. I am sure he could get invaluable help from Bergin also; but I gather from what Best says that he is not likely to ask for it. I have always regretted that Bergin could not be retained as editor: he would be an ideal man for the business. I am ready to do what I can, but it is not much, especially as I cannot possibly afford time to verify quotations etc; which seems from what you say to be very necessary. I can't imagine how you find leisure to do work of that sort for others. I have seen the *first* and *third* proofs of the columns you refer to; in the first I only noted things of some importance, thinking that M. or his assistants would set right a vast number of minor mistakes which I had observed: but I found that very many of these reappeared in the third proof: I marked what caught my eye.

Of course to make a satisfactory Dictionary there ought to be preliminary Durchprüfung of the texts, but that is hardly possible with the staff of workers available. I must try whether I can persuade M. to beg help more widely. I daresay Quiggin would help, perhaps some others. But your criticisms would be worth more than all the rest together, and I do hope that you will continue to give them, in spite of M's irritating ways ....

Sincerely yours
E.J. Gwynn[11]

Meyer had meantime gone to Baden in Switzerland and enjoyed a lovely sail round Zürich lake. He sent Gwynn's letter on to Best who was looking after a text Gwynn had prepared for *Ériu*. To Best he also sent his introduction to his *Älteste Dichtung*, telling him by way of news that Robin Flower had been appointed lecturer in Irish at University College London, for which post he fancied W.P. Ker had given the money.[12]

After a busy summer looking after the School and the comforts of Pedersen, Loth and other visiting scholars, Best took a holiday in the Lake District early in August. The first part of the Dictionary was published on 14 August 1913 and so the bequest of £1000 was saved. It was a fasciculus of 112 double column pages entitled *Dictionary of the Irish Language* and stated on the title page to be based mainly on Old and Middle Irish materials.

Osborn Bergin's first reaction was to write to Best on August 24, ten days after publication:

The great Dictionary is what we expected. It must have cost C.M. an amazing deal of hard work, and it will be most useful. But for real information it is 50 pages too long. I have collated numbers of examples, and have a fair list of howlers. Everything is edited, and to a certain extent normalized, by leaving out capitals and apostrophes and hyphens and stops. Then the result is not always trustworthy. [Bergin here gives examples] ... And of course there are misprints. I

hope the next part will not be rushed. By the way, if all proper names are to be treated like *Dáire* we may expect a special fasciculus for *Diarmait* or *Domnall* ....
Macte virtute!

With kind regards
Yrs always
O.J. Bergin[13]

This verdict of Bergin's, while in part critical, is overall one of approval, if we are to take his view that it was what had been expected and that it would be most useful. It appreciates the 'amazing deal of hard work' which it must have cost, and Bergin was not one who would give his judgement without some consideration. Why, then, did he fail to support Marstrander when controversy broke?

Best, relaxing in Ambleside, received in his post a large-paper copy of the Dictionary from the Printer, 'Presented at the request of the Editor.' He had to say it *looked* well, as well it might, since the paper was chosen by Praeger and himself and was certainly better than that of most dictionaries including the Thesaurus Latinus. 'I have sent C.M. a card acknowledging the colossal work, monumental, I added was quite inadequate to describe it. He must have worked like a Trojan to get it ready in time. As for the printer, *his* work is beyond praise. When I consider that it was still in MS in April, if I remember rightly, it was certainly a feat that it should be in the hands of the public in August.'[13a] He was greatly interested in what Meyer had to say about Hessen who was working on another Irish dictionary. As for the Dictionary, by which he meant Marstrander's, he did not intend to bother about it. Most of the illustrations in it served little purpose. 'A glorified O'Reilly is what we want at present'.[13b] This last remark was an uncharacteristic piece of nonsense from Best, who was surely aware of Whitley Stokes' devastating verdict on O'Reilly's Dictionary, against the use of which for scientific purposes the great scholar protested vehemently as it swarmed with errors.

One cannot help but think that Best trimmed his sails according to whom he addressed. He acknowledged his copy to Marstrander, not without some appreciation it would seem, or so Marstrander's reply suggests:

> Dear Best,
> Thank you for the beautiful card you sent the other day. What a charming spot to spend one's holidays in! I am very glad you like the appearance of the fasc. so well. As to the work itself, it is of course far from perfect – though as a whole it compares favourably with the Contributions.
> I shall probably be in Dublin in a fortnight or so. I am looking forward to see you again and have a chat with you at the D.B.C.! I may even [then?] go to the Blaskets for a week.

With kind regards
Yours ever
Carl Marstrander[14]

Fair enough on Marstrander's part, but we find Best, home from the Lake District, writing to Meyer that 'he [Marstrander] admits its defects but says it would compare favourably with the Contributions! Of course it should surpass mere contributions, which had no pretensions to be a

Thesaurus on historic principles. However modesty is better late than never. Perhaps it is too late for him! The damage is done. Bergin is loud in his denunciations, echoed by Fraser. Bergin was so disgusted that he wrote a strong expostulation to Gwynn, whose reply seemed to me rather weak'. Errors were inevitable in a work of this sort, no doubt, continued Best, but he did not think they could arraign Marstrander before the Council on errors. They could recommend a change in his methods. Regarding future parts Best proposed that in order to lessen the risks of error, proofs should be sent to Meyer, Thurneysen, Pedersen and Bergin, inviting suggestions. There must be no attempt to override Marstrander. Should he wilfully persist in error, he must be corrected after publication, in the interests of the Academy as the publishers. Marstrander said he was coming to Dublin in a week or so, noted Best, 'and in that case you will probably meet him. We could have a private talk with him, and also a Dictionary meeting. The second fasciculus should not be allowed to go forth until the proofs have been read in the way I suggest.'[15] Best, an adept in the ways of diplomacy, hoped to smooth out the difficulties and forestall acrimony. He failed. Writing from Freiburg on 20 September, Meyer made his refusal clear.

Hotel Victoria
Freiburg
20-9-1913

No, my dear friend; I have long ceased to consider myself a member of the Committee and have no intention to rejoin it. Nor do I wish to have anything more to do with the Dictionary. The satirical and insulting postcards which C.M. wrote to me in return for my services put an end once and for all to my taking part in a work which the R.I.A. has left without a single safeguard in M.'s hands. They – the R.I.A. or the Committee – should thank me on their knees for what I have done to the proofs at the eleventh hour. What if the sheet I sent you – which has passed through Gwynn's hands – had been printed off with all those terrible howlers and careless statements? I believe the Academy would have had to withdraw it. Let there be no mistake. It is not only Bergin and I, it is Flower, Pokorny, who have already expressed their astonishment to me, it is Thurneysen, Pedersen and in fact every one who can judge that will speak as we have done. They may not all care to tell M. so, or to write severely on his work – just as you and Bergin seem to have refrained from expressing your opinion to M.'s face. But it does not matter about M., whose conceit nothing can shake; the one thing that matters is the Dictionary itself and the money which the Academy has to spend on it.

It was my intention to send my slips from E onward to M. But I shall not now do so. He will not miss them, as it will take years before D is finished. With his method di – and do – alone will take up many instalments.

I shall now devote myself entirely to making Hessen's work as thorough as possible; he is a *candida anima,* and if he has not the genius of C.M., his character and temper are superior to those of our Norseman. And the older I get the less I care for constant friction and worry over the shortcomings of people in that respect. One must *salvare animam suam* and have peace in one's studies . ...

I arrived here this afternoon from Lucerne, where I spent two days with my brother and his wife. Yesterday we went (by rail) to the top of Mount Pilatus. ...

I must now go to the 'Römische Kaiser' to dine with Hessen.

Kindest wishes to your wife
Kuno Meyer[16]

Marstrander had no notion of the storm which was brewing. Criticism of the Dictionary followed the lead of Meyer who considered the scale of the work too elaborate and ambitious, in the light of the less than advanced state of existing Irish scholarship. His great influence and authority attracted the agreement to his views of other Celtic scholars. Bergin followed his lead. So did Best. There were exceptions, like Edward Gwynn of Trinity College who remained firm in his appreciation of Marstrander and, more than probably, John MacNeill. Marstrander attended a meeting of the Dictionary Committee of the Royal Irish Academy on 23 October 1913 – the proceedings of which have been described as stormy[17] – and defended the order and method of his work. Best and Bergin found themselves in opposition to the man whom some short years before Best, at least, had praised in almost extravagant terms. No doubt Marstrander had expected their support and it appears he had hard things to say to them. A curious feature is that there is no reference to that stormy meeting in what is available to us of Best's correspondence, leaving the question to be asked as to whether he discreetly edited his letters.[18] The Council of the Academy, accepting the criticisms of Meyer, pressed Marstrander to reduce the plan of the work for its future issues. This he declined to do. His equanimity generally held firm during this very difficult period and apart from some high tempered letters to the Academy one cannot but admire the moderation with which he describes the parting of ways between his colleagues and himself in his own summing up of the episode:

> As I have not succeeded in convincing the Council of the Academy as to the impossibility for cramming the treatment of the work within the narrow confines designed, I have with great reluctance come to the conclusion that it was my duty to relinquish all connection with the conduct of the Dictionary.[19]

Marstrander's vision of Irish language lexicography placed him in advance of his contemporaries in the field, great though their talents were. Meyer found it difficult to accommodate himself to the independence of the man whom he acknowledged, even in the stress of controversy, to be a genius. As an instance of Marstrander's individual and independent ways of thought we might consider the memorable statement of how he approached his task:

> The fundamental principles I have followed during the preparation of fasciculus 1 are simple and natural and will, I am convinced, be followed by those who take up the work where I leave it. My aim has been to create an Irish dictionary that would reflect the most important periods in the history of that wonderful language, basing my work mainly upon Old and Middle Irish literature. It was my intention to trace, not only every word, but if possible every characteristic expression on its way forwards, whether it be first met with in the hard lines of the ogam stone or in Keating's graceful style; to reveal the meaning of words solely by the aid of literary sources and the living spoken language. My work was therefore quite independent of Cormac, O'Mulconry, O'Davoren, O'Donovan, Stokes, Windisch and Meyer. I have always tried to see with my own eyes, and to face difficulties without flinching. Therefore ... I bring a great deal that is new. But fresh ground is hard to till, and no one could be more ready to admit that I have often been mistaken with respect to details.[20]

Few Irish language scholars would have the daring to write in the fashion of the foregoing paragraph. This was not due to temerity on Marstrander's part, but to his all-inclusive view of 'that wonderful language', capable as he was of surveying it in the full range of historical perspective. His claim to see with his own eyes, and to face difficulties without flinching, proclaim the assurance and integrity of his scholarship.

Time, and his successors in the work, have vindicated him. It is a pity that the Dictionary Committee of the Academy did not see proper to print the Preface he had designed for the first issue. The whole regrettable chapter was a victory for the men of caution over the man of vision, for the conservatives over the pioneer of adventurous and comprehensive yet soundly-based scholarship. Nor was there a word of appreciation of his immense labour.

Marstrander, who just before the publication of the fasciculus, had been appointed, with the support of Meyer in fact, to the chair of Celtic Philology in the University of Kristiania, now bade farewell to the Irish scene. We are left to speculate on the particular loss sustained through the severance of his immediate ties with Ireland. In his native land he entered on a new phase of a scholarly career that brought honour to his country through his brilliance in Celtic and diverse other fields. Any biography of Marstrander must be Norway-centred. There lay his main career and achievements.

One of his durable accomplishments was the foundation in 1928 of the *Norsk Tidsskrift for Sprogvidenskap* (Norwegian Journal of Linguistics) which stands to him as a monument, twenty substantial volumes of which he edited, providing a vehicle for the learned studies of Norway's leading linguists as well as for the bulk of his own scholarly output.

The second part of the *Dictionary* did not appear until 1932 and it continued to be produced in parts by various scholars until its completion in 1976 as one of the major achievements in Irish language scholarship, bringing to fruition the dream of Stokes, Todd, O'Donovan, O'Curry, and the other dedicated men by whom it was first projected in 1852. The distinguished author Frank O'Connor, writing in December 1964 while, with sixteen parts published, it was not yet complete, called it 'a project comparable in scale and possible importance to the Shannon Scheme ... a great undertaking greatly carried out.'[21]

In the Historical Note to the completed work, Dr. Ernest Gordon Quin, who was General Editor from 1953 to 1975, points out that 'in fact Marstrander laid down the lines for the arrangement of the material which have been adhered to ever since,' a vindication that justifies the faith in his vision of the great pioneer who was its first contributor. Carl Marstrander died in Oslo on Christmas Eve 1965. At his funeral the Irish Ambassador, Mr. Valentin Iremonger, spoke on behalf of Ireland an appreciation of his services to the Irish language. But we anticipate events.

After the acrimonious October meeting a distinct coolness developed between Meyer and Marstrander. Meyer sent no copies of his Wortkunde to Marstrander, 'who has broken off correspondence with me, and sent me no offprint of his contribution to Torp's *Festschrift*'.[22] However Meyer sent two copies of his Wortkunde to Macalister, 'who may if he likes forward one to Marstrander. After his behaviour to you and Bergin I will no longer, as I have told you, have any relations with him unless he apologises,' which suggests that Marstrander had said hard words to Bergin and Best. Meyer declined an invitation to write a review of the Dictionary for the *Berliner Literaturzeitung*, his intention being to reserve his review of it for the *Zeitschrift* which, when published in 1915, raised a storm of hostility against Meyer, for reasons that were quite apart from language and lexicography, as will be related presently.

NOTES

1. *Irish Glosses. A mediaeval tract on Latin declension,* Dublin 1860, p. 2. Dated at Caraig Breacc, Howth, August 16, 1858.
2. Quoted in R.I. Best 'On recent Irish studies in the Academy' R.I.A. *Preceedings,* Vol LI, Section C, No. 2 (1946) 20-21.
3. Meyer to Best, 25 Feb. 1910. NLI Ms No. 11002.
4. Best to Meyer, from 57 Upper Leeson St., Dublin, 18 May 1913. NLI Ms No. 11002.
5. Meyer to Best, from Charlottenburg, Niebuhrstrasse 11A, 23 June 1913. NLI Ms No. 11002.
6. Best to Meyer, date unavailable, probably first week of July 1913. NLI Ms No. 11002.
7. Meyer to Best, from Charlottenburg, Niebuhrstrasse 11A, 11 July 1913. NLI Ms No. 11002.
8. Meyer to Best, from Charlottenburg, Niebuhrstr. 11A, 29 July 1913. NLI Ms No. 11002.
9. Best to Meyer. NLI Ms No. 11002.
10. Meyer to Best, from Charlottenburg, Niebuhrstrasse 11A, 4 Aug. 1913. NLI Ms No. 11002.
11. E.J. Gwynn to Meyer. NLI Ms No. 11002.
12. Meyer to Best, from Grand Hotel, Baden, 17 Aug. 1913. NLI Ms No. 11002.
13. Bergin to Best, from 61 Leinster Road, Dublin. NLI Ms No. 11002.
13a. Best to Meyer, from Elder Grove, Lake Road, Ambleside, 18 Aug. 1913. NLI Ms No. 11002.
13b. *Ibid.*
14. Marstrander to Best, p.c. postmark Kristiania 4 Sept. 1913. NLI Ms No. 11001 (28).
15. Best to Meyer, 14 Sept. 1913. NLI Ms No. 11002.
16. NLI Ms No. 11002.
17. D.A. Binchy, 'Norse scholar whose Irish dictionary caused a furore', *Sunday Independent,* 16 Jan 1966.
18. In the ordinary course Best would have written a full description of this meeting to Meyer in Berlin. After her brother's death in 1919 Toni Meyer returned Best's correspondence but it does not include any reference to the meeting. Perhaps such a letter was not amongst those returned at all, but that such existed can hardly be in doubt. Meyer was Best's chief confidant in all such matters, to whom he would certainly have given full details. Neither has Best deposited any correspondence from Toni Meyer after 1932 in the National Library, except for a few stray items.

19. *Revue Celtique XXXVIII* (1917-1919), 4-5. Extract from Marstrander's article 'The Royal Irish Academy's Dictionary', pp 1-23, 211-227, in which he gives a full statement of the problems attending the Dictionary in reply to Meyer's criticisms in *Zeitschrift für celtische Philologie* (1915) 361-83. Marstrander's reply is dated Kristiania, December 15th.
20. *Ibid.*, p. 5.
21. 'The book nobody knows', *Sunday Independent* 13 Dec. 1964.
22. Meyer to Best, from Berlin, 12 Dec. 1913. NLI Ms No. 11002.
23. Meyer to Best, postcard postmarked Charlottenburg, 16 Dec. 1913. NLI Ms No. 11002.

Chapter 15

WHILE the Bests were holidaying in the Lake District Meyer was travelling central Europe, calling to Leipzig to see his old teacher Windisch, now very shaky and cherishing the one wish that he might live to finish his History of Sanskrit Philology. At Freiburg in Breisgau, where his stay was pleasant, he met Hans Hessen and his old friends the Creizenachs of Krakau. Hessen was a mere youngster, just twenty-four, awfully nice and full of the soundest knowledge, but Meyer learned that he would only work when told to or forced to and had deliberately chosen a librarian's career in preference to an academic one. Meyer's impression was that he was not strong. No, Hessen would not do for the School, this evidently in answer to Best's enquiry, because for one thing, he could not get leave and then all his leisure must for two years be devoted to the Irish Dictionary he had undertaken. Hessen's plan was to collect into a single work all the material hitherto scattered over dictionaries, vocabularies to particular texts, commentaries and older Irish glossaries. Sadly it was his fate to be killed in action in the war soon to envelope Europe with his task only part-accomplished. Meyer had a letter from Marstrander 'making light of my corrections', and as he was by now estranged from the Norwegian scholar, he left Hessen his interleaved copies of A-DNO and all his other lexicography material. A letter from Gwynn deplored Marstrander's obstinacy and proposed all sorts of things but what, reflected Meyer with resignation, could be done with the RIA's hopeless Dictionary Committee. Weather permitting he would visit the lovely isle of Reichenau and walk there in the footsteps of the Irish monks before going on to Baden-Suisse for curative treatment.[1]

Arrived at Baden he found all the hotels full to the garret but on a second visit he got into the Grand Hotel which was much to his liking. For 10 francs a day he had excellent board and lodging, the baths, the use of the Kursaal with roulette table and sundry other amenities. Most of all he liked the doctor who took a real interest in his case, was half a Celtologue and a reader of his books, and examined him by x-ray from which he hoped for good results. The hotel company was international, including English, some Fitzgeralds from Ireland and many French.[2] He met an old fellow student from Leipzig, Salvioni, an Italian, now professor of Romance languages in Milan but still with a distant interest in Celtic derived from Windisch's course in Old-Irish in 1881.

Meyer was worried about his historian brother who was laid up. He worked far too much. Having just finished the 2nd edition of Vol II of his *Geschichte des Altertums,* over 1000 pages, he plunged straight away into Vol III, using his vacation for the labour, this being his only free time. Berlin professors tried to do too much.

Meyer's doctor wanted him to stay four weeks in Baden to begin with. He had a touching letter from Gaidoz, typewritten, as his eyes had got very bad. He was arranging his library for sale after his death. It was wonderfully rich in monographs, separata and ephemeral literature. What Meyer described as 'a distressed card' about Marstrander's Dictionary had arrived from Bergin. He thought Bergin would have made a better thing of it.[3] But would he? There is evidence that what he tried of it did not meet with satisfaction. And granted that he took on the task would he, at his acknowledged slow rate of work, have finished it in the allotted time or have made much progress at all? Or finished it ever? Few scholars knew the language as well as Bergin but his production was slow and cautious, if in the final result close to impeccable.

Meyer was feeling fatigued with the cure, which meant early rising with massage at 6.45 a.m., bath and hot douche at 7.15, inhalation at 11, mechanical gymnastics at 3 p.m., electrocution (not the deadly kind) at 5 p.m., and five small bottles of radium per day.[4] He hoped nothing would interfere with a proposed visit to Dublin, but he had besides much to do in London and Oxford before going to Liverpool where the brethren wanted his advice and help in all kinds of difficulties that had arisen with the Council. A dead set had been made against poor old Mackay, whom he would advise to retire as soon as he could do so with dignity. What a tragi-comedy life was! He had finished reading *Les Dieux ont soif* by Anatole France, surely one of the finest, freest and serenest spirits whom the age had produced.

Perhaps it was the radium, or the severity of the cure, or the other pressures which beset him that caused the sleeplessness from which he suffered in the closing months of 1913. Writing to Edith Best after returning from his Dublin visit he described his situation. 'It is 3 a.m. and I am still up, for ever since I have come back here I suffer from sleeplessness, quite a new thing with me. It must be the difference of the air; for it is most mysterious. The other night I got up at 4 and went to a café which is kept open all night. It was full of people.'[5]

A note from Best discloses a readiness to conform to Meyer's view-point in a manner not at all in the vein we might expect from that estimable man: 'Bergin also continues to discover fresh Marstrandiana. From what you tell me of Pokorny's labours and your own in the same field this great North Sea bubble will be pricked and rent in a very short time.'[6] Unfair comment surely.

Following a teaching session in University College London where he had a class of fifteen Welsh, nearly all Cymry, and of ten for Irish, the latter group including W.P. Ker, Eleanor Hull, an Anglican divine, Robin Flower, a Dr. Burchardi and Miss MacNaughton, Meyer went to relax in the luxury of Allington Castle, Maidstone, as the guest of his old colleague, William Martin Conway, Lord Conway of Allington to be, who had graced the Roscoe Chair of Art in Liverpool during 1885-88. It was one of the oldest castles in England, dating from the twelfth century, rebuilt under Henry VIII and now brought up to every modern comfort and luxury by his old friend. The poet Wyatt lived there, so that it was the cradle of blank verse, while right opposite, across the Medway, was Dingly Dell and the pond on which Pickwick skated, providing for Meyer,[7] who appreciated his English literature, a wholly gratifying milieu of rest and reflection. Martin Conway was to remain through peace and war a steady friend.

He was getting used to sleepless nights which nothing, not even a hot foot bath, could cure, and the idea of drugs he firmly rejected. Gradually sleep returned, and he seemed in good spirits as he wrote to Best:

> I am glad to say that I am slowly mending. I am almost sure that it was radium which I imbibed, for I felt exactly as I did two years ago when I was inhaling it. But if I told a doctor he would deride it ... I went to see Shaw's 'Pygmalion' last night and was astonished to find Sweet (though a strong caricature) the hero of the piece. He is called *Henry* Higgins and can tell everybody as soon as he opens his mouth where he comes from. But the thing won't do in German. I had to translate it into English all the time. But the public – the house was crowded – liked it well enough. It has not been acted in England yet ... My *Kelt. Wortkunde* IV is now ready. ... It contains a severe criticism of Marstrander's treatment of proper names, referring to Pokorny for a full list of corrigenda.[8]

It might well be that the increased calls of social life helped his sleep to return. Dinner parties beckoned almost every evening. He had become a member of a dining club with Wilamowitz, Diels, his brother Eduard and about ten others.[9] His present attention was occupied with an old pagan prayer for long life which was to appear in Mackay's *Festschrift*. Sad news from Dublin was that Thomas P. O'Nolan, a good Irish scholar, had been taken by sudden death. A note from Best on 19 December told him that a copy of his long-delayed Bibliography of Irish Literature, one of the first in, was addressed to him officially that same day by T.W. Lyster on behalf of the National Library Trustees which he hoped Meyer would find useful, though, he modestly added, it was not without defects.

Acknowledging to Best the receipt among other gifts of Susan Mitchell's works Meyer remarked on the extraordinary interest taken in Germany generally in the new Irish writers. He should not wonder if translations of Yeats for instance were soon brought out. Moore of course and Synge were already translated. 'As for the Bibliography it is the most generally useful work that has appeared in Irish studies for a long time. It will be at every scholar's elbow constantly. Never mind about a mistake here or there. It implies an immense amount of work most conscientiously and splendidly done. I will write to Lyster acknowledging it. I have ordered a copy for my seminar.'[11]

He was going to Leipzig on the 26th and then into the Harz mountains for a few days with the hope of finally recovering his sleep there.

Best should make plans for visiting Berlin in the coming year which would be something to look forward to. He might himself visit England after the Easter vacation which began on 1st March. From the Central Hotel de Pologne, Leipzig, he wrote on 28 December:

My dear Best,

The old year is rapidly on the decline and nearing its end. I must not let it pass without wishing you and your wife a very happy and prosperous new one, which I hope will in its course bring about your long delayed visit to Berlin. I am once more writing from my old university town where I always like to go to see old friends and revive ancient memories. I constantly come across people whom I have not seen for thirty years and more. I found Windisch more improved in health. To the astonishment of his doctors, an open sore on his leg, which they were afraid was tuberculous, has completely healed and freed him from much pain and trouble. I spent all yesterday afternoon in his company and that of his wife, daughter and three stalwart sons. Among other things he spoke of your Bibliography as a most useful work which would often save him trouble. The evenings I spent with Sievers who was most eloquent and instructive on Irish metres and their melody as distinguished from the mere outward form (counting of syllables) and even from rhythm. His ear is so keen that he hears the whole thing intuitively. It is a pity that his knowledge of Irish is not deep enough.

I read in the English papers that Abbott has died. I had no idea he was so old (84). He must have begun his Irish studies when he was about 75. I found an old letter from Dowden to me amongst old papers, which I enclose as it refers to you. Perhaps you will keep it as an autograph. Mrs Green wrote me a long letter the other day and sent the Ballymoney pamphlet with her and other speeches. She tells me that W.P. Ker has suddenly grown alarmingly old and altogether changed. I noticed something of the kind last October. With a man of his physical strength, an inveterate climber, etc. and at his age (he can't be more than 58) it is most unexpected. It may account for his not having asked me for a course of lectures next spring as he promised he would. Mrs Green is greatly pleased with the last number of *Ériu*. How is Gwynn getting on with his text? Pokorny's grammar is now almost ready for press. I wonder whether it will supplant O'Connell's. Havers whom I had hoped to see here is unfortunately from home during the vacation. Mrs Sievers turned out to be a native of Drogheda which she left 30 years ago to marry.

I return to Berlin after to-morrow. ... My brother is going to lecture on the Hittites before the Emperor on January 11th. My sister and I have been invited.

With love to you both and all good wishes.[12]

Best thanked him for his kind words about the Bibliography. Warm acknowledgements had also come from Loth, Quiggin, Mrs Green and others. He found to his horror when writing to Baudis that he had omitted some folklore articles by Eleanor Hull, who 'will scarcely forgive me', but it was due to an error in arrangement.[13]

Mrs Green, generous with praise as with purse, wrote a letter of thanks to Meyer for another wonderful piece of work he had sent her, for even without Irish she could follow it in great part, and admire. It was good of him to send it to her, 'and you always are so good'. And what an enchanting translation he had given in *Ériu*![14] 'I was in Belfast when I first saw it, and Mr. Biggar was exclaiming about what you had done for Ireland – "more than all the Gaels put together," which is true. You have revealed a new world, and put into the right people a new enthusiasm'. She recalled how, a week since, she had been in Liverpool to give a lecture to the Welsh society and at the mention of his name there was a great outburst of applause, hearty, strong and refreshing.[15] The remainder of the letter included references to the Ulster gun-running, a rare incursion into political matters on her part, and some of the letter is missing.

Meyer was back in his Berlin flat on December 31, when he acknowledged Mrs Green's letter and pamphlets, all of which he had read with much interest, including that on the place of women, for Mrs Green was a great champion of womens' rights. He could not take Carsonism seriously, too unnatural a thing for the present century, but in order to supply the lack of historical knowledge prevalent in England and Ireland, he proposed that a good school of history at Belfast should at once be founded by the government. But who, besides herself, would they make professor? Meyer was cudgelling his brains about what they could posibly do 'for our poor Dublin School' next session, and thought of H.C. Wyld on Phonetics, but it was not a subject to attract. He was pleased with *Ériu* and went on to pay an unexpected tribute to Eoin MacNeill whose merits, contrary to his former view, he was now coming to recognise, doing as he was 'splendid work on the Annals and Synchronisms. What with his researches and the forthcoming second part of my *Älteste Dichtung* we are getting back well into the seventh century and into the sixth, which brings us near enough to the fifth/sixth century Gallo-Roman period, without which everything is inexplicable'. He had just sent off a very fine pagan prayer for long life, luck and fame, remodelled on Christian lines in the eighth century, as a contribution to the *Festschrift* being prepared in Liverpool for Mackay. His insomnia had cleared and he wondered whether it had been one of the evil effects of radium.[15]

Meyer had a long letter from Pedersen who wished Marstrander would not continue the Dictionary and this merely on the ground of Meyer's brief list of blunders in the proper names. What would he think when he saw Pokorny's huge Sündenregister? Quiggin had sent him the Ridgeway *Festschrift,* a magnificent volume.[17] Marstrander had evidently come to know that Pokorny was writing a review of the Dictionary and had written to him putting the blame for the numerous mistakes on the state of the slips. Meyer passed on this information to Best, adding 'This is of course not true. The mistakes are all of his own making.'[18]

One of Meyer's great pleasures was the enjoyment of music, which he shared with Toni, even though as if conscience-stricken at his indulgence, he describes the experience as 'leading a dissipated life, which however seems to agree with us,' writing in this vein just after coming back from a Mozart concert (at noon on Sunday) conducted by Fiedler. 'It was a luxury to correct proofs' (he actually brought them to the concert hall!) 'MacNeill's and Hamel's among them, to the strains of the S minor symphony. But when Lille Lehmann (now over 60) began to sing and Schnabel to play a concerto I had to put them aside'. Some dissipation!

He was due to give two lectures early in March at University College London.[19]

Meyer, on board the *Kaiserin Auguste Victoria* of the Hamburg-Amerika Line on his way to England, recalled to Best that it would soon be forty years since he first crossed the North Sea, 'a boy of 15 *bliadhna binne*', which seemed incredible, even though the captain of the *North Star* in which he sailed, an old seabear called Tait, then a young man, had retired only a few years since. Now he was travelling in state. His brother Eduard was urging him to go to America and Harvard wanted him to lecture so he thought he might go in October.[20]

'What a glorious morning!' This on 27 February. He was on his way to London where he gave two lectures, the second of which, helped by the good weather, was well attended and quite a success. 'Norman Moore was there, with whom Ker, Flower and I dined afterwards, O'Keeffe, Mrs Boothby, Dodgson the Basque scholar from Oxford, the insufferable Graves (who coolly proposed that his 'versions' of Irish poetry should be rendered (he hinted, by me) into German), a Japanese who is 'studying' Vallancey to find analogies between the Irish and Japs, and several other cranks.' He was reading Moore's *Vale*. Had Best no news yet from Berlin in connection with the presentation of the Leibnitz medal? He was off to Nantwich next day, there to put up at Brine Baths Hotel and have a few days rest.

The subject of the Royal Irish Academy's Dictionary came up for discussion. Pokorny had been going through Marstrander's work. It seems that there was an understanding between Pokorny and Meyer (and Bergin?) to assemble as complete a list as they could of what errors it contained and publish them in a composite effort. In Marstrander's defence it might be said that criticism, if it was to be fair, should contain, in addition to a list of corrigenda, a word of acknowledgement for work done, if not perfectly, at the very least well. But no scholar stood up to say so. And if Pokorny, excellent man, were to be compared on the score of Irish scholarship to Marstrander, if would not be difficult to say in whose favour the comparison might point. Was Meyer being wholly objective when he wrote:

> As to Pokorny's criticism, his (and my) object is not to show up M. and his work, but to make the Dictionary more useful by supplying such a list of corrigenda as M. himself might – and ought to – have added. This it was desirable to throw into a form which makes it easy for any student to find the corrections at a glance, and so the alphabetical order was adopted. I wish he had made the list fuller and indeed exhaustive, so as to save people from checking the quotations themselves. If M. replies he will only give himself away still more. I shall see that P. leaves out any doubtful etymologies or the like.'[22]

He was leaving on 22 March for Liverpool. He had many visits from old Liverpool friends, including H.C. Wyld and Edgar Browne the son of 'Phiz'. Near as he was to Ireland, the only thing that would make him change his plans and induce him to go to Ireland would be the outbreak of real hostilities, but he hardly thought it would come to that. He was glad to hear that Bergin, who had been ill, was now better.[23] Next day he was on his way to Weimar to attend the fiftieth anniversary of the foundation of the Shakespeare Gesellschaft, then to Berlin to resume lectures.[24]

John Redmond, leader of the Irish Party at Westminster, had expressed a hope on meeting Meyer that he would settle in Dublin, a hope which Richard Best did not consider to be feasible in the light of Meyer's crowded and honour-laden life in Berlin.

> You seem (he wrote) to be having a very busy time among your many friends and to be crowding your days with memorable incidents. How delightful it would be for all of us if Redmond could make it worth your while to settle down in Dublin, but this is too much to hope for now. You would hardly exchange Berlin, the Academy, and Red Eagles of the Imperial Government (on which hearty congratulations) for our lilliputian metropolis. Though your acceptance of a chair in the National University would have been a blessing to us, I am glad for your own sake you did not accept it. What would you have done in that examination ridden shop, which actually advertises its wares (scholarships!) in the public press?[25]

He thought Meyer would not have found congenial spirits there, apart from a few. As between London and Berlin, however, Meyer was very clear in his preference. He had greatly enjoyed his recent visit to London and was very sorry to leave. 'I have no real friends in Berlin and Moore is quite right in saying that there is no intercourse abroad comparable to what you get in London. It is stiff and formal in comparison.'[26] No doubt it was this state of affairs that prompted him to go about the foundation of a social club in Berlin University. There is an isolation which affects individuals in the world of scholarship. Perhaps Best felt it also. Certainly he found himself restricted in some ways.

> Notwithstanding that I live in a Library and see the foreign reviews and periodicals as they come out, my mind is getting rusty, and I feel it when suddenly brought into contact with strangers fresh from other fields of intellectual activities, e.g., with that charming Madame Orr. It is necessary to fight against this. Bergin and I talk of almost nothing but Irish matters. He has little interest in the world that Moore lives in, but he soaks himself with Shakespeare, and thus manages to maintain some sort of equilibrium.

Further on in the same letter Best refers to political proceedings in Ireland. It is needless to point out that no one could accuse him of being radical, but the strength of his views may come as a surprise to many. He wrote:

> Carson's speeches are preposterous. I have no patience with the airs he gives himself and his ludicrous army. What *is* the Government to do? Carson is to be allowed to muster an army to resist the application of a law when passed by Parliament and signed by the King. But if the Government makes the slightest attempt to move a battalion into Ulster, he breaks into denunciations of their damnable plot to drive a loyal people out of the Empire and into revolt!! I hope the Government will doggedly persevere to pass the Bill, and then without losing a day dispatch some warships to Belfast, and move a few regiments to Belfast and Derry to *prevent* any ill-advised outbreak of hostilities. They need not explain their action in the House. I think that was very weak of them. They have treated the Opposition with too much consideration. The Conservatives would have given a Nationalist Carson very short shrift …'[27]

The publication in 1913 of the *Bibliography of Irish Philology and of Printed Irish Literature* under the aegis of the National Library of Ireland marked an important advance in the progress of Irish studies. It was wholly the work of Richard Best and although his name does not appear on the title-page, in the anonymous tradition of the civil service, it is appended to the Introduction, so that and it has come to be known, familiarly and deservedly, as Best's Bibliography. It provided a succinct and thorough survey of all that had been accomplished, by print and fac-simile, in the field of Irish literature, from the second half of the six-teenth century when the first Irish printed works appeared, until 1912. There were omissions, as Best readily acknowledged, but they were few and trifling. E.C. Quiggin of Caius College, Cambridge acknowledged it as the most precious and useful Christmas gift to come his way while Alice Stopford Green spoke for many in saying 'It is a very noble ser-vice that you have rendered to Irish scholars, not the first and not the last, but one of the most extraordinary.' All over the world, students of Irish literature continue to be grateful to Richard Irvine Best.

Best was father confessor to many scholars as his correspondence attests and his role as counsellor to younger students at home and abroad has been remarked by Eleanor Knott[28] who wrote with appreciation of his devotion to the cause of learning. A scholar, one of many, who was grateful, Anton Van Hamel, addresses him warmly thus:

> All I can say is this: I have been in your debt for so many years, and if the debt has increased, it is only the natural consequence of your usual readiness to give your friends the benefit of your own accomplishments. I am feeling this very strongly in these days; I have always been grateful to you, and I am still more grateful today. There is no doubt many of us Celticists have to say the same thing to you, and many of us will express it better than I. Let my profound feeling of indebtedness make up for my poverty in words![29]

For his Bibliography, services to the School of Irish Learning and his valuable contributions to Irish literature in *Ériu* Richard Best received acknowledgement from the most prestigious body of learned men in the world, the Prussian Academy, which awarded him the Leibnitz Silver Medal, an honour announced to him by Kuno Meyer who we may imag-ine had some part in influencing the Academy's decision. He wrote:

Charlottenburg
Niebuhrstrasse 11A
19.2.1914

It gives me great pleasure to be able to tell you that at their meeting this afternoon the Prussian Academy, on the recommendation of Wilhelm Schulze, Brandl, Heusler and myself has awarded you a silver Leibnitz medal in recognition of your services both to the School of Irish Learning and to Irish scholarship. I send you the Vorschlagsliste so that you may see what company you are in and what has been said of you. I may add that the signatures of Schulze and the others are not a mere formality. As you will see, the other candidates are generally recom-mended by two members only. Schulze knows all your work, Brandl has ordered the Bibliography and Heusler has read your translations in *Ériu*. I do not know when you will get the official communication. Till then you had better treat mine as private. The ceremony of the Verleihung is on the Leibnitztag, i.e. July 2nd, when I hope you will be present to receive the medal at the hands of the President, old Waldeyer, or the Chief Secretary, Diels. It will be the first meeting in our new gorgeous buildings and altogether a brilliant ceremony and gathering. So you and your wife must come. Meanwhile let me congratulate you warmly on this well deserved distinction. The Prussian Academy prides itself on having its eye all over the world on men who are working for the advance of learning, and that you have bravely done for over a decade now. The beginning of July will be an excellent time for a visit to Berlin as you will find good weather, everybody still here and music etc. not quite over. My sister and I are both looking forward very eagerly to your visit. I shall not be very busy and quite ready to 'explore' – as Jane Austen uses the word – with you in all directions both by day and night. Meanwhile, with warmest regards to you both,

always yours
Kuno Meyer[30]

It was a highly elated Richard Best who wrote back:

My dear Professor,
   Your letter announcing the bestowal of the Leibnitz Silver medal upon me by the Prussian Academy has given me the greatest surprise of my life. Never did the thought occur to me that I should be the recipient of so signal an honour. The feelings of gratification with which I read your kind communication speedily gave way to those of depression as the consciousness of my utter unworthiness was borne in upon me. I am deeply sensible of the honour of being recommended by such eminent scholars, and I own to some confusion at the thought of Schulze and Heusler reading through my modest contributions to *Ériu*, which are set forth in such flattering terms in the Vorschlag. This list, which came this morning, has indeed made me realise even more fully how great the distinction is that you have obtained for me. The remembrance of it will ever be a source of joy to me. I shall not however regard it as a reward for anything achieved, but as a stimulus to further effort, and thus endeavour to realise, though in a small way, the object for which I take it this medal was instituted. I regard it also as something more than a personal honour, valuing it also as a recognition of our School by the most learned assembly in the world.[31]

Meyer's informal announcement was followed by an interval during which Best heard nothing further and as the days went by and no news came, Edith Best began to have misgivings. However a re-assuring message come from Meyer in the second week of June, on the heels of his latest *Wortkunde,* and for this Best was grateful. Edith was making preparations and Best himself was having a new morning coat 'built' (he believed that was the proper word) for the occasion, his older one having being built in the last century. Edith and himself were thrown into alarm by Meyer's announcement of parties and festivities, matters they would prefer to evade. He besought that they be kept to a minimum. For news he had that Bergin was working on lengthy and curious grammatical tracts and that Praeger told him a furious letter from Marstrander had reached the Academy, which was insisting that he curtail his Dictionary scheme.[32]

Presently the official letter from the Prussian Academy signed by Waldeyer was delivered to the National Library telling Best of the Academy's intention and expressing the wish that he should attend personally the sitting of July 2nd. This he acknowledged at once in careful German, saying he was much honoured and would be present.

Meyer wrote to wish them both a pleasant journey to Berlin. Toni and himself proposed to meet them at the Zoologischer Garten which was close to where they lived. He had news that Flower and Bergin had started for the Blaskets two days since, Flower being not at all well, incapable of work, with a steady headache for a fortnight, hardly able to see out of his eyes. Flower had a glowing account of his two German pupils, Miss Müller and Miss Harkampf. Meyer hoped his holiday in his beloved island would set him up again and wished he could give up his librarianship and lead a more leisurely life. He sent Best the programme for the Leibnitztag. Since there was to be no long oration the proceedings would be shorter than usual.[33]

An hour before the Best's arrival Meyer found leisure to write to Alice Stopford Green telling her that Richard would be the guest of the Prussian Academy on the coming Thursday, when he would receive the silver medal and be entertained to dinner by the members. 'It will be a formidable ordeal for his modesty.'[34] The Emperor however would not be present owing to the horrible outrage in Bosnia. Meyer was caught up in many duties, 'horribly busy' his exact words, not only lecturing, and seeing the *Zeitschrift* through the press, a double number in honour of Windisch's seventieth birthday, but making arrangements for the new University Club, his own creation, which was to be opened in October.

Mrs Green's letter gave him great pleasure in everything except the news that she too had begun to suffer from rheumatism. He put it to her that the best thing would be a short cure at the only right source, namely Pistyan in Hungary. The one chief regret of his own life was that he had not known of these baths when he had his first attack of rheumatism in 1892. It was only in 1904, when the disease had become chronic, that he discovered them, too late, for he was persuaded that he could have shaken it off wholly at an earlier period. It would be pleasant if she could join him in August, when they might profitably plan and discuss Irish work at their leisure. Think it over, he advised, it being his own intention to go as early in August as possible, probably on the 2nd or 3rd. He had become great friends with Professor Schiemann, a keen observer of the international scene who admired her writings, and looked anxiously to the future, believing as he did that in spite of Sir Edward Grey's denials there existed or was about to exist some sort of naval agreement between Russia and England which, did it come to exist, would have the effect of bringing about a further increase, on an enormous scale, of the German navy, for which the country was quite ready and willing to pay.

He could not find the time in term to work much at the third instalment of his *Älteste Dichtung,* which would be the most interesting and important as well as the largest.

It will carry us into the sixth century. One of the things that strike me in this early literature is the familiarity with a seafaring life. How little the Roman accounts have been utilised by Irish historians. Have you ever read Vegetius (about 380) on the Irish invasions of Great Britain? He wrote for Theodosius, who in 368 successfully repelled the Irish and Pictish attacks. Vegetius describes the Irish coracles – *scaphae* he calls them – as painted all over, ropes, sails and all, in a neutral tint so as to escape observation (like our hideous modern battleships); twenty oars a side; even the crew were dressed in grey (khaki!). A small *corpus* of all classical and early mediaeval references to Ireland would be a useful publication.

I hear that Mr. Flower has gone to his beloved Great Blasket Island; his health seems to have been very poorly; that Mr. Ker is not unlikely to be made the Warden of All Souls; that Dr. Hessen's concise Old-Irish Dictionary is progressing well; that Dr. Van Hamel, a most enthusiastic and able young Irish scholar, is going to be appointed professor of his native Dutch language and literature at Bonn and will thus strengthen Thurneysen's hands. Professor Mackay is leaving Liverpool for good this term and will get an enormous Festschrift volume, to which I have contributed a translation of an Old-Irish poem, which I will send you in due time.

Let me know what you decide about Pistyan.[35]

Richard Best received his medal to the acclamations of the Academy. They were, he told Eleanor Knott,[36] having the time of their lives. He had met most of the learned world, had talked with Hermann Diels, who proposed the health of 'unser Freund Best' at the Academy dinner in a most kind and friendly speech. The stars of classical learning and ancient history were there, Harnack, Wilamowitz, Waldeyer, Sachau, Eduard Meyer and a host of others. 'Yesterday [5 July] I had a touching interview with Ebel's widow who insisted on my accepting his photo (the last but one in her possession). She still has on her door "Professor Ebel".' Hermann Ebel, who died in 1875, might have seemed to belong to the far past, but his work, for Celtic scholars, endures. Best went to Kuno Meyer's seminar to hear his pupils read, and after to his public lecture, delivered in English. Edith and Richard then had a month of leisure in which to visit their favourite places of Germany. At Weimar they went to see Goethe's house, Liszt's house and the Garthenhaus to say nothing of a walk up the Caverna and through the town. Richard wished he knew Goethe better, as T.W. Lyster did, when every object would have had a tale to tell of him. Liszt's house was more familiar, thanks to a photograph of the Abbé at his writing table given him by Meyer. Pauline, their guide, showed them around, and he told her that Edith had seen Liszt in London and heard him play at the Novello's reception, and that he himself was a pupil of a pupil of Liszt's. By 9.30 p.m. he was pretty tired on his feet and rested in the Hotel Chemnitius.[37]

The Bests' visit took place at a time perilously close to the outbreak of the mighty war which was to envelope Europe. The 'horrible outrage in Bosnia' which had prevented the Emperor from attending the Leibnitz function at which Best was honoured was the murder on 28 June of Archduke Franz Ferdinand, heir to the Austrian throne, by a Bosnian student. A swift and fateful series of events followed. Austria-Hungary declared war on Serbia on 28 July, Germany declared war on Russia on 1 August and on France on 3 August, invading Belgium on the same date, and England declared war on Germany on 4 August. Italy for a time remained neutral while Holland almost miraculously preserved her freedom throughout the large scale conflict which followed.

With great armies on the move the concerns of individuals seemed of little moment now, as Robin Flower in the British Museum was to reflect with resignation, all his literary plans upset and postponed, lamenting that his cockleshell boat was powerless in the seas of adversity. He had been happy on his beloved island until one day the postman, arriving from the mainland, had greeted him with the tidings that a serious event had happened in the east, the murder of an archduke.

The Bests hurried out of Germany not a day too soon. Their trip, instead of taking them to Hanover, brought them to Lohne and round to Amsterdam and The Hague. They had a roughish passage to England but slept through it. Arrived in Dublin, Best had a talk on the afternoon of August 2nd with Mrs Green, just returned from Sir Horace Plunkett's 'where she exploded in righteous indignation over the attitude of the latter to the Irish point of view in the present crisis. It seems P. has become a Home Ruler (!) of a special brand.' She was greatly concerned at the thought of communication with Meyer being cut off, and so were the Bests. Edith had written to Toni Meyer and hoped the missive had reached her. And what would Meyer do for a cure? Would Italy be attainable, or the Canaries? And what of *Ériu*? Coming events would militate against Celtic publications. Already panic stricken householders were laying in stores. 'Our love and good wishes to you both', and as it turned out, the Bests had lain eyes on the person of Kuno Meyer for the last time.

The 1914 Summer course of the School was given by Professor Osborn Bergin, who lectured for two hours daily, Saturdays excepted, from 10 to 28 August, as a labour of love, loyally undertaken, on Early Modern Irish, particularly Bardic Poetry, a difficult regime of literature, reflecting social life from the thirteenth to the mid-seventeenth century, and common to Ireland and Scotland. The course was held in the shadow of the great war, which had just broken out, and was attended by twelve students, including one from the United States, and two from Scotland.[38] It was the thirteenth session of the School since its foundation. For the first time since its inception, the links with Europe were broken. The great days of the School were over.

NOTES

1. Meyer to Best by postcard from Freiburg in B. 10 Aug. 1913 (NLI MS No. 11002); and postcard from Zürich 15 Aug. 1913. NLI Ms No. 11002 (41).
2. Meyer to Best, 20 Aug. 1912. NLI Ms No. 11002 (38).
3. Meyer to Best, 29 Aug. 1913, from Grand Hotel, Baden. NLI Ms No. 11002.
4. Meyer to Best, 2 Sept. 1913, from Grand Hotel, Baden. NLI Ms No. 11002.
5. Meyer to Edith Best, 4 Nov. 1913. NLI Ms No. 11002.
6. Best to Meyer, postcard 12 Nov. 1913, from 57 Upper Leeson St., Dublin. NLI Ms No. 11002.

7. Meyer to Best, 19 Nov. 1913 from Allington Castle, Maidstone. NLI Ms No. 11002.
8. Meyer to Best, postcard postmarked Charlottenburg 29 Nov. 1913. NLI Ms No. 11002 (41).
9. Meyer to Best, by postcard 11 Dec. 1913. NLI Ms No. 11002 (40).
10. NLI Ms No. 11002.
11. Meyer to Best, by postcard postmarked Charlottenburg 23 Dec. 1913. NLI Ms No. 11002.
12. Meyer to Best, 28 Dec. 1913 from Central Hotel de Pologne, Leipzig. NLI Ms No. 11002.
13. Best to Meyer 30 Dec. 1913. NLI Ms No. 11002.
14. The reference is probably to 'The Guesting of Athirne', *Ériu* VII, 1-9, including eight poems.
15. Alice Stopford Green to Meyer, 21 Dec. [1913] from 36 Grosvenor Road, London S.W. NLI Ms No. 15122.
16. Meyer to Alice Stopford Green, 31 Dec. 1913, from Charlottenburg, Niebuhrstrasse 11A. NLI Ms No. 15091 (1).
17. Meyer to Best, 2 Jan. 1914 p.c. postmark Charlottenburg.
18. Meyer to Best, 24 Jan. 1914 from Charlottenburg. NLI Ms No. 11002.
19. Meyer to Best postmark Charlottenburg, 18 Jan. 1914. NLI Ms No. 11002.
20. Meyer to Best, 26 Feb. 1914. NLI Ms No. 11002.
21. Meyer to Best, postcard postmarked London 13 March 1914. NLI Ms No. 11002.
22. Meyer to Best, 16 March 1914, from Brine Baths Hotel, Nantwich. NLI Ms No. 11002.
23. Meyer to Best, 21 March 1914, from Brine Baths Hotel, Nantwich. NLI Ms No. 11002.
24. Meyer to Best, 23 March 1913, postcard from Weimar. NLI Ms No. 11002.
25. Best to Meyer, 6 April 1914, on NLI notepaper, NLI Ms No. 11002.
26. Kuno Meyer to Best postcard 12 April 1914, NLI Ms No. 11002.
27. Best to Meyer, 14 April 1914, from 57 Upper Leeson St. NLI Ms No. 11002.
28. *Ériu* XIX (1962) 123.
29. Anton G. Van Hamel to Best, postcard from Utrecht, 2 July 1932, NLI Ms No. 11004.
30. NLI Ms No. 11002.
31. Best to Meyer, from 57 Upper Leeson St., Dublin, 22 Feb. 1914. NLI Ms No 11002.
32. Best to Meyer, 11 June 1914. NLI Ms No. 11002 (61).
33. Meyer to Best, postcard postmarked Charlottenburg, 21 June 1914. NLI Ms No. 11002.
34. Meyer to Alice Stopford Green, from Charlottenburg, Niebuhrstrasse 11A, 30 June 1914. NLI Ms No. 15091 (2).
35. *Ibid.*
36. Best to Eleanor Knott, postcard postmarked Berlin 6.7.1914, R.I.A. 12 0 21.
37. Best to Meyer, from Hotel Chemnitius, Weimar, 18 July 1914. NLI Ms No. 11002.
38. *Report* 1914-15, in *Ériu* III, part I, 1915.

Chapter 16

IN mid-July 1914 Alice Stopford Green received a postcard from Meyer giving details about the Hungarian health resort Pistyan which he recommended as a place of treatment for her threatening rheumatism. His friend Professor Schiemann thought however that in a short time they would have the inevitable war, which would make travel impossible. 'Today' continued Meyer, 'the Emperor of Austria is going to sign an ultimatum to Serbia, encouraged by our Emperor, who in an autograph letter, which Sch. has seen, promises his help.' This was followed by further comment on the deteriorating international situation, all on an open postcard, addressed to Mrs Green who was the guest of Francis Joseph Biggar at his home Ardrígh, Belfast. This disclosure of high politics, at best an indiscretion, might have gone unnoticed had not Mrs Green mentioned it to Charles Trevelyan who in turn told the editor of the *Times*, Wickham Steed, who nearly had a fit, and pressed Mrs Green to let him publish its contents. She rejected his requests and was equally adamant in her refusal to bow to the Foreign Office to whose attention the matter was brought. A long and vexatious correspondence ensued, involving the offices of Lord Haldane and her nephew Sir John Simon, throughout which she steadfastly refused to commit a breach of confidence against one whom she did not hesitate to acknowledge as a friend and colleague in Irish studies, unpopular to the authorities though such an association was considered. Finally an honourable compromise was arranged with the Foreign Office, ending an ordeal from which she emerged with full credit.[1]

On 10 October 1914 the city of Antwerp, famed as a centre of the civilised arts, fell to the German army. On the same day Kuno Meyer, then staying at the Essener Hof in Wernigerode, finished and gave to the printer a contribution to the *Zeitschrift für celtische Philologie*[2] consisting of criticisms and corrigenda of Marstrander's Dictionary of the Irish language. Richard Best in his bibliography of Meyer describes it pithily as 'A critical notice of Fasc. 1. D-degóir'. But it was signed and dated by Meyer as *am Tage der Eroberung von Antwerpen,* 'on the day of the capture of Antwerp'. In thus breaching scholarly etiquette he angered and estranged many former colleagues. Vendryes in particular expressed himself vehemently. It was on Meyer's part a declaration of full commitment, if ever so unhappily indicated, to the Fatherland's course of action. He does not seem to have considered that he was giving offence to fellow scholars. Indeed he does not seem to have given the matter a passing thought and never made an attempt to explain it. The review itself was hardly impartial, influenced as it was by the regrettable differences between Marstrander and himself, and the views of many contemporary scholars on it corresponded with the later observations of Dr. D.A. Binchy who wrote – 'Although it included some valuable material, it was nothing more than a long list of *corrigenda* many of them indeed genuine, but some doubtful, some clearly unjustified, some trivial and some (though to be fair, most of these were not contributed by Meyer himself) just silly. And there was not a word of praise for the ingenuity and the wide learning displayed by the pioneer of this new advance in Irish studies.'[3]

The contributors to the list, besides Meyer, were Pokorny, and probably Pedersen. Two days later, Meyer wrote to Best from Wernigerode telling him of his present situation and that he had changed his Berlin address, from now on to be Wilmersdorf, Nassauische Strasse 48[11], a flat more central than the old one and convenient to Lichterfelde. He would be just in time for the wedding of his second niece Gertrud. His nephew Hans Eduard, son of his historian brother, would attend. He had made a marvellous recovery from a wound received in action, the bullet having been extracted by a great surgeon who alone of his colleagues had dared to operate. So unique was the cure that it would be published in detail. Lectures in Berlin were to begin on the 29th. Celtology had been receiving attention and a *Festschrift* for Windisch had appeared, with however only three Celtic contributions, by Thurneysen, Meyer himself and Mühlhausen. Meyer was still working a good deal on *Saltair na Rann*. He wondered how Priebsch, a former Liverpool colleague, was and would Best please find out. The woods were looking lovely in their Autumn foliage, his physical condition was much better after his cure and he was ready to plunge into the gaieties of Berlin. He advised Best when writing to try an open letter, which he understood was allowed, and to let him have as much news as possible. More cautious now, he signed the letter with his initials K.M., a circumstance caused by the ways of war.[4]

His next letter to Best went over much the same ground but hinted as well at a new departure which was to have important consequences and was only incidentally connected with scholarship. It speaks for itself.

Berlin-Wilmersdorf
Nassauische Str. 48[11]
4/11/14

My dear Best,

I will begin this letter now though I shall probably not send it off for some time. Next week I intend to start on a journey to Holland (where I shall visit Van Hamel) and perhaps to Belgium, as trains from here to Brussels and beyond have now begun to run regularly. It will be an interesting journey. I shall then post this letter which I hope will reach you safely as it shall not contain any 'contraband' matter.

We live here pretty much as usual. Lectures have begun and are, I hear, pretty well attended. Quite a number of Americans are among the students. I have got leave of absence as I want to travel. My health is fairly good, the mudbaths of Nenndorf – a charming place near Hanover – have done me good, though they are not nearly as potent as those of Pöstyén. I was there for about a month and then went for an after cure to Wernigerode where I stayed at the Essener Hof (the hotel where we had one of our many farewell dinners) and was very comfortable. Meanwhile my sister had moved to these new quarters which answer our expectations in every way. The rooms are not quite so large, but everything is very convenient and commodious. I have two studies, there are no draughts and no noise from railways or trams. We had a little party here last night, the Schiemanns amongst them. Their only son has been through all the battles against the Russians and sends his diary regularly. My wounded nephew has made a most successful recovery. The operation was performed with such skill that he will probably be quite restored to his ordinary health after a time. He is already back at Strassburg drilling recruits. The other 2 boys are both in the field. Sachau has lost both a son and son-in-law, Wilamowitz a son and Harnack a son-in-law. By the way Richard M. Meyer has died quite suddenly of a weak heart. You might send a note to the 'Athenaeum'. The date was October 8th. He was only 54 years of age. I miss him greatly. I have been working at small things and send you *Zur Kelt. Wortk. VI* for distribution. Heft 3 of the *Zeitschrift* is nearly ready. During my absence Thurneysen will look after the printing. I have contributed new Mitteilungen, the review of the Dictionary, and some minor matters. Thurneysen has a searching criticism of V. Hamel's paper on *Leb. Gab.*, Hessen a review of Pokorny's Grammar. I sent you some proofs through V[an] H[amel]. Hessen is a volunteer and hopes to go to the front in about a month. Havers is back in Leipzig, lightly wounded. The most interesting news is that Dom Louis Gougaud is a prisoner at Paderborn. He had to join his regiment as a sergeant and was taken at Maubeuge in August. The Emperor has ordered that all priests are to be treated as officers and so he is very well off. He wrote to me twice quite cheerfully saying that he is using the opportunity to learn German thoroughly. I am sending him books ... Miss Müller, Flower's pupil, wanted to join my classes. I am taking her privately and setting her some work during my absence. She is a clever little thing and a devoted student. If you should write to Flower remember me to him. If I settle anywhere abroad I will let you have an address to which you can write. But that may take some time. I had a letter from Miss Schoepperle who gave me news of the Summer school. Perhaps I shall see her soon. I wonder how you all are, and what is doing in Celticis. They at any rate must not be allowed to suffer under the war. I saw in the English papers that Traill has died, but I find nothing about his successor.

There is a continuation of this letter, dated 5.11.1914, on *Königlich Preussische* notepaper:

I am writing this at a meeting of the Academy while Einstein is reading a paper by Schwarzschild who is in the field... When I came home today from a visit to Schiemann, from whom I always hear the latest and also confidential news as he has direct dealings with headquarters, I found dear old Mrs Ebel at our house. She gave me a spirited account of your visit to her and commented on your youthful looks which contrasted with your 'Berumtheit'. A lady who is going to edit J. Grimm's correspondence also called and showed me letters from Siegfried (written in 1859), in which Stokes is spoken of as the coming man in Celtology. The most interesting part to me, however, was a confidential report on the Irish Dictionary of the Academy – exactly the same muddle as 50 years later ...

With many kind regards
Yours always
Kuno Meyer
Rotterdam 14/11

V.H. tells me that he forwarded your letter to me to my Berlin address ... He told me about the Dictionary and Marstrander. I send the commencement of my review.

K.M.[5]

Meyer's way of thinking naturally came as no surprise to Richard Best who, before this episode at all, had been holding communication with Robin Flower and apprising him of Meyer's absolute commitment to Germany's cause. Flower expressed his sadness that the military party had captured the whole intelligence of Germany. 'That Meyer, not a Prussian and so intimately acquainted with English life, should think these things is a staggering proof of the completeness of their success. One expected of course that he would support his country once in the war'.[6]

Throughout the conflict Flower never ceased his admiration for Meyer's scholarship and courage, defending him when necessary from critics like Sir Norman Moore who in the angers of war were not prepared to acknowledge his talents in learning. After reading a letter of Meyer's which Best had lent him he was generous in his comments:

> Dear Best,
> I am returning Meyer's letter with many thanks for having had the opportunity of reading it. Except for his use of the word 'gaieties' I don't find any strikingly forced note in it. That is, we who know Meyer and his indomitable spirit will expect him to face the situation with an unshaken cheerfulness and determination. And that is what I read in his letter. No German could trust his inmost thoughts to paper in these days ... Meyer will keep up his heart to the last, and one could not wish it otherwise ....
>
> R. Flower

Holland, practically in the territorial centre of the warring nations, was fortunate to remain free and neutral throughout the war. This enabled scholars in Germany to keep in touch with correspondents in Ireland and England, and vice versa, through intermediaries, and Anton van Hamel, the Netherlands Celtic scholar, was the medium through whom many such contacts were made. It also meant that ships of the Holland-Amerika Line could maintain their sailings to the United States, a facility that enabled Meyer to travel to America in November 1914 on the S.S. *Rotterdam* from which he penned a letter dated 18 November, addressed from 'Mid-Ocean' to Best:

> My dear Best
> I hope you got my letter from Rotterdam where I spent a day with Van Hamel. I shall probably stay in America until the end of the war and visit many places as far as San Francisco.
> I hope this cruise will do me good. I get up at 6.30, take a hot salt water bath, breakfast at 7.30 (grape-fruit, porridge and cream – how they manage to give a whole pot all to oneself I cannot imagine – bacon and eggs and fish - in short I am doing myself well). Then a constitutional tramp around the promenade deck, a siesta in a steamer chair, a game of cards in the afternoon, chess in the evening, letter writing and a page or two of *Saltair na Rann*. To bed at 10. We get of course no news, not even wireless ones, and have met no ships of any kind so far. At Dover we were boarded by an English officer, who made all the Germans and

Austrians sign a document that they would not fight against England. He also told the captain the safe route through the mines. When we were passing to the south of Ireland I thought much of my friends there. I wonder whether there will be a new chapter to the *Gabála Érenn*. Not unlikely from what I hear. Perhaps before I arrive in A. you will have heard yourself.

Give my love to your wife and remember me to all friends. Have the Macrans been let off? Who is the new Provost? Mahaffy after all?

Yours always
K.M.[8]

Contrary to usage, he signed only his initials to the letter. The new chapter to the *Gabála Érenn* he wondered about was a reference to a German invasion or incursion into Ireland which he expected to take place. Professor Macran of Trinity College, visiting Germany, had been cut off by the too swift advent of war and J.P. Mahaffy had indeed, 'after all', been appointed Provost of Trinity College. A week later he wrote again to Best, this time from Hotel Knickerbocker, 42nd Street and Broadway, New York:

My dear Best,
You did not I am sure expect this. But you know it had long been my intention to visit America and this is a glorious opportunity. For I can now do more than merely lecture on Irish literature. Unless they keep it out of the papers, you will soon hear of me. Meanwhile I have settled here in comfortable quarters.[9]

It had been a perfectly glorious crossing. Travelling on the same ship was the violinist Kreisler, limping from a leg wound.

This was a clear hint that his main purpose in visiting the United States was other than to lecture on Irish literature. Osborn Bergin was probably right in saying that Meyer, as a Berlin professor, had tasks thrust on him from which he did not shrink but which must surely have been uncongenial. He felt, and said at the time, that his lifework was ruined.[10] What then was his purpose in going to America? To make propaganda on behalf of Germany was the obvious one. As a member of the Prussian Academy he was close to the Emperor, both in his own standing and more so through that of his historian brother.

With his perfect command of English, his incomparable knowledge of Irish literature and tradition and his patriotic commitment to Germany, he was the ideal person to appeal to the sympathy and support for Germany of the large Irish and German population of the United States. He has been called a spy in some respected biographies of Sir Roger Casement but one might ask how a middle aged man with a serious physical disability, well-known in the world of scholarship, who made no secret of his coming and going, could be regarded as engaged in the underhand business of espionage.

Richard Best was careful enough to keep a copy of his answer to Meyer's letters of 18 and 25 November. It was a cautious communication, befitting the times, for Meyer's sympathies were an open book and his mail could be subject to scrutiny. Best expressed himself as not at all surprised at his visit to the States for he knew Meyer had a long standing invitation to lecture at Harvard on Irish literature. What a delightful experience he thought it must be to travel in these modern ocean grey-hounds and have a whole pot of cream to oneself at breakfast. If Meyer were to go to Illinois he was to visit the fair Miss Schoepperle. A pupil of Marstrander's had turned up in the R.I.A. to collate *Lebor na hUidhre*. With regard to Meyer's compatriots in England, Priebsch and Von Hugel had become naturalised Englishmen while Schaafs was still interned. Poor old Traill had gone over to the majority and J.P.M. reigned in his stead, claiming to be good for ten years. Macran was still in Berlin. Best hoped the dry climate of America would have a good effect on Meyer's rheumatism and signed the letter 'with our affection-ate greetings'. A postscript contained the real import of the letter. It read: 'P.S. I must wind up on a more serious note. I am sorry to hear that your mission is not merely the peaceful one of disseminating Irish learn-ing. For I think that everyone should stick to his part, and there are others who could carry on political propaganda. If that is your other task, I think it only fair that you should know, when writing to me, that my sympathies in this European crisis are not with Germany, but the other side. Mais vous ne m'en voulez pas. My admiration of German learning is undiminished. Therefore I pray you caution. Tell me nothing'.[11]

It was prudent advice. Best may have been aware of how Mrs Green had got into trouble owing to Meyer's indiscreet postcard message. Best's letter besides being frank and honest, provided as well something like a saving clause against any future inquiries.

There was a large German population in the United States. Great numbers had emigrated from their homeland in the second half of the nineteenth century and formed so important an element of the popula-tion that the influential *New York Times* published a German edition of its journal to cater for them. By the beginning of the first world war the German ethnic element had been augmented through first and second generation growth and now, at the outbreak of war between Germany and England, formed a very considerable segment of the country's citi-zens. Emigration from Ireland, on a vast scale, had continued since mid-nineteenth century and the influence of the Irish was powerful. They had the advantage of the German and other ethnic strata in that their knowl-edge of the English language, thanks to the Education Act of 1831, gave them access to political life from the day they set foot in the country, because one of the salient facts of the nineteenth century was that in multilingual America English became the dominant tongue. Language was the sole gift the Irish took from England. Otherwise their historical inheritance imbued the American Irish with a hostility to English rule that gravely embarrassed Britain. Insofar as his individual persuasion could, it was Kuno Meyer's task to influence these two powerful forces to work their moral influence in favour of Germany.

Meyer was delighted with the quality of American life and became integrated into it almost at once. In little more than three weeks he had begun to lecture in Columbia University and had so many other engage-ments that his programme was full up till June of 1915. Gertrude

Schoepperle had arranged for a long stay at Urbana University in Illinois, which seemed to be the most active centre of Celtic Studies in America and he had promised to work there with a small class of students, all of whom were able to read Irish. He declared that he could live in America altogether, so pleasant was everything. Europe was indeed behindhand in the amenities of life. The telephone which he used to hate had become a friend, but then it was admirably managed. The combination of sittingroom, bedroom and bathroom all to oneself was most comfortable. The climate suited him very well. He was to spend a day at Oyster Bay with Roosevelt. Prominent Irish people he had met included Yeats *père*, John Quinn, Padraic Colum and his wife Mary. On 11 December he had dinner on the *Vaterland*, the most magnificent vessel he had ever seen, now lying idle in the dock at Hoboken. An old Hamburg friend who was a director of the Line lived on board like a hermit. They had a gorgeous dinner in the grand saloon at which sixteen people sat down. He hoped a letter from Best was on its way and he wanted news of all and everybody.[12]

Meyer had no doubt that his mail was being intercepted. After a month in America he had not had a single letter from Germany or England. He asked Best to address his letters to K.E. Meyer so as to have his identity merged in the thousands of his American namesakes. Early in January the Gaelic League was going to give him a great reception. He had spoken often at Irish, German and academic meetings. He had been dragged into a paper war himself owing to all sorts of false statements in the Press.

> I continue to like America greatly. I constantly meet men and women of a refinement and intellectuality that we hardly know in Europe, more especially women. I spent my birthday among a circle of poets and poetesses, as pleasantly and congenially as possible. These, like all genuine, honest and intelligent folk are mit Leib und Seele Deutsch. Among them was the Irish-American wife of the Turkish Consul-General here, perhaps the most fascinating woman I have ever met.[13]

Meyer, an ardent theatregoer, thought the genuine American farces about the only thing in theatre worth seeing. The opera had many famous stars, but the ensemble and orchestra were poor. The Rosenkavalier after Berlin was almost insufferable. Urbana was expecting him next semester and Miss Schoepperle promised him at least four serious Irish students, with whom, should he go, he would read and translate *Saltair na Rann*. Meanwhile he was to lecture at all the universities around except Harvard, which had treated him badly[14] He dined out almost every evening and kept horribly late hours, which was the custom. 'I may say that I have never had as stirring and full a time in my life as now, nor such audiences, so large and sympathetic. On January 27th I am to deliver an oration on our Emperor (it being his birthday), when 3,000 German-Americans will listen to me. I would send you papers, but they would not be let through.'[15]

What Meyer had hinted to Best, that he would presently hear of his activities in America, become true in a manner that was far from welcome to some who had hitherto been his admirers. He had turned political propagandist and it was in the nature of things that he must as such lose friends. One of his early essays in this controversial field was his address on 6 December 1914, at Long Island, New York, to a meeting of the Clan na Gael, the American Irish nationalist organisation in which John Devoy was a leading influence, in the course of which he referred to an Irish Brigade being recruited from prisoners of war in Germany with the aim of fighting England. Extracts from the address were reprinted in the *Times* (London) one of which reads:

> For 30 years I have resided among the English, with many of whose prominent and leading men, not only in literature, science and art but also in politics, I am united by ties of long standing friendship, which nothing, not even the present enmity between our two nations, shall sever, so far as I am concerned. Three years ago I returned to my native land, where I have lived in constant touch with well-informed and influential political circles. From all these circumstances, I may say that I have perhaps had better opportunities to become acquainted with the events that have brought about this war and with the issues now at stake than most people outside the sphere of professional diplomats and politicians.
>
> From 1896, when the first distinctly threatening note was sounded in England that Germany was the arch rival who must at all costs be crushed, I have followed closely every step that brought us nearer to the inevitable issue, carefully noting everything in my diary. It was in the summer of 1911 that I lost all hope of peace between England and Germany.

He went on to say that he believed an invasion of England and Ireland would take place sooner or later and that the restitution of autonomy to Egypt and Ireland must be one of the conditions of peace, Germany being victor.

The *Times* gave voice to the reaction felt in England at Meyer's address. He had, it said, lived in England for thirty years, for a whole working life had eaten the bread of England, had been befriended by many of its most brilliant scholars and had made there the reputation which lately won him the succession to the chair of Zimmer in Berlin. It was no reproach to him that after all this he remained entirely German at heart. But that he should use the position he had attained in Celtic scholarship for the purpose, futile as his efforts would be, of stirring up sedition in Ireland and endeavouring to stab in the back the country to which he owed so much, was quite another matter.[16]

Meyer replied to the *Times* from the City Club of New York on 27 December in defence of his position.

> Your censure of my present attitude towards England in your issue of December 24 has been cabled across here to your namesake in this city. Allow me to reply briefly to it. I regard all you say as another indication that England has not even realised what this war means to her and to Germany. You talk cheap sentiment and false morality while two mighty Empires are engaged in a life and death struggle. In this struggle it behoves every member of the two nations to take an honourable part to the best of his ability. But you say that my indebtedness to England should prevent me from doing so. My answer is that we, Germans, are not fighting that England which many thousands of us from the Emperor downward

have loved truly and well but a misguided, iniquitous England, bent upon the destruction of an inconvenient rival. As for myself, I am but continuing what I did when I lived among you, when I fought by the side of some of England's noblest and, to me, ever dear sons and daughters for freedom, truth and justice against oppression, falsehood and wrong wherever we encountered it. That is how I have served England while eating her bread. As sure as I write these lines the time will come when all honest Englishmen will feel ashamed of this war, and abominate it as much as ever they did the Crimean, the Opium, and the Boer wars. As for Ireland, Germany is but holding out a friendly hand to a nation betrayed by her leaders, and naturally unwilling to shed its blood for those who have oppressed its liberty, as they are now trying to deprive us of ours. That constitutes our common cause, and you cannot, after all I have said, blame me for endeavouring to help this cause to victory.

Meyer had formed the resolve almost on arrival in America, to sever all association with his former University of Liverpool, where as late as March 1913 he had delivered a notable lecture on his hopes for the University's future. If the severance was painful he kept it to himself. But he compounded the break by including with his resignation some polemical comment envisaging a German invasion of England and other animadversions. His letter of 3 December 1914 to the Vice-Chancellor of Liverpool University, Alfred Dale, has not survived but it seems was tantamount to his resignation from the Honorary Chair of Celtic which he held in the University. It also contained references to the German occupation of Belgium and the forthcoming German invasion of England to all of which the Vice-Chancellor sent on 23 December what was, all things considered, a fair and firm reply.[17] Earlier, on 15 December, the University Council passed a resolution treating Meyer's letter as the equivalent of resignation and recording its acceptance.[18]

Meyer's attitude and his controversial actions in America provoked outrage in the city and University of Liverpool. Angry letters were written to the press. Alderman Harford, described in press reports as leader of the Liverpool Irish, denounced him as a spy and the accusation was taken up far and wide. His portrait by John which hung in the University Club was threatened with destruction by irate members and was removed to a cellar. Some odd stories about him circulated although few people might be as credulous, or as imaginative, as Ramsay Muir who in his *Autobiography* conjured up a stream of goosestepping students of Celtic sent by Meyer to the Aran Islands and other places to institute fuel depots for German submarines. On 26 January 1915 the University Senate resolved:

> That the Senate desire to place on record their strong condemnation of the action of Dr. Kuno Meyer, lately a Professor of the University and indebted to our country for hospitality and honour during a period of thirty years, in acting as an agent of sedition and in imputing treason to loyal Irish soldiers now prisoners in Germany. The Senate also record their satisfaction that Dr. Meyer has ceased to be a member of the Senate and Staff of the University.

The University Council recorded likewise. Meyer writing on 9 February from the Congress Hotel, Chicago, published his reply in the *Times:*

'Allow me to say that I regard the resolution as lacking both common-sense and logic. It speaks of my being an agent of sedition as though I were a British subject. It assumes that my indebtedness to England for hospitality and honour should have made me disloyal to my native country when she called upon me in her hour of need. It denies a fact about the truth or untruth of which none of those who voted for its adoption can have any knowledge.'

On 24 December 1914 Edmund Cosby Quiggin, of Gonville and Caius College, Cambridge, wrote to the *Times* – Sir: Amongst the numerous honours conferred on Professor Kuno Meyer in our islands, he received a couple of years ago the freedom of two Irish cities. What attitude are the Corporations of Dublin and Cork going to adopt in this matter?

Kuno Meyer never forgave him. In correspondence with Best he represented Quiggin as a mean-hearted person whom he remembered with diminished affection since the time Quiggin had the impertinence to correct his English (Meyer was proud of his English, with reason it might be added). Best used his diplomatic talents to try and soften Meyer's attitude and defend Quiggin but Meyer's antipathy was unyielding.

It did not take Dublin Corporation long to react. Foremost among those who pressed for some action to be taken was Alderman David A. Quaid who, in a letter[19] to the Lord Mayor, alleged that Meyer was fomenting in the United States a movement among Germans and an irreconcilable section of the Irish against the Empire of which cognisance should be taken. He published correspondence from Herbert A. Strong, Professor Emeritus of Latin at Liverpool University, a former colleague of Meyer's, alleging that Meyer used to think the Irish a silly and useless nation and that Meyer's influence on the University was thoroughly bad, being all for germanising it and that he had put in an assistant who was found to be a very dangerous spy and imprisoned.[20] The debate raged on both sides of the Irish Sea. John Sampson, once a close friend and fellow-adventurer into the Gypsy haunts of Wales, wrote to the *Times* on January 1915, that as a colleague for twenty years of Professor Meyer he had constant opportunities of hearing his opinion on most subjects, such as that his devotion to Celtic studies did not extend beyond the older language and literature and that the cult of Old Irish and modern Ireland were things apart, while of native students of Irish, with the signal exception of the late Whitley Stokes whose supremacy in this field he fully recognised, he spoke with the contempt of the scholar for the dilletante. The Irish themselves he regarded as an ill-balanced, emotional race, unfitted for any form of self-government, and, by reason of their incurable tendency to romantic and impracticable ideals, a danger to stable rule and a constant thorn in the side of the British Empire. Augustus John, his portraitist and another old friend, expressed to John Quinn of New York his conviction that throughout his years in England and as an honoured Celtic scholar Meyer had been spying and sending home reports of English weak spots.[21] But Quinn liked and admired Meyer as a companion and scholar.[22]

Judgements like these were formed in the tempers of war. Meyer did not lack advocates in Ireland. Ella Young, poetess and friend of Maud Gonne, wrote to the *Irish Times* on 12 January 1915:

> In justice to Kuno Meyer, whom I have known for several years, I would like to say that the thing that struck me most when I first met him was the interest which he took in Ireland and in the struggle her people were making for national expression. Interest, indeed, poorly describes his attitude, which was one of warm, living sympathy. He had more than the interest of a scholar in our literature – he had a pride in it. He resented aspersions on it as an Irishman might do – as many Irishmen have not done.
>
> Once, speaking of the old manuscripts and the fine work of continental scholars, he said: 'I should like to see a number of Irish scholars fully equipped to work on these manuscripts. I would like the honour of research work to go chiefly to the country to whom the literature belongs'.
>
> .... He was not eager to speak evil of anyone. I find it hard to believe that Kuno Meyer spoke scornfully of the Irish.

At a meeting of Dublin Corporation held on 15 March 1915 Kuno Meyer's name was expunged from the Roll of Freemen by thirty votes to sixteen after a sharp debate. Cork Corporation acted likewise by twenty-four to three. In Dublin Councillor William T. Cosgrave made an earnest appeal against the motion in an eloquent letter to the City Council setting out in detail the work on behalf of the Irish language and nation achieved by Kuno Meyer. 'Dr. Meyer has done more for Irish scholarship and Irish national glory than any other living man'.[23] In vain. Dublin Corporation however redeemed itself at its meeting of 12 April 1920 in accepting, unanimously, the motion of Alderman W.T. Cosgrave M.P. 'that the name of Dr. Kuno Meyer be, and it is, hereby restored to the Roll of Honorary Burgesses'. Many things had happened in the interval. But Kuno Meyer did not live to see his honour vindicated.

For all that he espoused the cause of Fatherland with full heart and nature, the sundering of friendships that this entailed must have been painful to Meyer. One of the unhappy episodes of his American visit was the abrupt ending by George Moore of their association. Meyer wrote a short, cordial letter to his former friend asking him for a 'nice long letter' and to address it c/o F.N. Robinson, Longfellow Park, Cambridge, Mass., where he was going to deliver some lectures. He expressed his liking for America and its ways, and hoped to remain for a year at least and go as far as San Francisco. He moved much in Irish circles and had met Yeats *père*, John Quinn and many others. He thought there would be a new chapter to add to an old Irish book called 'The Invasion of Erin' and 'meanwhile, my dear old friend and new enemy, I remain in peace or war, yours always sincerely'. It was addressed from the City Club of New York and dated 8 December 1914 .

Moore's reply, dated 4 January 1915, must be reckoned to stand high in the annals of ungraciousness. A long and hostile address ended with the words 'It is hardly necessary for me to add that I am taking leave of you for ever, but not because of the German that is in you, but because of the man that is in you.' He then gave the correspondence to the press. Even for something uttered in the tempers of war it was ungenerous and Moore lived to regret it. Of Meyer's own reaction we have no record, but his sister Toni did not forget it easily.

NOTES

1. NLI Ms No. 15119 (1) to (6); McDowell, *A Passionate Historian* 101-2.
2. ZCP X 361-83.
3. *Sunday Independent* (Dublin), 16 Jan. 1966. 'Norse scholar whose Irish dictionary caused a furore'.
4. Meyer to Best, from Essener Hof, Wernigerode, 12 Oct. 1914. NLI Ms No. 11002.
5. NLI Ms No. 11002. The confidential report on the Irish Dictionary of the Academy may correspond to the document printed in R.I. Best, 'On recent Irish studies in the Academy'. RIA *Proceedings* Vol LI, Sect C, No. 2, 31-34 (August 1946).
6. Flower to Best, from Dept of MSS, British Museum, 30 Sept. 1914. NLI Ms No. 11000.
7. Flower to Best, from Dept of MSS, British Museum, 13 Nov. 1914. NLI Ms No. 11000.
8. NLI Ms No. 11002.
9. Dated 25 Nov. 1914. NLI Ms No. 11002.
10. *Freeman's Journal* (Dublin) 18 Oct. 1919.
11. Best to Meyer, 14 Dec. 1914. Note on letter by Best – 'Copy of my answer to K.M.'s letters dated 25/18 Nov – 1914.'
12. Meyer to Best 12 Dec. 1914 from the City Club of New York. NLI Ms No. 11002.
13. Meyer to Best 23 Dec. 1914 from the City Club of New York. NLI Ms No. 11002.
14. The *Gaelic American* (New York) of 26 Dec. 1914, gives a full report of a speech given by Kuno Meyer on 17 December at the Irish Volunteer meeting at Terrace Garden, New York, from which the following extract will explain his reference to Harvard:
    'The other day, at a Clan na Gael meeting, I spoke freely before a friendly audience of Irish-Americans how delighted I was that the course of events had brought Germany and Ireland together ... I sent a copy of the report of my address to a friend at Harvard, where I was under an engagement to lecture on ancient Irish poetry. My good friend, distressed, I do not know at what, took the paper to the President, who at once decided that my engagements must be cancelled as, after the delivery of that address it would be violating the spirit of neutrality ... to invite me to speak at Harvard ... I am glad I sent the paper. I could not live or breathe in an atmosphere so close and vitiated as that which seems to prevail at Harvard.'
    Copy of *Gaelic American* in NLI Ms No. 11002 (70).
15. Meyer to Best, 23 Dec. 1914. NLI Ms No. 11002.
16. *The Times* (London) 24 Dec. 1914.
17. Thomas Kelly: *For advancement of learning; the University of Liverpool 1881-1981* (Liverpool 1981) 174.
18. *Ibid.*
19. Dated 28 Dec. 1914 from 9 & 10 Eustace Street, Dublin.
20. David A. Quaid, letter dated 2 Feb. 1915 in *Irish Independent* 3 Feb. 1915. Seems to be a reference to G. Schaafs who was interned in England.
21. To John Quinn, 3 April 1915. Cf. B.L. Reid: *The Man from New York: John Quinn and his friends* (New York 1968) 226.
22. *Ibid*, 117.

23. Councillor Cosgrave's letter appears in the Minutes of an Adjourned Monthly Meeting of the Municipal Council of the City of Dublin, 15 March 1915. It is dated Feb. 8th 1915 from 174 James' Street. It is reprinted in *The Vital Issue* (New York) Vol III, No. 3, 17 July 1915, 5-6.

Chapter 17

ON his way to America Meyer broke his journey at Rotterdam where he spent some days as the guest of Van Hamel at Nieuwe Haven 93. He planned to remain in America until the war was over, lecturing as he called it, but on what Van Hamel had his suspicions. Meyer looked quite vigorous and his rheumatism was not half as bad as it used be. Van Hamel was able to talk with him easily, found that he was not at all fanatic and thought that he suffered much under the present rupture between Germany and England.[1] During his stay with Van Hamel Meyer sent Mrs Green a postcard from Rotterdam[2] the message on which was innocent enough. Amongst the English in Berlin there were, he told her, a number of friends, including the Macrans of Trinity College, also the Knight of the Ships, all of whom were well. Neither of those were English. Henry Stewart Macran, professor of Moral Philosophy in Trinity College, had failed to get out of Germany in time. The Knight of the Ships was Sir Roger Casement. Meyer promised to write again, though Mrs Green does not seem to have received that particular message. She did receive his next letter, dated three days later from S.S. *Rotterdam,* Atlantic Ocean, but posted from New York, and her reaction was one of surprise and near alarm, embarrassed as she had been by his previous indiscreet message. Meyer wrote:

S.S. "Rotterdam"
Atlantic Ocean
17 Nov 1914

I hope you got my few words from Rotterdam which I wrote just before embarking. The chief purpose was to let you know that our friend the Knight of the Ships had safely though after great dangers arrived in Berlin, where we met repeatedly. He has burned his ships behind him and is embarked on a new course, or rather one as old almost as the Old Woman herself, at least since she has fallen upon evil days. He will get every assistance that he and she stand so much in need of. Everybody is interested in him. He spent an evening at the Schiemann's and wished you had been there with us. By a curious coincidence Schiemann had just translated his last pamphlet which showed that wonderful insight into coming events.

As you see I am myself embarked upon a venture. It had long been my wish to visit America, where I have many friends. Now is a very favourable moment, which I must not let escape. I shall probably stay as long as the war lasts. I go to New York first, but hope to visit every place where there are German and Irish friends, as far as San Francisco. I am also using the opportunity to give courses of lectures on Irish Lit. at the universities.

Now both our friend and I are very anxious that you should come over as soon as possible. Leave England to the English and the Germans and await the end in a quiet country. We could do much together. Of course you know the country better than I and will be able to judge better. At any rate consider the matter well.

I shall probably stay with Mr. John Quinn to begin with. At any rate letters addressed to his care (31 Nassau Str., New York) will always find me. I leave everything else till I can talk or write more freely to you.

Our voyage so far has been very pleasant, except for three hours while the boat was being searched by the English. Some Germans and Austrians on board had to sign a document saying that they would not fight against England! At one time I thought they were after me but they soon departed telling us which route to take to avoid mines..

Perhaps I shall add a word or two before I send this off from New York.

K.M.[3]

It is interesting to speculate on the import of Meyer's invitation to join him in America. Was there something more than politics in it, something personal, perhaps? 'We could do much together.' Or was it purely political? Mrs Green clearly did not consider it other than political, as her comments confirm. She noted on the letter:

> This letter was a great surprise to me. I had no tidings of Kuno Meyer after the war began, and knew nothing of his political position. I do not remember ever speaking to him on a political subject until March 1914 – when we talked of Carsonism and its exaggerations and I wrote to him once in June on that subject, only to protest against any rumours of civil dissension. ASG[4]

Mrs Green felt bound to reply and state her position, relative to her own aspirations, to her friend Sir Roger Casement, and most important of all, in the changed circumstances, to the necessity for Meyer of severing his connection with the School of Irish Learning. She obviously discussed the matter of his resignation with Best and the Governors of the School before sending him a letter which she must have found very difficult to write:

> My dear Dr Meyer,
>
> In your letter from the steamer "Rotterdam" you refer to a letter you wrote me from Rotterdam itself. This letter I never received. I know nothing of Berlin and what happened there except what has appeared in the papers.
>
> The tone and substance of your letter from the steamer did indeed fill me with amazement. We have long been associated in the work of Irish learning and history, an intercourse in which I have ever been grateful for your unfailing help and sympathy, and for the stimulus that was always radiating from your mind, incessantly at work. Politics in all these years never entered into our talk. I was the more surprised therefore at the sudden change in tone in the correspondence, when the old staple of our intercourse hitherto is replaced by political suggestions never before mentioned between us.
>
> Now that we are separated by the catastrophe of war, there can only be silence between us on every political subject. I cannot discuss with you an action which you as a German take in the service of your Government. My motives and hopes and aspirations are altogether different from yours. Nor can I discuss with you the subject of my friend Sir Roger Casement though your references to him force me to express the profound and heartfelt sorrow I feel at the political course he has been unhappily led to adopt wholly unknown to me.
>
> You will certainly agree with me in one thing, regarding the School of Irish Learning in which from the first we have been closely associated – that under the circumstances it must be impossible for you to retain the Directorship of that School, founded by you in happier days on lines of pure learning apart from

politics. Such a separation is one of the evils of this disastrous war, which brings calamity down even to our small community. If in the future the evil can be repaired it will bring to no one greater relief and comfort than to myself. But you will now recognise that it would be an act of justice and consideration on your part voluntarily to set the School free from a compromising position.

I write in great sorrow, which oppresses me heavily.

Let me wish for your success in the work of spreading the knowledge of Gaelic Learning. In Ireland for the moment all progress in that learning is arrested, to our immeasurable loss. In the cause and in the memory of old days

I am yours still sincerely
Alice S. Green[5]

Owing to the irregularity of the mails, delays in transit, the opening of letters no doubt, and the upsets of communication caused by war, the sequence of correspondence became erratic. Meyer did not receive this letter of Mrs Green's until 1 January 1915. Two days before that he had sent his resignation to Best, as Secretary to the School, in a brief note which reads:

The City Club of New York
29/12/1914

My dear Best,

Your letter – the first since the outbreak of the war – has just reached me. I think it will be best to resign both the Directorship of the School and the Editorship of *Ériu*, which might henceforth be conducted by Bergin and you. I have already resigned my honorary Liverpool professorship. Please see to this.

It is no use writing on anything else. Perhaps when the war is over you may see things in a different light. With kind greetings to your wife.

Yours as ever
Kuno Meyer[6]

This note carried an acknowledgement of Best's letter of 14 December in which he had explained that his sympathies in the present European crisis were not with Germany, 'but the other side', Meyer's observation on which was unusually curt, implying a German victory which might cause him a change of mind.

His friendship with Mrs Green had been long and sincere and her letter of December 15 had clearly distressed him. But he had no hesitation in accepting its message that he must sever all connection with the School. He wrote:

The City Club of New York
1/1/1915

My dear Mrs Green,

Your letter, which reached me this morning, was a sad opening to the New Year. I will not attempt to reply to it, or to excuse and defend myself; but only write to thank you for its kind tone, and to tell you that some time before you wrote I had myself come to the conclusion that it would be right to sever all official connexion with England and Ireland. So I sent in my resignation both of my honorary Liverpool professorship and of the directorship of our School and of the editorship of *Ériu*, which Mr. Best and Bergin may well carry on together. The feelings and thoughts that come to me again as I write this to you I must not now attempt to express. As you say, silence should now reign between us for awhile, if not for ever.

I will only add one word more. The man who in 1911 wrote 'Ireland, Germany and the next war' was bound to go to Berlin as he did.

Whatever you may read or hear about me, try to remember that I shall always remain

Yours as ever
Kuno Meyer[7]

It was a tense and troubled time for Mrs Green which made heavy demands on her character. Deserted by former friends she was left isolated and obliged to rely on her own great moral resources of learning and intellect. But she valued Kuno Meyer's past achievements and friendship too highly to let the present crisis sunder them and in that spirit she wrote, paying him a tribute that he richly deserved and holding out for herself the hope that the ideals they both cherished might flourish yet:

My dear Dr. Meyer,

I was much touched by your letter. Pray do not think of me as one ready to let slip our long friendship. My thoughts often go back to the first days of the School of Irish Learning – that bleak stormy Autumn, the days and nights of rain, of the in and out of trams in the dripping tempests, on your devoted way to lectures and classes, our one open restaurant, dinner of the unfailing chop and back again in the rain to the hotel where in the empty smoking room you lay on the sofa and had your first rest and warmth. How vividly I remember your patience and fortitude. You were alone in believing a Dublin School could be formed. You rode down all doubts and criticism. And you carried through your work triumphantly. Now we suffer a great loss. All I can hope is that there will remain a little band of scholars to carry on your tradition of Irish learning. Help from England for such work will be farther off than ever, if possible. We shall still have to remember our real fellowship with the scholars of Europe, and wait for re-union of friends in better days. It is impossible at this time to write with any freedom. Letters are opened and every phrase is liable to be misinterpreted, even the simplest. At least I should like to assure you that I look with indignation on words that have been written by those who owed you much, and who have shown no loyalty or fidelity but to themselves, even in this crisis, as in all past ones.

I agree entirely with what you say about the pamphlet.* That is all I can now say. I have been practically separated from my former friends. I use the time to read and think, and I have begun some new history work which I will pursue earnestly. Out of discouragement and trouble there can still come a renewed purpose.

I am yours sincerely
ASG[8]

* Regarding the pamphlet mentioned in the letter Meyer adds a note at the end saying 'This refers to my saying that the author of "Ireland, Germany and the next War" was bound to go to Berlin', the author being Sir Roger Casement.

A meeting of the Governors and Trustees of the School of Irish Learning was held on 12 January 1915, at which the Chair was taken by William P. Geoghegan. Present also were Douglas Hyde, Osborn Bergin, Eoin Mac Néill and the Hon Secretary R.I. Best. The business of the meeting was to consider a letter from the Director, Dr Kuno Meyer, offering his resignation. The following resolution was unanimously adopted:

We, the Governors and Trustees of the School of Irish Learning, wish to record the deep regret with which we find ourselves obliged to accept Dr. Kuno Meyer's resignation of his position as Director of the School and Editor of *Ériu,* owing to the unhappy circumstances of the present European conflict. He was the originator and founder of the School, and since its establishment twelve years ago he has

179

laboured ceaselessly to promote Irish studies and to bring the School into direct association with fellow-workers abroad. To the School journal *Ériu* he lent the prestige of his name, and to his unrivalled knowledge and experience is in great part due the honourable position it now holds. To the workers in the School Dr. Kuno Meyer has been a faithful friend, always ready with encouragement and assistance, and the resolve to secure recognition of a wide-reaching kind for good work done. It is impossible in this time of sorrow to rehearse calmly the very signal services rendered to Celtic learning by Dr. Meyer, and more particularly his rare services to the Irish community of scholars. It is with sorrow that we contemplate this separation as one of the catastrophes of a war which has for a time divided nations and severed natural communications. We still hope that among the reconciling forces of the future none will be more powerful than the loyalty of scholars to one another and to their common service of truth.[9]

It was a warm, sensitive and sincere tribute and its wording was admirably independent in the circumstances, when Meyer was little in favour with the powerful interests of the hour. The drafting of it was probably the work of Best, with some help from Mrs Green.[10] Meyer, in New York, had expected an earlier reply than the postal system, such as it was, could provide, and wrote again on the 21st a letter which gave a character of finality to his decision:

> Hotel Willard
> 252-256 W 76 St
> New York
> 21/1/15

My dear Best,

I had hoped to have heard from you by this that my resignation has been accepted. I am anxious to sever all official and public connexion with England and Ireland. It is the only right way. All others who are free agents have done so (Freund, Lehmann-Haupt, Holl, etc) and though at first I hoped that the effects of the war would not be felt in international domains like those of scholarship and science, I see now that it must be so, as personal and private relations are bound up with it. The English chapter of my life is closed, never to be continued I am afraid ...

> Kindest greetings to your wife
> and yourself
> Always yrs
> K.M.[11]

The severance, then, was made complete. In a way, it might be said, Meyer was the School. He was the bridge between it and Europe. It was by his influence and urgings that the most distinguished continental scholars came to the School to lecture. He it was who introduced the courses in Welsh. The great inaugural lectures contributing to the School's prestige were mainly his. Of the energy, the correspondence, the social and personal contacts that promoted the growth of it, he was largely the source, not to speak of the enterprise, faith, commitment and optimism by which from the first day he was actuated. With his resignation the sovereign link was broken. It was a tragedy that he was obliged to put his talents to use on behalf of his country in the cruel circumstances of war.

One has to admire the way in which Robin Flower championed the achievement in scholarship of Kuno Meyer despite the differences between them caused by war. One of Meyer's hostile critics was Dr. Norman Moore, a medical man of Irish parentage, Birmingham born, who had learned his Irish in London and possessed a fine Irish library, had translated Windisch's textbook of Irish grammar from the German, and was, besides many other things, the author of a history of St. Bartholomew's Hospital. His knowledge of Irish language matters and personalities was extensive, and we are indebted to him for valuable contributions to the Dictionary of National Biography, including biographies of Whitley Stokes and William Maunsell Hennessy. A collector of Irish manuscripts, he was thought to possess what was reputed to be the archetype of Brian Merriman's *Midnight Court*.

Of especial value and interest to Irish scholars was his long contribution in the form of a letter to the *Times Literary Supplement* of 28 October 1915 outlining the career of Standish Hayes O'Grady who had recently died. In the course of this he referred to the criticism by O'Grady of Kuno Meyer's text and translation of 'The Battle of Ventry' which had been printed in the *Anecdota Oxoniensia,* adding a biassed comment which Flower, with a true sense of fair play, replied to in the TLS of November 11 under the heading 'Irish Scholarship':

Sir, – In a letter from Dr. Norman Moore in the *Times Literary Supplement* of Thursday, Oct. 28, with which in all its says in praise of Dr. O'Grady I am in enthusiastic agreement, a reference is made to Dr. O'Grady's paper on Dr. Kuno Meyer's 'Battle of Ventry'. Dr. Moore goes on to say: - 'Those who in recent controversies have spoken of Kuno Meyer as a profound Irish scholar can hardly have read this paper.'

Now I submit that in recent controversies Dr. Meyer's Irish scholarship has not been in question. His political conduct has been much – and justly – criticised. But those among us whose business it is to have an opinion in matters of Irish scholarship will hardly allow that opinion to be changed by a reference to ancient criticisms of the first publication of the scholar concerned.

As a matter of fact, if criticism of detail is to be fatal to a scholar's reputation, then Dr. O'Grady himself would be in a parlous state. For Dr. Meyer's review of his 'Silva Gadelica' was infinitely more shattering than his own criticism of 'The Battle of Ventry'. But all students of Irish know perfectly well that in this field the reputation of both men is secure. O'Grady's inspired translations and brilliant interpretations of the spirit of Irish literature, Kuno Meyer's accurate textual work, his invaluable lexicographical translations, his delicate and beautiful translations, and the inspiration of his teaching; Irish scholarship would be infinitely the poorer wanting either of these.

The facts of Dr. Meyer's political action are known to the general world. And let the world give judgment on them. But the achievements of his scholarship are known only to a few. And, if British scholarship is to maintain its integrity, it is the duty of those few to protest when those achievements are called into question.

Yours faithfully
Robin Flower
(Lecturer in Irish in the University of London)

Nor could Norman Moore refrain, in his otherwise valuable account, from having a fling at German Celtic scholars by remarking that 'The foundation of O'Grady's knowledge of Irish was quite different from that of "The German School of Keltologues, who derive no assistance from the ear," as he himself once said, as a remark of definition not of denunciation.'

Mrs Green had nothing complimentary to say about Norman Moore.

> I was delighted, (she wrote) that the excellent Robin Flower answered the very mean paper of Dr. Moore; I always think that there is nothing too shabby that one can expect of a man who has resigned nationality and retained sentiment without feeling. What wars and disasters these people are guilty of!
>
> I find that Dr. Moore is not in contact with a single one of the modern scholars, and takes no interest in meeting them, neither Dr. Ker nor Robin Flower. It is wonderful what a part vanity plays ...[12]

Hard words. But to anyone removed from the stresses of the time and the feeling that war generates, the judgement on him of Mrs Green, sincere and dedicated person though she was, appears unduly harsh. It would be unfair to dismiss Dr. Norman Moore in her terms. He had given services to the Irish language which deserve that he should be remembered with gratitude.[13]

NOTES

1. A.G. Van Hamel to Best, p.c., p.mk. Rotterdam 20 Nov. 1914. NLI Ms No. 11004.
2. Addressed to 36 Grosvenor Road, Westminster, 14 Nov. 1914. NLI Ms No. 15091.
3. NLI Ms No. 15091.
4. *Ibid.*
5. A.S. Green to Meyer, 15 Dec. 1914. NLI Ms No. 15091(2). This letter appears to be a copy or a draft. In Mrs Green's correspondence there is a letter of 22 Dec. 1914 to Best saying: 'I wrote to Dr Meyer suggesting that he should resign from the School during the war.' NLI Ms No. 15114(23).
6. NLI Ms No. 11002.
7. NLI Ms No. 15091(1).
8. A.S. Green to Meyer, 28 Jan. 1915. NLI Ms No. 11001(2).
9. *Ériu* VIII, pt. 1, 1915. Report on the work of the School 1914-15.
10. Mrs Green's correspondence with Best includes the following undated letter which refers to the drafting of the resolution:

36 Grosvenor Road SW1

Dear Mr Best,

   I don't know how to put it in a 'resolution' – too rigid a form for such a situation. Could it be proposed to accept with sorrow the resignation – and to add to this bare statement a message from the School 'in remembrance of a long and remarkable association with Dr. Meyer, and of the services so freely given us.'

   I enclose what I would like said. I am disgusted by the virtuous Moores and all the rest of the lot, shouting out their own (much-needed) praises and flinging their smart stones. Dr. Meyer must be suffering acutely. We at least need not join the hunt. Use or reject or correct what I write. It has been hammered out of me with such sorrow. And when (where?) sorrow is so deep it is often of no use to any one else.

   I hope to enclose in this a personal letter, and ask you to send it with your resolution. Don't you feel for me that it was I who had to write that resignation letter. He has of course never answered me.

Yours very sincerely
ASG

NLI Ms No. 15114(8).
At the time of writing she had not received Meyer's letter of 1 Jan. 1915.

11. NLI Ms No. 11002. C.F.F. Lehmann-Haupt had been Professor of Greek in Liverpool University since 1910. He was out of England when war broke and resigned at once.

12. A.S. Green to Best, from 36 Grosvenor Road, Westminster, 2 Dec. 1915. NLI Ms No. 15114(25).

13. For details of Sir Norman Moore's interest in the Irish language see Pádraig de Brún and Máire Herbert, *Catalogue of Irish manuscripts in Cambridge Libraries.* (Cambridge 1986), Introduction XIV-XV, XXII-XXV, 85, etc.

Chapter 18

RICHARD Best duly received on 17 November 1914 the two letters from Meyer begun in Berlin and completed in Rotterdam, followed next morning by a proof of his *Zeitschrift* review of what Best, in one of his less admirable moments, was pleased to call 'M's folly'. He was delighted to see Meyer's familiar hand, but expressed surprise that he was on his travels again. He wrote back all he had of news, much of which was tragic, inevitably, for war was taking its toll of friends and scholars. Séamus Geoghegan, serving with the Inniskilling Fusiliers, was killed the other day. He was the son of Sam Geoghegan, brother of W.P., Trustee of the School of Irish Learning, and his sister Fanny, and Mrs Geoghegan's nephew Captain Stack, a second cousin of Best's wife, had fallen in battle. Several others whom they knew had lost sons or brothers. Among the scholars whom he heard had lost sons were Windisch, Sachau and Wilamowitz-Moellendorff. A casualty of compelling sadness was Joseph Déchelette, author of the *Manuel d'Archéologie*, the foundation stone of Celtic archaeology, who had fallen at the head of his company, a regiment of Territorials, near Soissons, leaving his great work unfinished. A devoted patriot, he need not have volunteered, being over age. On his memorial plaque the nobility of his life and death is recorded in majestic Latin – *Galliae reliquias illustravit, pro Gallia miles cecidit*. The sender of the sad tidings was Joseph Loth. Best also had a letter from Henri Gaidoz, whose object in writing was to obtain news of Meyer and to send him his *sentiments d'amitié*. Poor Gaidoz, his sight was getting worse and his writing was difficult to decipher. Best was happily able to re-assure him about Meyer's well-being.

Best reported that things were pretty much as usual in Dublin. Celtic matters could hardly be said to flourish. They were being pestered by young ladies in quest of subjects for M.A. degrees in Modern Irish, some editing MacCurtin, others MacCuarta, while the excellent Hyde would speak of their work with bated breath and gravely aver that they had actually discovered copies in MSS! What a farce it all was! Best thought it a pity that Meyer could not incorporate Bergin's list of errors in the Dictionary notice. He had not seen Bergin that day or he would have passed the proof on to him. It is doubtful if Bergin would have relished being involved in the review that came to be dated so questionably. Marstrander had definitely resigned. All the Dictionary slips and material were in Christiania where they might remain until the coming of happier days. 'But between ourselves, there are some members of the Academy who would be greatly relieved if a (shall we say, friendly) torpedo sent them to the bottom of the North Sea. It would solve once and for all this eternal Dictionary question' . Surely an unkind thought for some members of the Academy to harbour, and do we find Richard Best himself partaking of it? He was dividing his spare hours between the *Times* and *Audacht Morainn,* all the versions of which he had copied, and some of which was beyond him. Yes, Dr. Traill was dead and he had heard privately that Mahaffy was to succeed him as Provost of Trinity College. Que devient Marstrander? asked Gaidoz, et le fameux Dictionnaire, oeuvre de Sisyphe, ou plutôt plusieurs Sisyphes? Best hoped Meyer would continue to write, as he would likewise do and if his letters were stopped, that need not discourage Meyer. 'With our love to you both'.[1]

Best's letter of 18 November, having gone first to Berlin, reached Meyer in New York on 29 January 1915. Meantime Meyer had received from him directly the resolution of the Board of Governors of the School of Irish Learning regretting his resignation and acknowledging his services, in the drafting of which he recognised Best's friendly hand. He thanked Best for the wording and asked him to convey his thanks to the Board. This was one matter which had been dealt with gracefully, with credit to both parties. Meyer was making farewell visits to New York, as he was going West. The Boston meeting was a great success, with an audience of Irish, Scots and Germans. He was presented with an illuminated address from the Boston School of Irish, dated an Seiseadh lá fichead Januar 1915 which expressed as its hope 'Tá dóchas mór againn as do Thuras don Tír seo'.[2] It amused him to think that at the same time Dublin would strike him from its roll of Freemen. Poor Yeats *père* was so wild about Moore's ungenerous letter that he meditated a reply to the papers.

Every mail brought Meyer abusive and admiring letters. He remained unshaken in his certainty that Germany would win the war. 'When I compare the divided state of England with the perfect unanimity of Germany and her imperturbable resolution, I can have no doubt where victory will be found'.[3] However, there was no chance of an end to the war before another year, so he prepared for a long stay in America. He was making arrangements with Harvard for the Autumn course and in June would go to San Francisco. Because of his Terrace Garden speech, however, Harvard made known to him it would not entertain his lectures. For the present, he had an engagement to lecture in Urbana at the University of Illinois, where his arrival was anxiously awaited by Gertrude Schoepperle, who went to meet him at the train accompanied by Professor Sherman. The latter, before setting out, had read George Moore's account of Meyer to brief himself as to what kind of man to expect. They returned to Sherman's where they talked for hours. Miss Schoepperle was utterly captivated by Meyer, who was charming beyond her greatest hopes. Even Sherman, whose mind was anchored to the eighteenth century, was moved almost to the point of taking up Celtic studies.

Meyer spoke of Best and Bergin and all his Dublin friends with the highest appreciation. The war had not changed him. He spoke about it with the greatest sanity and tolerance. The Shermans, violently anti-German and uneasy about his coming, were completely set at rest by his civilised outlook. He told Miss Schoepperle that the talk about his being a German emissary was quite untrue and he had officially assured the President of the University of the fact. Quite obviously, Miss Schoepperle was thrilled with her distinguished guest and the prospect of working with him. She had organised three classes, one of twenty five in Celtic Philology and Literature (through English), one of six beginning Irish (with Thurneysen's textbook), and a third small class of three translating *Saltair na Rann,* the marvellous collection of Early Middle Irish poems, edited without a translation by Whitley Stokes. Graduates and undergraduates formed the first class; members of the English, German and Romance faculties the second and third. The moment Meyer opened his mouth they were at work in earnest. Miss Schoepperle foresaw a very valuable semester. But she was perturbed and no doubt over-attentive, as the next part of her letter shows:

> Poor Meyer. He has suffered torture physically, what with the discomfort atten-dant upon adapting himself to fixed hours for meals, steam heat, college regula-tions, etc. He is patient and gentle in the extreme. When he left Friday noon to spend the weekend in Chicago I could have wept at my ill-success in making him comfortable. Please, I beg of you, write me some advice as to his personal pecu-liarities. Poor dear man! Imagine him here – dying for thirst because he can't, or won't, stoop over the fountain, which in our 'sanitary' mad Urbana one must drink from in the University buildings lest one get a contagious disease from a tumbler! When I discovered his difficulty I had infinite pains running around the campus between his two classes trying to get him something to drink from, the janitors infinitely disgusted at my making so much fuss to 'cater to' such a for-eigner's idiosyncrasy.
> I thought I had everything fixed up for him ...

She had prepared an office with all the Celtic books together, with just his desk and her own in it. To do this, she had to move the head of the department out, and another member and herself around. One wonders if those others were pleased. But she didn't believe Meyer cared for the arrangement in the least. She thought he would like living at the University and she had got all her friends to help her decorate his rooms and finish them, but there was something wrong with them, she did not know what. He was angelic about it, but could not sleep or eat. She wished the Bests were there to tell her how to look after him. He seemed to like to chat with her, and he was so helpless about finding his way, and getting food, that she was constantly taking him off to tea in the afternoon and in the evening after class to hot chocolate. 'Do you think he will get too bored with me? Of course I am doing everything possible to introduce him here.'[4]

On the 25th she wrote again, this time to say that Professor Meyer, after a week, had found himself in such ill-health that he had to abandon his work. He suffered from the climate and the spartan living conditions and the weight of anxiety and long distances of travel had been too much for him. She was deeply impressed by his noble spirit.

> He is the one person I know here who in the midst of this terrible time preserves undiminished the critical and dispassionate historic sense. Whatever the newspapers may have said, do not fail, I beg of you, to believe that his friendship with you and his love for his friends in England is as warm as ever. His heart is with Germany, of course, and the tendency of his mind is, as I imagine it has always been, aristocratic and conservative.[5]

Miss Schoepperle herself loyally took on the undergraduate lecture course on Celtic Literature for which he was scheduled and this in addition to her regular work placed a heavy burden on her. She was also trying to continue the translation of *Saltair na Rann* along with Dr. Blondheim, Meyer having agreed to help them by correspondence.[6]

Writing a few weeks later from Buffalo, Meyer told Best of his experience in Urbana:

> Miss Schoepperle will have told you that I left Urbana after an unsuccessful attempt to m'y acclimatiser. It is a very primitive place, almost a village, without any comforts or (according to European notions) even the decencies of life, and the climate did not suit me at all. A horrid black oozy Prairie soil striking the damp through you. But everybody was kindness itself and they fully understood the reasons for my sudden flight. I keep in touch with Miss Schoepperle and Dr. Blondheim.[7]

The visit was a dismal failure. It must have been a serious disappointment for Gertrude Schoepperle.

There existed a firm union of sympathy between Meyer and Sir Roger Casement. Casement is the author of a long letter, the beginning of which is missing, signed R.C. and dated Berlin 12 November 1914, written obviously to Kuno Meyer, although his name does not appear. Casement advises him about what American people to contact for his lecture tour and suggests that John Quinn would 'get you the names of proper men for running it – and introduce you to some of the right people ... Your status as a citizen of Dublin and Cork and your University honours are themselves all the credentials necessary. Can you take with you some copies of the (1st) small edition of 'Four Old Irish Songs' ... Perhaps one of your best introductions to the American public might be of reciting that wonderful old nature poem and telling them something of the world of Celtic life and aspiration it reveals.' Nearly all the rest of the letter, over 30 pages, is taken up with 'the facts, in outline, of the Christiania case' and Casement's charges against Adler Christensen.[8] There are occasional references to Sir Roger Casement in Meyer's letters to Joseph McGarrity of Springfield Avenue, Philadelphia, a prominent leader of the Clan na Gael. They are brief; sometimes he is Sir Roger, sometimes 'our friend', and they usually indicate his mood or state of mind according as his hopes fluctuated. 'I hear from Berlin that our friend is not at all well, much depressed, and at present in a sanatorium near Berlin. I trust that as our arms are more and more victorious his good spirits will return ... Did you see Mr. Kommer's excellent article on Sir R. in the *Vital Issue?*'[9]

He wrote to Casement to cheer him up, told him he was in correspondence with Mrs Green and in touch with John Devoy, 'the Old Man', Nestor of the American Irish nationalist organisation, and with his colleague McGarrity, both of whom were his allies in trying to influence public opinion against supporting Britain. A pencilled note on top of the letter indicates that it was addressed to Professor Schiemann:

A chara dhil agus a aonphósta agus solás na hÉirenn (Gaelic characters)

I hear from my sister that you are not in good health and spirits. May I soon have better news! I hope you will not despond because things are not going as rapidly as our impatience wishes. They are going well, everywhere, so *sursum corda!* All your movements are closely followed here and your name is spreading in ever wider circles that do not conceal their sympathy. I enclose a German version of my friend Kommer's article on you. By this time you should be a good German scholar.

I may say that I am doing much here in a quiet way. It is easier here than in New York. My sister will have told you of my doings. I hear little from Ireland itself. I am in correspondence with my friend an Bhantigherna Uaine. Schiemann keeps me well-informed as to all that is going on in Berlin. I am planning another descent upon New York where the Stimmung is now much less hostile than it was some months ago. Gt Britain has overdone it and overreached herself. The false news about the great successes in the Dardanelles was generally received with shrugs of the shoulder and incredulous smiles. Write to me about yourself to c/o L. Guenzel, 332 So. Michigan Avenue, Chicago. Letters get through safely now. I remain in touch with the Old Man and friend Joseph and am to speak in Philadelphia in May on the 'two Irelands'. The relations between the Irish and my countrymen here are getting closer every day. I am to address a meeting of both to-morrow, in Buffalo.

Slán agus beannacht leat!
go fíorbhuan
K.M.[10]

On 16 March, after returning from what he described as 'a splendid Irish-German demonstration in Buffalo', Meyer had news, just come from Berlin, that Sir R. appeared to be in better spirits. The article on Casement in the *Vital Issue,* a publication supporting Germany, was written by a good friend of Meyer's, an Austrian journalist named Kommer. A German version had also appeared.[11]

Meyer spoke at Powers' Theatre in Chicago on Sunday 21 March, where he had a great reception, with the platform full of representative men, who had all come to assure him of their disapproval of Dublin's action in removing his name from the roll of Freemen. He told them he well knew it was not the true voice of Ireland, whereat there was mighty cheering. In the course of his speech he made a plea for the establishment of a library and museum of Celtic literature and art in Chicago for the purpose of making the city a centre of Irish learning, the funds to be provided by wealthy Irishmen. 'I have again heard from Berlin and am glad to say that our friend was then reported to be quite cheerful. I suppose he has his ups and downs like all of us'.[12]

188

Meyer had prepared two lectures aimed specifically at an Irish-German audience entitled (1) England and Germany before the War (2) The two Irelands. There were others, none written out formally, as he spoke from notes, 'scraps of paper' and a well stocked memory. For these lectures he received a fee as was normal, since travel and hotel expenses had to be met. Evidently McGarrity was persuading him to have the lectures published and he did intend to publish them sooner or later, 'but not just yet, as I would deprive myself of good lecture material, and it is essential that I should go about lecturing. It would be easy to change the titles of my various lectures, but not the substance'.[13]

His schedule, a wide-ranging and busy one, made considerable demands on his stamina and obliged him to take an occasional rest.[14] The following letter to McGarrity, written from Milwaukee, gives a sample of his activities:

'Your letter of the 2nd has just reached me here, where I am to address an Irish gathering to-night on ancient Irish literature. I had a very successful meeting at the University of Minnesota last night and am going from here to Cornell University. I hope to stay in Philadelphia over the 7th and should be delighted to meet your countrymen at a friendly dinner. But I must leave on the 8th early, as I have to travel all the way to Cleveland to lecture there on the 10th.

My next address will be New York, at the Knickerbocker Hotel (till about the 14th), but letters will always be forwarded. I may have to go to Baltimore on the 15th.

I was greatly pleased to get the resolution of the Ancient Order as well as one from Wexford in similar terms. I feel that I have the Irish people behind me as always.[8]

Yours alys sincerely,
Kuno Meyer

I met a fine old Fenian here, one Mr. Quinn from Limerick, 83 years of age.[15]

An Bhantighearna Uaine was Mrs Green, to whom Meyer wrote in the beginning of June:

My dear Mrs Green,

I have been so busy and travelling about so much that I have had little time for correspondence. I meant to go westward, but some engagements to lecture in the neighbourhood have brought me to the East once more. I spent many weeks in Chicago, where I moved much in Irish circles. Padraic Colum and his wife were there also, as guests of the widow of an American poet, Vaughan Moody. He lectures and writes a good deal on Ireland. Wherever I go I try and stir up the interest in Celtic studies. I am to lecture at Berkeley in California in July, where President Wheeler is an old friend of mine. Next week I go to Providence on a visit to Professor Burgess, who has just brought out a splendid book on the causes of the war. When in Washington the other day I saw Mr. Wilson. If as I fear I have lost some of my old English friends I am making many new ones here. In Baltimore I spent two delightful days in the company of Sir Walter Raleigh, just as in old times. He at any rate has remained true to me, and so have Prof. Mackay and Conybeare. Have you any objection to my sister translating your book *Irish Nationality*? A certain friend is going to write a preface to it and my brother will add a final chapter. Write to me at 134 E 58th Street, New York City, where letters will always be forwarded.[16]

Meyer corresponded a good deal with Dom Louis Gougaud, author of *Les Chrétientés Celtiques,* now a prisoner in Germany and, because the

Emperor had ordered all priests to be treated as officers, comfortably housed in a Benedictine Abbey in Westphalia where he was putting his time to use by becoming a good German scholar. Meyer's youngest nephew was missing, a prisoner in French or English hands, while another was storming Przemysl. His brother Eduard had published a book on the causes of the war, in which he predicted a century of conflict, punctuated by armistices and generally forecast a pessimistic future. Meyer himself was finishing a study on the tenth century *Saltair na Rann*, which Miss Schoepperle was translating under his supervision.[17] All this he communicated to Mrs Green who was a sympathetic recipient of everything which concerned him. The translation of Mrs Green's *Irish Nationality* into German with preface by a certain friend, most probably Casement, and the final chapter by his brother, would have made a unique historical document which fate decreed was not to be.

Meyer's notion that Sir Walter Raleigh, his colleague for ten years, 1889-1900, in the University of Liverpool, had remained true to him following the outbreak of war, has to be qualified by the observations of Raleigh made in his correspondence, published in 1926 after his death. In a letter to H.C. Wyld, a former Liverpool colleague of both, Raleigh comments that 'Old Kuno', as he familiarly calls him, 'has been going it,' in reference to Meyer's breach with his former university, and goes on to say that the morality frankly expounded by Kuno was the German morality since Frederick the Great. Still Kuno talked and thought of his English friends more than of anything else. 'There is nothing else that he is so much attached to, by what heart he has. I suppose every German of parts is a Govt. agent. All that I gathered from Kuno is that he is not a paid agent (he has his Chair of course) and that he does not report to his Govt. The last may be a lie, which German morality makes it a duty to tell'.[18] Nevertheless we must surmise that Raleigh, critical though he was, had a warm spot in his heart for Meyer, suppressed for the present time of war. Toni Meyer refers to a friendly letter which Raleigh wrote him after it was over.

Meyer's own family was not untouched by the ravages of war. His youngest nephew, son of his brother Eduard, a boy of twenty, who had volunteered in the autumn, was killed at Ypres in his first battle.[19] Two weeks later his brother bore another loss when the fiancé of his youngest daughter, a fine young scholar, was killed in the great Carpathian battle after having taken part safely in the whole Russian campaign. 'These continuous losses of our best youth are terrible. And to think that so many of them fall fighting those lousy swinish poxed Russian hordes!'[20] Upset though he must have been at grievous family losses, one feels that Meyer's dignity lapsed for a brief moment. The tidings about Casement continued to worry Meyer. There was bad news, he told McGarrity, of their friend in Berlin, who was almost desperate for the reason that only sixty out of four thousand Irish prisoners had volunteered for the Irish Brigade he was trying to raise, a number so small that nothing could be done.[21] Little of what he heard from Berlin from then on was re-assuring but he was not prepared for the news of Casement's arrest, which caused him grave disquiet, as he communicated to McGarrity:

> This is dreadful news about our poor friend! though we do not know the whole truth. But I fear there can be no doubt about his being in the enemy's hands. Another Irish patriot made away with before he could accomplish anything – no, fortunately not anything this time. For the rising in Dublin and the German sub-marines between England and Ireland, and I fancy also a supply of arms must after all be the beginning of greater things to come. Poor Sir Roger! They will keep it all from him and he will eat out his heart in his lonely prison. They will not dare to execute him, I think. If I had been in Berlin I would have dissuaded him from risking his own life so prematurely. But his impatience was no doubt too great, and everything seemed to promise well ...[22]

The tragedy of Sir Roger Casement, who was hanged in Pentonville on August 3rd 1916, caused a wave of shock throughout Ireland and Irish America. Meyer was in Fish Creek, Wisconsin, when he heard the news on the following day, first from a Limerick girl who had seen it in the early papers and immediately afterwards from Joe McGarrity. He wrote at once to McGarrity:

> My dear friend,
>
> I received your letter this afternoon, about an hour after I had heard of the last act of the tragedy from an Irish girl who only left Limerick about 10 weeks ago and had read an account in the morning papers at Sturgeon Bay. So our brave and noble friend has joined the ranks of the martyred hosts of Ireland, surely not the least brave and noble among them. I shall cherish his memory to my dying day and make it an object of my life to pay him all the respect and honour due to him both in private and in public. The fact that he was not in favour of a revolution just now was entirely new to me, but from his view and character, I can well understand it. We must do something to clear his memory from all the false and grotesque charges made against him; but it is probably only when I get back to Berlin that I shall know the whole truth. Meanwhile I am going to speak on his life and work to a sympathetic audience of German-Americans here, and shall take every opportunity of doing so again.
>
> My movements are very uncertain. I may be back in N. York before the month is out. Perhaps we shall meet then. Kindest greetings.
>
> Yours always sincerely
> Kuno Meyer[23]

Mrs Green was deeply distressed by the tragedy of Casement. She had spared no effort to secure his reprieve but her task was hopeless. His fate had a profound effect on her and was one of the factors which influenced her to support the rising nationalist movement in Ireland, while remaining a constitutionalist, and to change her place of residence from London to Dublin. How acutely she suffered was felt by Meyer, who wrote her in words of understanding and sympathy, years after the event, from Germany:

> My dear Mrs Green
>
> Often and often during the past years I have thought of you and what you must have suffered. Centuries of history which we used to read and think far removed have been pressed into the space of a few years and have entered our lives with their worst horrors. But few of the tragedies that have been enacted have so shaken me as that of August 3rd, and how you find the strength to live through it

is a marvel to me. A poor Irish girl here took her own life when she knew that it was all over, and my sister who had become warmly attached to him has never had a smile since. We read your wonderful poem, which must have been a last great solace to him. You will be interested to hear that quite a literature has sprung up about him in this country.[24]

NOTES

1. Best to Meyer, 18 Nov. 1914. NLI Ms No. 11002.
2. NLI Ms No. G685.
3. Meyer to Best, 29 Jan. 1915, from Hotel Willard, New York City. NLI Ms No. 11002.
4. Gertrude Schoepperle to Edith and R.I. Best, 14 Feb. 1915, from Urbana, Illinois. NLI Ms No. 11001(19).
5. G. Schoepperle to Best, 25 Feb. 1915, from University of Illinois, Urbana. NLI Ms No. 11001(19).
6. *Ibid.*
7. Meyer to Best, 15 March 1915, from The Lafayette, Buffalo. NLI Ms No. 11001(19).
8. NLI Ms No. 5459.
9. Meyer to McGarrity, 13 March 1915, from Congress Hotel, Chicago. NLI Ms No. 17465.
10. NLI Ms No. 13085 (22). Letter dated 12.3.1915. Head of writing paper bears medallion device of University Club of Chicago.
11. Meyer to McGarrity, 16 March 1915, on headed paper of Illinois Athletic Club, Chicago. NLI Ms No. 17465.
12. Meyer to McGarrity, 24 March 1915, on headed paper of Illinois Athletic Club, Chicago, enclosed with which is presscutting of *Chicago Tribune* of 22 Mar 1915. NLI Ms No. 17465.
13. Meyer to McGarrity, 21 June 1915, from Fort Pitt Hotel, Penn Ave and 10th St., Pittsburg, PA. NLI Ms No. 17465.
14. Cf. Meyer to McGarrity, 12 April 1915 – 'I go to Baltimore on Wednesday, just for a day or two, to meet a friend; then south to Florida for a little holiday. I had very successful meetings in Minneapolis among the Germans and the academic body and in Milwaukee at a large Irish gathering. But they tell me the young Irish are all pro-English! In Ithaca, I spoke before the University on Irish studies. If you have any relations with Pittsburg, Cincinnati and other places in the neighbourhood, I might go there from Cleveland in the second half of May. You know my subjects and my terms. My address in Baltimore is c/o Prof. Nitze, 4 Bishops Road.' Written from Hotel Knickerbocker, New York.
15. Meyer to McGarrity, 7 May 1915, from Hotel Pfister, Milwaukee, Wisconsin. NLI Ms No. 17465.
16. Meyer to Mrs Green, from Hotel Willard, New York City, 2 June 1915. NLI Ms No. 15091.
17. *Ibid.*
18. Raleigh to Wyld, from Tregenna Castle Hotel, St. Ives, Cornwall, 30 May 1915. *The letters of Sir Walter Raleigh (1879-1922),* ed. by Lady Raleigh. 2 vols, London 1926. II 425-6. There are interesting references to Meyer in these volumes, some friendly, pre-war, some critical during war.
19. Meyer to McGarrity 7 June 1915, from Hotel Willard, New York City. NLI Ms No. 17465.
20. Meyer to McGarrity 21 June 1915, from Fort Pitt Hotel, Penn Ave and 10th St., Pittsburg, PA. Part of this letter is quoted above; cf note 13.
21. Meyer to McGarrity, 3 Aug. 1915, from Hotel Robins, Post Near Jones, San Francisco. NLI Ms No. 17629.

22. Meyer to McGarrity, 26 April 1916, from Plaza Hotel, Chicago. NLI Ms No. 17629.
23. Meyer to McGarrity, 4 Aug. 1916. NLI Ms No. 17465.
24. Meyer to Mrs Green, 13 July 1919. NLI Ms No. 15091 (3).

Chapter 19

MEYER'S lecture tour was suddenly interrupted on the 9th of September when he was severely injured in a railroad collision between Corti Madera and Alto in California. He was taken to the San Rafael Cottage Hospital, 20 Nye Street, San Rafael, where he was laid up for more than five weeks. Some big muscles of his neck and back were badly sprained and lacerated and recovery was slow. Luckily no bones were broken and only a few flesh wounds incurred which after five weeks were almost healed. On October 18 he was removed to the German Hospital, San Francisco, which he feared would be his address for a long time to come. All his engagements for October and November had to be cancelled and in his present state he found it hard to imagine that he should ever be able to move about again as usual.[1] But his resilience was marvellous. He later sued the railway company for damages and after long and tedious proceedings a settlement was come to between them which left him with scant recompense for his trouble and injuries.[2]

The news of his accident first reached Ireland through press reports which put the event in the gravest light. Anxious and distressed, Richard Best wrote to Mrs Green in London who was thrown into something like alarm. She put her feelings in a letter:

> My dear Mr Best,
>
> I am very grateful to you for writing to me though the news is even worse than I expected.
>
> What a terrible thing it must be to be in that critical state away from all friends and natural advisers and helpers.
>
> I shall wait with great anxiety to hear when you next have news. Meanwhile I most heartily share your distress. He has already left a place that nothing else can fill among us and this gloomy tragedy is appalling.
>
> Yours very sincerely
> A.S. Green[3]

Edith Best sent a worried query to Toni Meyer, addressing it through Anton Van Hamel, and got back a reassuring reply:

> Thank you so much for your kind inquiries. Fortunately the newspapers have exaggerated a great deal, and although he was laid up for a few weeks, there was no cause for anxiety, I am thankful to say. Of course it has been a great shock to us all, and I feel most keenly not being able to be with him and look after him, but under the circumstances it would not be advisable – at least so he says – and I would only be in the way. He has the best of doctors and nurses and everything he wants. I just had a long letter from him dated September 29th which came in at

194

the same time as yours. I am glad to hear you and your husband are keeping well. With much love to you both, always yours T.M.[4]

The reply came back through Van Hamel who added a brief message:

Dear Mrs Best,

Your letter gave me a terrible shock, and I was greatly relieved when I understood Dr. M. was not in so bad a case as you supposed. Many greetings to you both. V.H. – Bonn 31/10/1915.[4]

Meyer's accident was a prelude to romance, swift in developing, an account of which he wrote in simple and unromantic terms to Joe McGarrity who was probably very surprised to hear of it.

Arrowhead Springs Hotel
Cal.
19/XII. 1915

My dear Mr McGarrity,

You will excuse my long silence when you learn that I was married on Dec. 10th. My wife and I have come to this lovely spot in Southern California, where we are spending our honeymoon. She was a Mrs Lewis, née Youngblood, a Nebraskan of Scoto-Irish descent. She is only 27 years old, so that there is a difference of 30 years between us. She was head nurse or Superintendent at the Cottage Hospital in San Rafael, where I was taken after the accident. Through her I have become the father of a little 9 year old girl, who is being b rought up in a Catholic convent in Berkeley, though my wife is a Protestant.[5] My health has greatly improved, and the good mountain air and sunshine and the baths are doing me a power of good. I hope to be able to take up lecturing once more in January. Our present intention is to spend the winter in California, and then when the fine season begins to drift gradually eastward, when I hope we shall meet again.[6]

Someone had sent the Bests a newscutting from a Californian paper and they were no doubt as astonished at the news as anybody. They were not therefore taken unawares when they received in January 1916 a card stating that:

MR KUNO MEYER
and
MRS FLORENCE LEWIS
announce their marriage
on Friday, the tenth of December
One thousand nine hundred and fifteen
San Bernardino, California

As in friendship and courtesy bound Richard wrote at once to Meyer offering warmest congratulations and all good wishes for his happiness, adorning his greeting with an old Irish aspiration.

Among Best's papers are some newscuttings. One of these, wanting date but marked 1915 in pencil and originating from San Bernardino, 12 December, two days after the wedding, gives details. It says that Professor Kuno Eduard Meyer who occupied the chair of Celtic Languages in the University of Berlin, was on his honeymoon in San Bernardino with his bride of three days, whom he had met as a nurse when he was taken to the San Rafael Cottage Hospital, after having been injured in a wreck on the Northwestern Pacific Railroad, three months previously. The bride was Mrs Florence Luella Lewis, of Creighton,

Nebraska. She was twenty-seven and a divorcée, Meyer fifty-seven. Meyer is reported as saying:

> After I was carried unconscious from the wreck, I awoke one day in the hospital at San Rafael to be fascinated at the vision who was acting as my nurse.
>
> I fell in love with her at first sight, and when I was able to leave the hospital and carry her away everyone in the place wanted to scratch my eyes out.

The words, as quoted, are more likely to be a journalist's embellishment than Meyer's own, and the account continues in romantic terms that Mrs Meyer, seated on the arm of her husband's chair, in the veranda of the Arrowhead Hotel, smiled at his enthusiasm, while she radiated happiness and admitted that she was very much in love with him.

Mrs Green also received in the post the card announcing Meyer's wedding. 'Startling news', she called it. Best had sent her some news-cuttings which she received in no mood of joy or congratulation, but which for her threw a brilliant light on the subject. 'The poor man! How I do hope that the lady will not experiment on him as she did on the first husband. It is such a danger and would be such a horrible catastrophe. I know that there was an old and desperate love affair, which was only confided to Mr Whitley Stokes. I should be glad to think that in a strange country and in the solitude which he must feel there was some solace for all his suffering'.[7] Mrs Green, a widow herself and gifted with intuitive powers which are particular to the feminine province, had forebodings, it would seem, which were realised at an early stage only to the extent that Meyer trimmed his familiar beard to a shape more in accord with his wife's wishes. She would prefer him without it, America being a land of the clean shaven where beards where the property of no respectable persons.

It would be of surpassing interest to know something about the old and desperate love affair which Meyer kept a secret from all but Stokes. Who was it he loved, how did it begin and when end? Was its end related to the change in his physical appearance when, from being 'the handsome, upright figure, fresh from his military training' which his pupil Eleanor Hull called to mind,[8] he became the bent and crippled figure that rheumatism left him? Or was there some other circumstance, now unknown to us, which may yet be brought to light in his diaries, which it is to be hoped have survived the vicissitudes of war and chance. It is an important chapter of Meyer's life, for the present secret from us and as far as we are aware, left unrecorded by Whitley Stokes, who alone could tell.

Anton Van Hamel, now lecturing in the University of Bonn, wrote to Best in high praise of his colleague Rudolf Thurneysen and his wife and wished Best could meet them. Van Hamel, visiting Berlin, called on Toni Meyer who showed him a picture of her recent sister-in-law, who appeared to be one of the loveliest creatures in the world. 'She is really handsome. He must be very happy in his married state. They passed their honeymoon in a lovely cottage near San Raphael in South California'.[9] Now they were returning to Frisco, where Meyer wanted to resume his lectures, 'on Celtic, of course' added Van Hamel innocently. Van Hamel surmised that the whole thing must have been a heavy blow for Toni, who however was courageous enough not to show any disappointment but partook of his happiness. It was tragic news that Hans Hessen, a promising young Celtist, had been killed the previous September. Pokorny went on etymologysing as always.

Van Hamel was probably right in thinking that Toni must have been disappointed at her brother's marriage. She was very close to him since his arthritis had set in about 1892, providing for his comfort, travelling with him everywhere, sharing his musical and literary interests. Van Hamel, at the crossroads between the warring nations, received and despatched much correspondence. He was bewildered at the behaviour of the 'National Volunteer', by whom he appears to mean John MacNeill. 'Poor man! Is this the result of a harmonious scholarlike life?' Fancy K.M. collaborating with Larkin! Who would be the next ally! This in reference to the activities in America of James Larkin and Meyer who, unlikely brethren, were united for now in their propaganda campaigns.[10] Meyer seemed to be in love with the New World. 'My happiness would be complete but for the war', he wrote to Van Hamel.[11]

Among those who wrote to the Meyers after their marriage was Gertrude Schoepperle of Urbana, whose admiration for Kuno was unbounded. Her letter, which is not available, was answered by Kuno's wife:

Dear Miss Schoepperle

The very first thing I shall do is to scold you for being so self-depreciative. ... My husband joins me in this 'scold' too and says you are not nearly as stupid as you would like to paint yourself. I can well believe it for it must take tremendous courage, perseverance, and no small amount of brains to decipher this almost dead language that you and Dr Meyer are so interested in and I am sure from all my husband tells me you will win some laurels yet. So, courage. As for me, I fear I can be of little help to my famous husband other than making him comfortable. Perhaps that will help some. When one is comfortable in mind and body I am sure one can do better work.

I too have led a very busy life and can well understand your not finding time to write.

You perhaps know I was a nurse for several years and that is indeed a very full life but very different from the one in which I now am placed. I am still slightly bewildered at the sudden change. You see I have always been a worker and now to be placed in a position of comparative idleness is, if not overwhelming, something to which I will have to adjust myself.

We expect to be in California perhaps a month longer. Will be in Chicago by the fifteenth of March where Dr Meyer will make his headquarters and then no doubt I will have the very great pleasure of meeting you and thanking you for your kindness to a stranger in a strange land.

Sincerely yours
Florence Meyer[12]

Later in the year Florence Meyer departed for Germany, taking her daughter with her. Presscuttings of early January 1917 tell us she was safe in a field hospital in Rumania, serving with the 9th army of Von

Mackensen, while her ten year old daughter was at school in Berlin. Meyer wrote to McGarrity:

1046 Lake Shore Drive
Chicago, Ill.
Oct. 8. 1916

My dear friend,
   My wife has gone to Berlin, where she intended to work under the Red Cross. I have no news from her since she cabled from Gothenburg in Sweden that she has safely arrived there.
   Postcards from Berlin written early in August and only arriving now speak with consternation and heartfelt sympathy of the tragic fate of our friend, who had made many warm friends there, especially among my family. Indeed my sister writes almost heartbroken, and says if I had been there I might have dissuaded him from his rash adventure.
   I have made Chicago my headquarters for the fall and till January, when I shall have to go to San Francisco. Is there any chance of a lecture or address in Philadelphia before that time? I subjoin a list of subjects, one or the other of which might suit.
   Let me hear from you. The Irish here are working splendidly hand in hand with the Germans.[13]

The list of subjects was -
The Life and Death of Sir Roger Casement
Ireland past and present
Germany and Ireland
The Golden Age of Irish civilisation
England and Germany before the war

It is interesting to speculate as to why his wife left him for Berlin after being married for less than a year. There may have been a variety of reasons. She could be of no practical help to him in his lectures and certainly shared none of his devotion to Irish literature. She may have found his unsettled state of life in going from one city to another difficult to adapt to. There was her young daughter, from whom she may not have wished to be separated and to whom the experience of moving from place to place would be upsetting. As one used to activity, she may have found it irksome to be placed in what she called a position of comparative idleness. Her nursing abilities would be useful in Germany. At any rate the change seems to have been made by mutual agreement. One cannot but think, however, that their time together was incongruously short.

Woodrow Wilson, not a man of war, on his re-election for a second term as President of the United States late in 1916, renewed his appeal to the belligerent nations for a negotiated peace, in which neither side would be victor. Neither side was willing to give way but on American relations with Germany taking a turn for the worse, Wilson broke off diplomatic contacts on 3 February 1917. Meyer touched on these events in writing to McGarrity on 25 March from Arrowhead Springs, California, where he was relaxing:

I have almost ceased to take any very excited interest in politics ... I often hear from my wife, who writes most cheerfully and confidently. Neither she nor I believe in a possible war between America and Germany. As to the feeling in

198

Germany she writes (imitating Lloyd George's pugilistic slang): 'Everybody in Germany prayed for the rejection of the peace offer. They are not ready for peace yet, not until they have licked the stuffing out of England.' It was as I expected and as I feel myself. I could not help telling Lloyd George of this (he is an old acquaintance of mine); he has humour enough, as a Welshman, to be amused at it ... This is a lovely place and a beautiful climate. I shall stay as long as possible, but must be back in St Louis for a lecture to the Irish there on April 21st. After that I shall again make Chicago my headquarters (1046 Lake Shore Drive).

Kindest greetings
Yours always sincerely
K.M.[14]

Meyer could not bring himself to believe in the break-off of diplomatic relations, not to speak of war, and declared to McGarrity that the German answer would 'take the wind out of W's sails'.[15] However the break-off was followed on 6 April 1917 by the entry of the United States into war, following a memorable speech to Congress by President Wilson. 'We are now about to accept gauge of battle'. No doubt Meyer was not relating fiction when he claimed to have sent a jocose comment to Lloyd George but equally Lloyd George was not amused to receive it and Meyer was presently to utter his conviction that he had to leave America through the intervention of the Welshman. Before leaving he wrote a final note to McGarrity:

1046 Lake Shore Drive
Chicago
April 28. 1917

My dear friend,

Just a line to thank you for your letter and to tell you that I have obtained safe conduct from the State Department to leave for Germany with the Austrian Embassy. Farewell, remember me to your wife and children, may we meet again in happier times. I carry away with me the pleasantest memories of your good will and kindness towards me, which I shall always cherish.

Yours ever sincerely
Kuno Meyer[16]

He was back in Germany in May. What had he accomplished by his stay in the United States? He had won a wife and step-daughter. The University of Illinois had published his *Miscellanea Hibernica,* a fifty-five page collection of brief texts, philological notes and explanations of Irish language terms. Whether his lectures on Irish literature bore fruit in the encouragement of students thereof does not appear. But he helped to some degree in the formation of a distinguished work of scholarship, *The Sources for the early history of Ireland,* and its author James F. Kenney has acknowledged his help: 'The late Kuno Meyer read a large part of the manuscript while it was still in relatively crude form. His kindly approbation is a treasured memory, and his suggestions and recommendations have contributed materially to the making of the book'.[17] This was certainly a service of value. His political propaganda achieved no success, patriotic though he was in the cause of his country, and his time and energy on it were a waste of his valuable talent. It is doubtful if he was happy at it.

NOTES

1. Meyer to McGarrity, 16 Oct. 1915, from San Rafael Cottage Hospital. NLI Ms No. 17465.
2. Meyer sued the Northwestern Pacific Railway Company for damages to the amount of $39,750 dollars. He alleged that because of the shock he sustained by being hurled against the wall of the car, an affection of the spine became aggravated. Because of the injuries he received there had resulted an immobile condition of the spine and neck, besides sustaining a monetary loss of $37,500 which he might have earned from lectures. A large amount of the damages asked for pertained to mental anguish and physical suffering caused by the train wreck. Meyer was represented by the firm of Sullivan, Sullivan and Roche.
   (Source: copy of American newscutting, no date or place, in envelope addressed to R.I. Best, National Library, Dublin, Ireland. NLI Ms No. 11,002 (69))
   The outcome of the proceedings is told in the following letter to McGarrity:

   > Arrowhead Springs Hotel
   > Arrowhead Springs
   > California
   > Mar 25th 1917

   My dear friend,
   I was so busy and worried with lawyers and doctors in S. Francisco that I have shamefully neglected my correspondence. At last, after many weary weeks, the Railroad Co. consented to a compromise and paid me 4000 dollars, of which sum 1,000 go to my lawyer, while the doctors behaved much more reasonably. I am glad to be done with it and have come here to enjoy a little rest and quiet and to take the baths. (NLI Ms No. 17465).
3. 5 Oct. 1915, from 36 Grosvenor Road, Westminster. NLI Ms No. 15114 (25).
4. By postcard 27.X.1915; Absender: A. Meyer Berlin-Wilmersdorf, Nassauische Str. 48. She sent the card to Van Hamel who wrote the additional paragraph dated Bonn 31.10.1915 and had it posted from neutral Rotterdam where it was postmarked 6.X.1915. It was addressed to Mrs Best, 57 Upper Leeson St., Dublin. NLI Ms No. 11002 (46).
5. Meyer was a Lutheran by faith. He mentioned this in a postcard to Best, reference to which has been regrettably mislaid.
6. NLI Ms No. 17629.
7. Mrs Green to Best, 26 Jan. 1916, from 36 Grosvenor Road, Westminster. NLI Ms No. 15114 (24).
8. *Irish Book Lover* XI, No. 5, Dec. 1919.
9. Van Hamel to Best. Postcard postmarked Amsterdam 24.11.1916. NLI Ms No. 11004.
10. Cf. Meyer to McGarrity, 9 Dec. 1914 – 'We had a great meeting at Brooklyn the other night, when Mr Devoy and Mr Larkin spoke splendidly. I am trying to gather some representative men to found a daily paper on the lines that Judge Cohalan suggested'. NLI Ms No. 17465.
11. Van Hamel to Best, 24 Feb. 1916. NLI Ms No. 11004.
12. Florence Meyer to Gertrude Schoepperle, undated but from internal evidence written February 1916, on headed paper of Hotel Stewart, San Francisco. NLI Ms No. 11001 (19).
13. NLI Ms No. 17629.
14. Meyer to McGarrity, 25 March 1917, from Arrowhead Springs Hotel, Arrowhead Springs, California. First part of this letter quoted earlier. NLI Ms No. 17465.
15. Meyer to McGarrity, 24 April [1917], from Plaza Hotel, Chicago. NLI Ms No. 17629.
16. NLI Ms No. 17629.
17. Kenney, *The Sources for the early history of Ireland: Ecclesiastical* (Columbia University Press 1929), Preface ii.

Chapter 20

KUNO Meyer was back in Berlin on 20 May 1917.[1] The war still raging, he resumed his activities on behalf of the Fatherland, visiting the front repeatedly, especially German headquarters in France, giving many lectures all over Germany and Austria, only retiring from the scene when Germany surrendered and signed an armistice on 11 November 1918. It was now a contrast to the euphoric days of November 1914 when he had set out for America. The Emperor whom he had looked up to and in whose honour he had as a student composed poems of praise had abdicated and taken refuge in Holland. Nearly two million Germans had been killed in the war and millions more wounded. The Allies continued to blockade Germany long after the conflict had ended, causing starvation, further death and widespread misery.

The Irish-German aristocrat Count Harry Kessler has recorded in his fascinating diary the scenes and spirit of the times. One reads in the entry for 4 August 1919: 'Five years ago!... Only five years ago, but a century lies between then and now. A different world'.

Berlin in 1919 was a grim and cheerless place, cold, hungry, miserable, racked with influenza. Society was shattered by the impact of military defeat, and deeply divided against itself. The capital witnessed strikes, demonstrations and other turbulence. Minor civil wars were fought in the streets. Two million soldiers had marched back from the field into the milieu of a stunned and confused country. The armistice terms were harsh and crippling. Mutiny broke out in the navy. There was revolution in Munich.

It was against this background that Kuno and Toni Meyer resumed correspondence with their friends, especially the Bests and Mrs Green, towards mid-1919, communication up to then being impossible owing to the blockade. Meyer had persistently been trying to get messages through, via Holland, Switzerland and Scandinavia, without success.

At last one of his letters, dated 11 April 1919,[2] got through to Best. The news he told of himself was that he had settled down to regular work again. A reference to Marstrander was cool. His book on the Hittites was received critically by learned colleagues of Meyer who considered its author too hasty and eager to obtain a result where none was to be had as yet. Ernst Windisch had died peacefully. Only the day before his death he was busy with the proofs of his History of Indian Philology. Toni was staying with old friends, the Boedikkers, near Hamburg. His brother Eduard's great study of Caesar and Pompey, out since Christmas and already in a second edition, was being avidly studied, and annotated, with reference mainly to recent events, by 'a certain august personage' now taking a holiday in Holland.[3] His wife would probably visit America and he might go with her, once the way was open. Of his wife's industry he had much praise. She had translated into English no less than three large novels of Gustav Meyrink,[4] a cousin of his own whom he describes as 'illegitimate', besides having taken singing lessons from a good master. Summer term in Berlin University would begin in May. He expected huge classes.

Mrs Green was a favourite correspondent with whom he could be always relaxed. He wrote to her London address, unaware that she had gone to live in Dublin, sending the letter through Van Hamel's Rotterdam address, 246a N. Binnenweg, and hoped for a reply. The news he had for her was of a kind that she would cheerfully receive, for he was now busier than ever before at his Irish studies. She for her part had always believed these were his true metier. He promised to send her what he had published when the ways were open again. He was now printing his 'Fragments of ancient Irish lyrical poetry', a large collection of poems of the most varied contents, laudatory, satirical, laments, nature and religious, which would comprise two volumes, with translation and notes.[4a] His students were mostly interned at Ruhleben, a racecourse used as prison camp, not far from Berlin, where they established a little School of Celtic Learning. One of them had since been made lecturer in German at Birmingham. This was David Evans, who spoke of many kindnesses received from Meyer during his internment, and was to say that 'We Celts have lost part of our soul if we do not acknowledge him for the man he was'. Meyer proposed to write to Mrs Green again when he heard that this had safely reached her. 'With kindest regards and remembrances'.[5]

At the end of July he was surprised to find on his table a letter in Best's familiar hand, the first for a long time, which had reached him, unbelievably, in four days. Relieved and happy he answered it at once, confessing that he had often felt like Noah sending out the dove in the hope that it would return in the shape of an acknowledgement, so many letters and pages had he sent through various countries to Best of which next to nothing seemed to have reached him. He forwarded Best's letter to Toni in Hamburg, knowing that she too would be delighted. He had a long letter from Gertrude Schoepperle who had left Urbana. German-Americans were coming over in large numbers. He would ask Best to remember him to Vendryes, but he did not know if 'the old man' was friendly.[6] Vendryes indeed was not friendly, far from it.

Best replied on 8 August by postcard which reached Meyer on the 11th. Meyer answered at once with a discursive letter.

My dear Best,

Your card of the 8th came today, which is even quicker than last time and almost like pre-war times. As I have just finished a paper on old-Irish river names etc. for a Festschrift for my old teacher Wilh. Braune at Heidelberg, and my wife

has gone to Switzerland on a visit to a niece of mine at Bern (she is at the Embassy there), I feel particularly well disposed for a long letter, which you richly deserve. I do not know how many of my missives from America have reached you nor whether any of my cards sent via Holland and Scandinavia have been allowed through; it does not seem likely, as the papers have been held back. Some of these I now send you. If you have them already give them to Hyde or MacNeill ....
Thurneysen is also in Switzerland at present. Windisch's chair was a purely Sanskrit one and has been filled with some one whom neither you nor I know. The younger generation of scholars I have not kept up with. My brother has just been chosen Rector of the University. He will have a very busy and controversial year, as many reforms are imminent. Fortunately it will also be a very remunerative one. As this is going to be a gossipy letter, there will not be much logical sequence in it. I should be sorry to see such a low cad as T.L. in an important chair. When you write again you must tell me what has become of O'Malley, O'Keeffe and others. I am more disappointed in Marstrander than I can tell. His conceit I was familiar with, but I thought he would do brilliant work. Instead of that it is cheap, unsound to a rare degree, and wasteful. Everybody here laughs at the presumption and absurdity of his Herbitic (?) book. I am going to write to the R.I.A. tonight to propose the continuation of my 'Contributions'. Perhaps when they meet after the holidays they can decide at once. For I am determined to go on with it one way or another. The Berlin Academy will give a grant if I ask them, and Niemeyer is also ready to go on. By sitting up late, which seems to agree with me, I contrive to do a lot more work than in my best years. But one must make hay while the sun shines. I am president of two important political societies and have a good deal of work to do in connexion with that, also to write for the press, both in German and English, with the assistance of my wife. And at present I am overrun with American visitors, both friends and friends of theirs who come with letters of recommendation. That Miss Schoepperle has given up Urbana I think I told you. America is not the country for her. As to the young lady who wishes to come to Berlin, I should be very pleased to have her as a student, though she must not expect regular courses, which I have almost given up. My best student now is also a lady, a Miss Miller, who before the war began her studies with Flower. She translates very prettily from Modern Irish and has brought out several books, for which there is an incredible demand in Germany, as indeed there never has been such writing of books as just now. Miss M. is working at the *Agallamh Beg* (Book of Lismore) ... When I was in France in 1917 I gave a carefully planned lecture on Ireland, which the Crown Prince attended and which I have since often held throughout the length and breadth of Germany and Austria, but not yet printed, as I intend to do shortly.... My sister, who sends your wife and yourself her kindest regards, will probably make her home in Hamburg, where she is very happy with plenty of relations and old friends. My brother and his wife are going to visit her this week. I have to stay here till the house question is settled. We have to move on Oct 1st and do not yet know where, as there is great difficulty in getting a suitable flat.

Here I was interrupted and cannot go on. But I will write again soon ...

Yours always
K.M.[7]

He wanted to consult Best about the two portraits of himself, one by Siegfried Wiens and the other by Augustus John, both his rightful property but now in the keeping of the University Club in Liverpool to which he had left them on loan. He confessed he did not care for either of them, nor did Toni, and he would willingly part with them, by gift if no way else, but preferably by sale.[8]

The letter to Mrs Green, which he had speculatively entrusted to the post, arrived in due course at her Dublin address. She, who admired him so much, was no doubt delighted to get it and wrote back on 11 August a letter which took ten days to reach him and put him in a happy frame of mind for having picked up again a valued thread of his former life. Unfortunately her letter is not available. But Meyer's acknowledgement, immediately written, is and gives an account of his interests and projects, among which one notes again his offer to the Royal Irish Academy to continue his *Contributions to Irish Lexicography.*

My dear Mrs Green,

Your letter of August 11th reached me this afternoon just as my old friend Prof. Schiemann was sitting with me, who participated in my delight at seeing your handwriting once more after so long a time, and learning that you are as active in your studies as ever. He begs to be remembered very warmly to you. He has just brought out his last (4th) volume of the life history of Nicolas 1, and is now engaged in writing his memoirs.

That you have exchanged London for Dublin (like Geo. Moore) was news to me. I would give much to be able to look in upon you and my friends there, as well as upon the Mss. It is a great thing that the transcripts of Wh. Stokes, about 70 volumes, are now deposited (by Windisch's bequest) in the Library of Leipzig University. At the beginning of the war an Irish society was formed here, who have published a wide series of literary and historical tracts, also translations from the Irish. I am one of the presidents and mean to develop it still further next winter. But I am afraid our youth here have other things to study and work at now. The classes at the University here are full as they never were (we had 13,000 students last winter) and my course, delivered in English, on the races and languages of Gt. Britain and Ireland was very well attended. But not a single s u-dent turned up for Welsh grammar, which I had announced, and I am afraid it will be the same with Irish. I am glad to hear that R. Flower is working at the history of Irish Literature. Thurneysen has a vol. ready on the Cuchulinn saga (its literary tradition) and is active in other ways too. See that *Ériu* comes out regularly. I wonder what the R.I.A. will do about my offer to continue the Contributions. I could easily get funds for it from the Academy here who have just had an enormous legacy (M175,000) from Emil Fischer, the famous chemical professor who died not long ago. I shall also try to interest the newly founded University of Hamburg (my native place) for Celtic studies. So you see there is plenty to do. My wife has learned to sing Irish songs to perfection – she has got a strong Irish strain in her – and will sing publicly next winter at various concerts. For a lecture on Ireland which I have prepared I should like a good collection of slides, which is not easy to be had here. Perhaps later on Best or some other friend may procure one for me.[9]

Further letters to Richard Best indicated that his life was in no way immune from the hardship of the times:

My dear Best,

Your letter written on Goethe's birthday reached me this morning and it would seem that you also got my various missives, so that one can write you with greater confidence. We are at present in a somewhat unsettled state, but I must snatch a few minutes to answer your questions. As to the portrait, nothing would please me better than your proposal; but the thing is at present in the hands of a gentleman called, I believe, the public receiver, which has also got hold of all other property of mine, amounting to about £1,200, just as my American money and that of my wife is in the hands of a similar functionary there. This is a terrible loss to us, amounting to over 200,000 marks at the present rate of exchange, and that will explain to you why I want to sell. But there is no hurry. The thieving will probably continue for a long time. It has, as you know, already extended to copyright. I shall therefore publish in Germany only, even English books, and bring out among other things a new edition of my 'Ancient Poetry' here. So make whatever arrangement you can with the University Club, Liverpool, where the 2 portraits are stored, I believe. That they were removed to the cellar or garret at the outbreak of the war I was duly informed by good friends ...

No, I have not seen the edition of *Leb. Gab*. Bergin continues to be a great disappointment to me. I suppose it is physical. I am sorry you had such a poor holiday. We have now made up our minds that my wife and daughter go to Switzerland (Bern, where I have a niece), for the winter, while I go into lodgings or stay with by brother, making the Academy, which has placed a room at my disposal, my workshop. The furniture will be stored, and partly sold. By the way, for people with English and American or indeed any other money Germany is now a paradise of cheapness. One dollar is worth at least 16 marks, so that even the big prices here seem ridiculously small to an American ... Berlin is of course the dearest place. We pay 23 marks for a pound of butter, which you can get for 16 marks elsewhere, and still cheaper in the country ....

Kindest greetings
K.M.[10]

I must write again about the portrait. I hear from our Govt that there is a law in England which makes all transactions or even correspondence about the property of alien enemies illegal. That is the reason probably why my bankers, publishers and other debtors don't answer. Find out and act or don't act accordingly. All these things are very bewildering and to a layman unintelligible, besides America follows again a different plan, it seems.... Gaidoz has just sent me his long necrologue on Rhys, a very gossipy and feeble performance. Heaven preserve me from falling into that fault in my old age! So far I only notice the tendency to repeat myself, but through underfeeding the memory has suffered even with men like my brother, who had a most retentive and ready memory before. My wife has already got her passport for Switzerland, and I have secured a perfectly beautiful room at the Academy, or rather two, so that I can both work and sleep there, with a balcony and every modern comfort. I shall convey my whole library there, which I hope, if the Spartakists[11] should storm the building again as they did last year, will be spared. There is a fixed belief that we are in for another revolution, as conditions are intolerable, another reason for sending my wife and daughter away. As I pointed out in an article to the only English paper appearing in Germany, our enemies by crushing us so mercilessly have destroyed the bulwork that has for centuries preserved Western Europe from the lawless eastern hordes. That lawlessness and brutal ferocity are now rapidly spreading in a country hitherto lawabiding, peaceful and orderly par excellence. Berlin is of course its hotbed, but Leipzig, Munich, Halle, in fact most larger cities, Hamburg and Bremen especially, are quite as bad, and as our army is now going to be reduced to a ridiculous number, we shall be at the mercy of these elements. So do hatred, revenge and ignorance blind to the most glaring facts. Fortunately the card is full.

K.M.[12]

To Edith Best he wrote that his sister Toni's address was Haller Strasse 16, Hamburg.

She will indeed be delighted to hear from you. She is much depressed and still suffering from the shock and grief of Aug 3rd, 1916, which was the death blow of her hopes in more senses than one. They had become very fond of one another, and she blames herself for many sins of omission. If I only had been here! Things would have taken a very different turn. For my influence over him was great.[13]

205

Her husband's letter of 24 August had only come that morning, with its description of Wicklow scenery which made him long for a visit to Ireland. The literature on Ireland published in Germany in recent years was immense. Amongst others, Pokorny had written a good sketch of Irish history. Meyer promised to collect what he could and send it. He wished to be remembered to the Geoghegans, both families, if they didn't mind, to Miss Purser and other good friends, also of course her brother and his wife, who must have suffered much.[13]

He wrote to Best thanking him for his delightful long letter which he was unable at present to answer as fully as he would like because he was sorting out his library, part of which he was going to sell. He was preparing to pack up. Things in Germany looked pretty calm at present, but as soon as the army was dissolved there would be worse doings than in November and January last and it behoved them all to prepare for it. His wife and daughter were going to leave Berlin for Switzerland by the end of the month, though that meant a terrible drain on his income, as they had to pay four marks for one franc. However, by selling most of the furniture, etc., they would manage to live a little longer from hand to mouth, which was the only thing they could do now. He had just heard that the public receivers of stolen goods both in America and England would not again part with their spoil. 'Knowing what caused this war I had not really supposed they would do so.' He had letters from Joseph Dunn and several other American friends and Robin Flower had sent him the *Dánta Grádha,* a pretty little volume.[14]

A letter from Best of 5 September reached him on the 9th, giving him heart that a regular correspondence could be carried on once more. He answered it at once, while his daughter Margaret was busy playing an easy Beethoven sonata and his wife was mending socks that had been mended a dozen times before. Margaret and his wife were leaving by the end of the month to get into Switzerland, if possible, and if not, to Bavaria where they would stay with Meyer's novelist cousin Gustav Meyrink. 'You ask about my health. On the whole the spare dish has done people with rheumatism and gout good, but at times it got too spare and one lost weight and strength appallingly. Whoever fell ill in that condition, no matter from what disease, was a dead man.'

Things had now improved somewhat. Curiously enough he was able to work hard, and by preference late at night until 1 or 2 p.m., after which he always slept soundly. But his wife had lost weight terribly and would have to try and recover under better conditions. His sister and brother never felt better physically than during the war. Such different effects it all had.[15]

NOTES

1. Cf. biographical essay by his brother Eduard Meyer in *Irische Korrespondenz* (Berlin, October-November MCMXIX), p. 4, col. 2.
2. NLI Ns No 11002.
3. The reference is to Kaiser Wilhelm II.

4.   Gustav Meyrink was the pseudonym of Gustav Meyer, novelist, b. Vienna 1868, d. Starnberg 1932. He lived for many years in Prague and became a convert from Protestantism to Buddhism. Writer of grotesque fantasy tales, his best known novel is *Der Golem* (1915), based on his Prague experiences. Kuno Meyer, in his letter of 9.9.1919 to Best, says his wife has been translating his books and was looking out for an English or American publisher. 'His novels have passed through countless editions (*Der Golem, Das grüne Gesicht,* etc.). I will ask Niemeyer about the price of back volumes.'

4a. Only one volume of this project appeared, the *Bruchstücke der älteren Lyrik Irlands,* containing 167 fragments, with translation by Meyer, Berlin 1919.

5.   Meyer to Mrs Green, 13 July 1919. NLI Ms No. 15091 (3). The beginning of this letter, referring to Sir Roger Casement, has been quoted earlier.

6.   Meyer to Best, 30 July 1919, from Nassauische Str. 48 II. NLI Ms No. 11002.

7.   Meyer to Best, 11 Aug. 1919 from Nassauische Str. 48 II. NLI Ms No. 11002.

8.   Meyer to Best, 17 Aug. 1919, postmarked Wilmersdorf, Berlin, NLI Ms No. 11002.

9.   Meyer to Mrs Green, 21 Aug. 1919, from Nassauische Str. 48 II. NLI Ms No. 15091 (1).

10. Meyer to Best, 2 Sept. 1919. NLI Ms No. 11002.

11. The reference is to the Spartakusbund, a radical socialist movement formed in Berlin in November 1918.

12. Meyer to Best, by postcard 5 Sept. 1919. NLI Ms No. 11002.

13. Meyer to Mrs R.I. Best, National Library Dublin, by postcard postmarked Berlin 5 Sept. 1919. NLI Ms No. 11002.

14. Meyer to Best, 6 Sept. 1919. NLI Ms No. 11002. The *Dánta Grádha* referred to was the earlier, Dublin 1916, issue, edited by Thomas F. O'Rahilly, with an Introduction by Robin Flower.

15. Meyer to Best, 9 Sept. 1919. NLI Ms No. 11002.

Chapter 21

KUNO Meyer missed the friendly pre-war society which he so relished, and there was a sense of yearning in the many efforts he made to get in touch with former friends in his desire to re-establish something of the old carefree companionship. He was not exaggerating when he said he lived as much in the past as in the present and it was this past which he tried to recover. An old friend of Liverpool days was John Smyth MacDonald (1867-1941), a distinguished member of the University Medical Faculty, to whom Meyer wrote in nostalgic vein, remembering the times that were and contrasting them with present realities:

> My dear Mac,
>   It was just such another gloriously fine September a quarter of a century ago when we went agypsying in Wales. As I live quite as much in the past now as in the nauseating present, my thoughts often go back to that time and the friends with whom I spent it, some of them my friends no longer. They did not adopt old Mackay's maxim when the war broke out which was 'Politics apart – friendship as ever'.

He enquired about former colleagues. Was Mair still alive? Edgar Browne and H.A. Strong he believed were dead. Did Sampson, Wyld, Raleigh, Elton lose any of their sons in the war? He wished to be remembered to any other friends who might care for him.[1]

Jean MacDonald remembered well the day the above letter arrived, at breakfast time, and her father's sense of helplessness on reading it, not knowing what he wanted to do or what he should do. 'I think the discovery of Kuno Meyer's political activities was one of the greatest blows he had suffered. Not because he disapproved of them, but because he had no idea they were going on.' Her father used to say that he thought the Meyer of New York and California was different to the Meyer he knew in Liverpool. But he was unshaken in his admiration for Meyer, no matter what the circumstances. 'He was a man.'[2]

The world was opening up. More letters were arriving, renewing former links. One from Douglas Hyde told of the death of Father Edmund Hogan, compiler of the *Onomasticon Hibernicum,* whose labours on the great repository of Irish placenames, virtually a companion to Holder's *Altkeltischer Sprachschatz,* was highly praised by Meyer, leaving him now with regret that he never had the opportunity to let Father Hogan know his appreciation. A project of his own was to print in the next *Zeitschrift* all the remaining poems, an enormous batch, from Laud 615. Looking through old papers he saw from a diary of his first visit to Ireland in 1879 that he wrote some verses in the visitors' book of the Dublin University Philosophical Society, where he had been introduced by the president, Mr. Green. In going through his Celtic books he found a large number of duplicates, of which he proposed sending Best a list as they might be useful to students forming a library. Martin Conway, now Head of the War Museum and M.P. for the new universities, had just written him a splendid letter. How differently did the war affect different people.[3] Himself and Florence were getting ready to leave Nassauische Strasse 48[II] which had been their home in Berlin. 'We are now beginning to pack up.'

They were to move on the 28th and 29th September, after which Meyer's address would be Lichterfelde, Mommsen Strasse 7/8. He was selling a huge quantity of English literature, including hundreds of Tauchnitz editions. They were giving some little farewell parties which were very cosmopolitan. His wife would go to Munich to stay with Professor M. Bonn, as Switzerland for the present would be out of the question owing to the rapidly devaluing mark. Meyer planned to travel a little in October as he had not a holiday in a long time.[4] He enclosed with his letter for Best a short article of his own from the *Continental Times* of 16 September 1919 entitled 'The treatment of German missionaries by the Allies' which might interest Catholic Ireland, a copy of which he had sent to his 'old friend Lloyd George.' It contained the accusation that Roman Catholic priests, lay brothers and sisters engaged in peaceful and sacred work in Africa and the South Seas had been imprisoned throughout the war and had their property and effects confiscated. Meyer indicted 'professing Christians like Lloyd George and Wilson' as being responsible while he praised the Society of Friends which alone had come to their rescue and help.[5] Maud Joynt had written him and he mentions a charming letter from Mrs Green. In his few leisure moments he was working on *Tochmarc Treblainne*.

Richard Best had grown a beard. He sent Meyer his photograph. Youthful, thought Meyer, but critically, more characteristic without and, talking about beards, his wife and daughter who, as true Americans, connected beards with the riffraff of their nation, or emigrants just arrived, always wished him to lay aside his. He was planning many works, both in German and English, but it would take too long to speak about them now. The most interesting letters he got came from America, where the German element was making every effort to recover its position, politically and in other ways. In Germany numerous newspapers and periodicals were being started and they all wanted him to write for them and the fact was he could make a living as a pamphleteer. He had just written for the *Norddeutsche Allgemeine Zeitung* an article on the present situation of the Irish problem, in his capacity as president of the Deutsch-Irische Gesellschaft. Henri Gaidoz had written him, a touching postcard, dictated, as he could not see, and was awaiting an operation for cataract. Why Vendryes should not continue to be friendly with Thurneysen, for instance, passed Meyer's understanding. Surely one should distinguish. A fellow like Quiggin he could give up easily. 'I always thought him a poor, mean, low creature. When he first called on me at New Brighton, he lay in wait for the first mistake I should make in English, and when (as he wrongly thought, showing he did not know his mother tongue) I had made one, he actually jumped up in glee from his chair and told me so!'[6] Best would try and soften Meyer's antipathy to Quiggin.

A letter just arrived from Mrs Green had much praise for Eoin MacNeill's *Phases of Irish History* of which Meyer hoped to be sent a copy.[6a] Meyer, in reply to an observation of Best's, wished he could get workers for an Irish dictionary on the same scale as Erman had for the Egyptian. Theodor Schiemann, at present on the isle of Rügen and wonderfully active for his 74 years, had just finished the 4th and last volume of his Life and Times of Nicholas I, of which Meyer had read the proofs for him. There was a pressing problem about the attitude to Germany of the foreign Academies and Institutes which had broken off relations with her, refused to exchange publications, wanted back the money deposited with Germany as the headquarters of the international Cartel and forbade German learned bodies to work on their territory. This hit very hard at geologists, astronomers and geographers, making much useful work impossible. Hermann Diels, the great authority on the presocratic philosophers, presided at the Academy discussion on the problem which challenged even his genius. 'The worst cases are those in which our enemies have simply stolen our collections, instruments, etc. Fancy if that had happened to me'.[8]

His wife was looking forward to her villeggiatura in Switzerland, where he felt sure she would recover soon. They had found the means for her to stay there rather than in Bavaria after all. She wrote splendid English, but like George Moore she lacked grammatical training. 'Warmest greetings to you both'.[8]

With five minutes to spare he answered a card just arrived from Best, promising to send him all duplicates once he had settled in at the Academy, and leaving himself in Best's hands with regard to the portrait by John. Toni was due from Hamburg on the morrow (25 September) and on Sunday his wife and daughter would leave for Munich. His English friends were beginning to write to him again, not only Flower, but Sir Martin Conway, Walter Raleigh, Mr Muspratt and others.[9]

Two days later he wrote to Mrs Green what turns out to be his last message and testament to Irish Celtic scholars.

My dear Mrs Green,

I am waiting to hear from Miss Bo'Acher(?)[10] to whom I wrote at once, before I shall send off this letter. It does look as if she were dead or gone somewhere else, or I should have heard before this. But my letter has not been returned.

We are packing up. I believe the result of my homelessness will be that I shall once more lead a wandering life. That my work does not suffer under it I think has been shown by my output of various papers during my American trip and the constant travelling since my return here. All my notes on *Saltair na Rann* I wrote on American railroad cars from New York to San Francisco and back again, and the lyrical fragments I translated on similar journeys here to headquarters in France and back to the East front or to Vienna. The circumstance that there is no other Celtologist in Berlin, and that I find it hard to get students, who have more important things to do, also makes me eager to get away from Berlin to Giessen where Professor Hirt has taken up Irish, or to Bonn, to chat with Thurneysen or to Vienna where Pokorny represents Austrian Celtology in solitary grandeur or confinement. When I was in America Roosevelt, who believed then that the war would soon be over, talked of a Celtic campaign with me and was really in earnest about it. But now poor Miss Schoepperle has been driven from Urbana, and all her and my plans for a great Celtic library, museum, etc., have come to nothing. They may say what they like, but Wissenschaft is only understood and honoured in Germany by the people, and as a matter of course; but now that the nation is thoroughly unsettled, half paralysed, uncertain of the morrow, and largely demoralised, it will not be easy to keep up the tradition.

As to the slides, what I should like is (1) ancient remains of all kinds (2) architecture and (3) a few samples of scenery thrown in. Can you let me have Mrs Boothby's address? What has become of Annie Stokes, I wonder? Early in October the first cargo boat from Hamburg starts for Ireland, but it has to touch England (Falmouth or Bristol); I should like to go disguised as a steward or coalie, but they would not let me land.

If you could influence the little band of Irish students in Dublin to publish and translate more from the Mss than they do, that would be the most valuable service you could render them. They somehow all need some one to I wont say enthuse them, but to make them work a little more systematically – Bergin above all, but also Miss Knott, Miss Joynt (who might do much good work), Best, O'Malley – indeed every one of them. Hyde is the only one who in spite of diffidence in matters philological is not afraid to go into print. Why should the others?'[11]

Thurneysen had a big instalment of an Abhandlung on the tradition of the Cuchullin saga nearly ready. Pokorny was working at an Old-Irish Reader much needed for teaching and private study. 'I have more plans than I can put down in a letter, and hope that some of them will mature next winter and spring'.[12] He would not begin lecturing in Berlin until January, as a Zwischensemester was devoted solely to the needs of 'our returned warriors, of whom there will be probably something like 18,000 at our University alone'.[13]

Before posting the above Meyer waited another day, hoping to hear from Miss Bo'Acher, but nothing had come. When he found time he would have inquiries made at the address. Mrs Green's card of the 24th came promptly that morning to Lichterfelde, whence Toni had just brought it. 'I must close now in order to devote the whole afternoon to packing'. The date was 29 September.

Toni Meyer had come from Hamburg to help in the task of moving. When that difficult business had been finished, and Kuno's wife and daughter had set out for Switzerland and Kuno himself, badly in need of a holiday, had set out for Weimar, Toni sat down and wrote to Edith Best a letter which tells us beyond any doubt of a state of unhappiness that existed in Kuno Meyer's household.

211

My dear Edith

I was so glad to hear from you again after this long sad interval of enforced silence. My thoughts have often gone out to you and it is a relief to know that both you and your husband are well. I have just gone through a very harassing time as I came here to help winding up our old household. Thank God it is over now, and Kuno has gone off on a ten days holiday to Weimar. His wife and her little daughter are on their way to Switzerland where they are going to stay with a niece of ours. I am afraid this marriage has been a very foolish affair and it has spoiled more than one life. But fortunately it has not crushed his spirit and he is very keen on going on with his work. I wish I could say as much of myself. My life is very unsettled and so far I do not know yet what sort of work I am going to take up. I mean to go back to Hamburg at the end of this month where I have many kind relatives and friends, especially a dear cousin who is left alone in her old age in spite of being a mother of eight children....

As you will gather from my address, I am now staying with my brother Eduard who has been appointed 'Rektor' to the University for the ensuing year. He is going to take up his new duties on October 15th, and I hope to be present at the ceremony. It will be a very busy year for him, but he is in very good form, I am glad to say ....

With kindest regards to both you and your husband.

Yours affectionately
Toni Meyer[14]

The sad, serious, truth was revealed. Kuno's marriage to Florence Lewis was a total failure. Perhaps after all Mrs Green had divined from the outset that the union was imprudent and not destined to survive. How too are we to explain the virtual separation which took place in the United States within less than a year of their marriage? Far from friends, in a strange country, recovering from the shock of injuries and cared for by a nurse who possessed physical attraction to a high degree, Kuno Meyer found himself in an emotionally vulnerable position to which resistance, in the circumstances, was beyond his capacity or will, to which, indeed, he gave acceptance with a happy mind. It is easy in the aftermath to consider it hasty and ill-advised. Even so mature a heart as his was not amenable to cool reason.

Yet in the whole of his correspondence, there is not the veriest hint, not the shadow of a suggestion, that the marriage was other than a happy one. References to his wife, her singing ability, the quality of her English, and other things, are such as might be expected from a domestic milieu in which all was harmony. The real state of affairs was thoroughly concealed from the outer world. It must have made for tension and unhappiness. Toni speaks of being through a very harassing time as she came to help winding up their old household. One can imagine the stresses felt by all and understand Toni's fervent 'Thank God' when it was over. If further confirmation is needed, it will be found stated, briefly and clearly, in a letter to Richard Best from Meyer's former German assistant Schaafs which, though written at a later time, may suitably be quoted from here – 'Do you know that K's marriage had never been a very happy one and that his wife's departure for Berne was a step preliminary to a divorce? It is a sad thought that the last months of his noble life should have been filled with anger and sorrow'.[15] One cannot easily associate anger with Kuno Meyer but that he had sorrow to endure cannot be in doubt.

NOTES

1. Meyer to John Smyth MacDonald, 10 Sept. 1919 from Nassauische Str. 48 II Berlin. NLI Ms No. 3890.
2. Jean MacDonald to Professor Gerard Murphy, 18 Feb. (1950) from Heronhill, Hawick, Roxburghshire. NLI Ms No. 3890.
3. Meyer to Best, postcard, postmark Berlin-Wilmersdorf 11 Sept. 1919. NLI Ms No. 11002.
4. Meyer to Best, by letter, postmark Berlin-Wilmersdorf 11 Sept. 1919. NLI Ms No. 11002.
5. Copy of article in NLI Ms No. 11002 (70).
6. Meyer to Best, 23 Sept. 1919. NLI Ms No. 11002.
6a. There was occasional correspondence between Meyer and MacNeill originating as far back at least as the early years of the Gaelic League. Meyer tells MacNeill he expects the first number of his new review to be out in December (1895), a slightly premature expectation, and MacNeill thanks him for *Imram Brain,* the Voyage of Bran, which he would 'commend strongly to his readers' of the *Gaelic Journal.* 'I am glad' MacNeill writes, 3 Dec. 1908, 'you are going to review *Duanaire Finn*' edited by MacNeill for the Irish Texts Society. 'So far, I have seen no intelligent criticism of it. You will let me know when you have reviewed it and where, and remember I am in nowise thin-skinned and can manage to care for nothing but elucidation' (MacNeill Papers, NLI Ms No. 10882). Meyer in his review in the ZCP (VII) 524 was in fact critical, as he was in a position of authority to be as editor of *Fianaigecht,* a text with introduction of basic importance to students of Fiannaíocht. While Meyer did not live to read MacNeill's *Phases of Irish History* his appreciation of MacNeill's learning grew with the years and he remarked on receiving many pages of learned correspondence from MacNeill his wonder that MacNeill did not entrust such important matter to print. The following letter from Meyer is the kind of commerce that passes only between scholar and scholar:

Verona
Hotel Londres
29.3.1911

My dear MacNeill,

Your interesting letter of the 16th came at a very busy time, or I should have answered it at once. I have just read it again, and after a morning spent in seeing the sights of Verona and before I leave for Padua I cannot employ the interval better than by transporting myself into the early centuries of Irish history, a chaos which I hope you will soon clear up for us. Meanwhile what Zimmer has achieved is I think shortly the follow[ing].

(1) He has shown that the Roman and Greek [accounts] of British and Irish customs are not mere travellers' tales about imaginary barbarians – as Rhys once called them – but *mutatis mutandis* to be accepted as founded on facts.

(2) He has further shown that these accounts refer in the first instance not to the Celt, but to the non-Aryan aboriginal population.

(3) He infers from early Irish tradition as shown in the heroic sagas that some of these customs had entered into Irish civilisation. Here he might have chosen far better examples, but his reading was almost wholly confined to TBC., F.B. and a few other similar texts. I look upon his investigations only as the beginning of much fuller work on similar lines. Thus, to mention one thing, he has never touched upon the custom of fosterage, which is the necessary concomitant of polyandry.

So far, I imagine, you agree. How far the Irish went in adopting any of these foreign customs remains to be seen. For many reasons it would have been natural that they should have done so. Had not the Ptolemies, in order to establish themselves on the throne of Egypt, to adopt from the Pharaohs the custom of marriage with the sister? And this brings me to your point of breeding domestic animals as a model for such adelphous or other incestuous matings. Is it not rather the idea that the highest and best born can only mate with their absolute equals? And if you confine this idea to the clan or the family you get of necessity incest.

I am now looking through Zimmer's *Nachlass*. Many ideas are unfortunately only thrown out. Sometimes you have to guess from a single word what was in his mind. Thus in connection with matriarchy he quotes the Welsh *rhieni* 'parents' = Ir. rígnai, i.e. the notion 'parents' developed from the queen-mother. I wish I could find out the exact meaning of derb n., gen. deirbe (once in Tigernach), later der, dar. It still eclipses in Derbhforgaill, also dergertne (Ferchertne mac Dergertne, Tochm. Ferbe). Derbráthair and derbshiur must be much older than the use of bráthair for a monk. …

Lately I have been busy with Irish metrics and found a lot of new things, which I hope to embody in a pamphlet. Two are of greater importance. First, I have found a number of very old poems standing half-way between the oldest alliterative rhythmic poetry and the later syllabic metres. They are alliterative and rhythmical, but rhyme. No definitive number of syllables is required. Fortunately they are all on the whole well preserved. Secondly, I discovered that for so-called assonance or consonance (as Thurneysen would have us say) or secondary rhyme (as Strachan called it) or *uaithne* (as Molloy says) the chief requisite hitherto wholly overlooked is the agreement of the assonating words in the *quantity* of their syllables. This enables one to correct mistakes in almost every poem hitherto published, notably Fél Óing., Gorman etc.

But I must end. That Mrs Zimmer has cashed the cheque you will have heard.

Marstrander will I hope soon leave for Riviera where I shall meet him after having finished a course of mud baths at Battaglia (Hotel delle Terme) presso Padova, where I am going for 3 weeks to-day..

With kind greetings
Yours always sincerely
Kuno Meyer

(MacNeill papers. NLI Ms No. 10882).

7. *Ibid.*
8. *Ibid.*
9. Meyer to Best, by postcard 24 Sept. 1919. NLI Ms No. 11002.
10. Miss Bo'Acher. The reference may be to the manageress or proprietress of a hotel at which Meyer planned to stay.
11. Meyer to Mrs A.S. Green, 26 Sept. 1919, addressed from Berlin-Lichterfelde, Mommsenstrasse 7/8. NLI Ms No. 15091 (1).
12. *Ibid.*
13. *Ibid.*
14. Toni Meyer to Edith Best, 3 Oct. 1919. On back of envelope – Abs. A. Meyer, Berlin, Lichterfelde, Mommsenstr. 7/8. NLI Ms No. 11002.
15. G. Schaafs to Best, 15 Jan. 1920 from Rothestrasse 14[II], Göttingen. NLI Ms No. 11003 (20).

Chapter 22

S HORTLY before leaving Berlin, Meyer wrote to Richard Best, 'My dear Friend', to say that Toni was delighted to receive Edith's kind letter, which had described conditions in Germany with such extraordinary accuracy. Moving house, which had been a strain, was now completed. All his books had been taken to the Academy, but it would be a long time before they were unpacked and sorted. He was setting out on Saturday for Leipzig and Weimar, feeling badly in need of a change. They were having a golden autumn, or fall, as his wife would say, who had left with little Margaret on Sunday and was now staying with Professor Bonn at Munich. Arrived at the station she had given her hand luggage to a porter, who at once vanished into the crowd with the bags, a symptom of the demoralisation which prevailed. Expenses were worrying. Meyer had to pay 170 marks in tips alone for the removal men, the whole business coming to a costly 1100 m.

He was very sorry to hear of the death of Lucius Gwynn, whose life must have been one protracted suffering. He remembered seeing him ill in Dublin in 1913.

> Poor mother! What has become of Stephen G[wynn], I wonder. He has played a sorry part. When I think how he and Dillon and the unspeakable T.P. [O'Connor] entertained Schiemann and me at dinner in the House after the second reading of the Home Rule bill and our talk then, and all that has happened since, it is as if one lived in an unreal world, a feeling I had almost immediately upon the outbreak of war, especially at night, or when I wake up in bed. And now indeed one moves through the world as if it had nothing to do with one. And yet there is a young generation eager to live and enjoy life, as we used to do. I will write to you again from Weimar.[1]

This postcard is the last item of an historic correspondence. Richard Best received it on Saturday 11 October. Kuno Meyer died that morning at half past six in a Leipzig nursing home. He never got to Weimar. It was a few days before the Bests were to know of the tragedy, which was announced to them in the following letter from Toni Meyer:

Leipzig
October 13th, 1919

> My dear friends,
>
> With a heavy heart I am sitting down to tell you the overwhelming news that my dear brother is no longer among the living. The whole development has been so sudden and unexpected that I can hardly yet realize it. He left us on Saturday the week before last to spend a few days in Leipzig and then he meant to have gone on to Weimar. But fate decreed otherwise. Some food he had with friends early in the week did not agree with him. No doubt he made light of it in the

beginning, but when matters did not improve, he went on Thursday into the private nursing-home of a professor whom he knew. They operated upon him on Friday for stoppage of the bowels and everything went well until Saturday morning at about half past six when without any previous warning he suddenly collapsed – probably a clot of blood in the lungs. On receiving the telegram which just contained the bare intimation of his decease – we did not even know that he was in hospital – my brother Eduard and I hastened there by the last train and learned all the sad particulars late at night. You expressed a wish to have a recent likeness of his, but oh my friends, I could not wish you to see him as he is now, emaciated and with the marks of suffering engraved on his face. Only his brow, that noble brow of his, is as imposing as it always was. To-morrow all that was mortal of him will be delivered to the purifying flames. How gladly would I have laid down my head if I could have saved his valuable life. He was so full of plans and projects for the future and his indomitable spirit was not to be broken by the vicissitudes of life.

Monday night

I was interrupted this morning and I have been on my feet ever since. Now all the arrangements are made for the last ceremony. It will be short and simple as he would have loved it. This morning they had a post mortem examination which showed that inflammation of the lungs had set in and the immediate cause of death was heart failure. In the afternoon I was present when they laid him to his last rest. He looked lovely, the painful expression had gone from his face and he appeared much younger. I put three red roses into his hands as his life had been given up to Dark Rosaleen. Now he spends his last night on earth in the cemetery cell near the Volkerschlachtdenkmal which you must have seen five years ago. We mean to take his ashes with us if we get the necessary permission and I am most anxious to have a beautiful urn made for his remains. Perhaps you could help me in getting some Irish design for it. It need not be done in a hurry.

At ten o'clock I am expecting my brother Eduard's wife and her soldier son who will be present at the ceremony, which is to take place at 1 o'clock tomorrow. My brother is prevented by his new duties as Rektor of the University to come over to-morrow. It is very hard on him and on Wednesday he has to deliver his inaugural address under these trying circumstances.

No more for the present. This time it is not war but grim death which stops our correspondence just begun again, but I hope that you will continue writing to me. Knowing that everything that concerns you will interest me greatly.

With fondest greetings
Your old friend
Toni Meyer[2]

For Toni Meyer the blow that fell, and the memories that came in its train, were more painful than words can describe. She who was closest of all to her brother and had looked after his comfort with such solicitude for so long, was unable to see him except at rare intervals over the last two years, while aware of his unhappiness. She recalled the last time they were together when he was storing his books in the Academy.

I remember so well when I was there with him during the last week to arrange the books, that he said: I suppose they will remain here till the end – who would have thought then that the end was so near! To me it is an everlasting regret that his last two years on earth were such as they were and I could do nothing to brighten them. Our various meetings at Frankfurt, Kreuznach, Giessen and on the Rhine stand out as bright spots in my memory. This last year he was to have come to me in Hamburg at Whitsuntide, but he was so afraid of the possible hardships in travelling that he gave it up altogether. For the last two summers he had not been

216

away from home and now that he did go for the much needed change, it proved to be fatal![2a]

To Edith and Richard Best it was a stunning and unexpected blow. They wrote at once to express their sympathy and distress. Their association with Toni and Kuno had been so close that the loss was akin to a family one. 'Beloved friend and teacher' was how Richard would remember him.

It seems that Meyer had special reasons for visiting Leipzig. No doubt some were sentimental. It was his old university town, where he had studied under his much respected master Windisch. There was also someone in hospital there whom he wished to see. An American friend, who under the initials H.G.S. wrote his obituary in the *European Press*[3] quotes from a card written to him a few days previously by Meyer who said he was leaving for a short holiday, probably in Thüringen, but would stop off at Leipzig 'to see Mrs. M.' This was an Irish lady who lay ill at a sanatorium. In a necrologue of deep feeling, as the loss was personal, the writer laments the end at the age of sixty-one of a life full of noble spiritual and intellectual enterprises and adventures. 'So falls one of the brightest pillars of German learning.' The writer placed special emphasis on Meyer's identity with the life and learning of England, embodying as he did all that was best in both nations, and numbering among his friends and acquaintances the greatest thinkers and writers of Germany and England. He would at times recollect those with whom he had talked, lived, travelled, worked, corresponded, George Borrow, George Meredith, Stevenson, Tennyson, Gladstone and many more, nor was there scarcely an eminent poet, scholar or statesman of the day, in England, Germany, Ireland, America and other lands, with whom he had not come into personal contact. His was a chain or rather a network of memories and associations which caused one to regret he did not live to reach the age when men write their memoirs. In a memorial full of feeling and regret the author pays tribute to his eminence as a Celtic scholar, and to his integrity as a German. 'Germany has lost one of her noblest sons, Ireland one of her most devoted lovers.'

It was one of many fine appreciations. Osborn Bergin's is particularly striking. Even though Meyer had often expressed his disappointment with Bergin's slow rate of work, he never made a secret of the fact that he had the highest regard for the Cork scholar's unrivalled knowledge of the Irish language, while Bergin for his part held Meyer in admiration on account of his manifold abilities and vision. In as near an approach to emotion as his reticent nature permitted, he opened his tribute by saying that 'One of the most melancholy tasks that can confront a man is that of writing an obituary notice of an old friend. Words are futile. One feels vaguely conscious of an incredible void.

　　The odds is gone,
　　And there is nothing left remarkable
　　Beneath the waning moon.

Such are the thoughts to-day of many who knew and loved Kuno Meyer in the old days. They cannot speak coolly and critically of the man himself. Let me attempt a less trying task, to set down my impressions of what he stood for in Irish scholarship'.[4]

Douglas Hyde, in coupling the names of Canon Peter O'Leary and Kuno Meyer, whom Irish cities had honoured a few short years before, said it was reasonable to mention them in the one context because each in his own way did work for Irish nationalism through the medium of Irish literature which he believed nobody else could have done. 'Kuno Meyer, like Father Peter, one of the most lovable men who ever existed, and himself undoubtedly in love with Ireland, called the attention not only of the world, but what was perhaps harder, the attention of Irishmen themselves, especially those of them who regretted that they were Irish, to the value of Irish literature in the evolution of Western European thought from the sixth century onward'.[5]

To Robin Flower the loss for Irish scholarship was irreparable. Neither can Flower have been free of emotion. Meyer was godfather to one of his children. Early in the war they had a difference of opinion caused no doubt by Meyer's controversial attitude, and Flower was much distressed at his accident in California. Writing after an interval when the shock must have softened, one is still sensible of how deeply he was affected.

> It will be long before we have so vivifying, so enriching an influence in all the branches of Irish work. I think we shall feel the lack of him more and more as time goes on and we miss that energy and enthusiasm that make him more than a fine worker himself, the source of fine work in others ... I think we can serve his memory best by carrying on the work as far as possible in his spirit and to the ends designed by him. He was a great scholar, and this is the service to their memory that great scholars most desire. But I wish we had him back again. When I seem to myself to have made some small discovery or to have come nearer to the understanding of some text, I always find my mind turning insensibly to him, I wonder what Meyer would have thought, and I feel his loss again in realizing each time that he is beyond our question. It is a loss we shall never make good.[6]

Pokorny[7] and Thurneysen[8] contributed worthy epitaphs. Vendryes' necrologue was mixed. He found himself unable to forgive that impulsive item of rhetoric about the capture of Antwerp, though he rightly pointed out that Meyer founded a School in which the pupils had now become the masters.[9] Eleanor Hull, a pupil, remembered him as a brilliant teacher.[10] Richard Best's memoir, which appeared in *Ériu* IX (1923), 181-86 was an impressive and finely modulated tribute. It is difficult to find him praised in English sources and his name does not appear in Bailey's *Times* index. The journal of the German-Irish Society of Berlin, *Irische Korrespondenz,* dedicated its October-November 1919 issue to his memory. 'Der treueste Freund des irischen Volkes ist in das Grab gesunken'. It includes the important factual survey of his life by his brother Professor Eduard Meyer and a sensitive appreciation by Julius Pokorny.

Most touching of all was the tribute of the Dutch Celtic scholar Anton Gerard Van Hamel. Simple, compassionate, straight from the heart, it can be said to stand for the views of all who acknowledged the services to Celtic learning of Meyer, although by none was it uttered so well. It is given fully here, as written to Richard Best.

Rotterdam
246 N. Binnenweg
Oct 18, 1919

My dear Best,

So he has left this world of care. Never until now I knew how much I loved him. There were things in his exploits in later years I could not approve. The campaign in America was a disgrace, and until very short[ly] before his death he pursued political objects that were an abomination to me. For all this I never became less attached to his amiable person. I readily forgave him what I considered as wrong. To be on less good terms with him, is an idea I could never have suffered. Besides, let no one interfere between a man and his country. If he transgressed the laws of divine morality, he has suffered for it, for he shared his country's fate. And now all is over.

Love may be unreasonable, and I loved this man for many things, great and small. He was a fine man, genial and yet distinguished. Everything was warm and living with him. His interest in us all was unrelenting. I liked his inviting smile, his sparkling eyes. I like to think of the way he used to welcome us in his house. I liked the way he pursued his Irish research. There was nothing of the common type of a professor in him. For his study he never made a holocaust of his soul. What I admired in him is that he always remained a man, never became a machine. His image remains before my eyes: the curved neck, the stiff arm, the bright eyes, and the face almost beaming. Too young he was to leave us. There are many of us who owe him a great deal.

Poor Keltology! She cannot spare so many of her foremost champions. Kuno Meyer occupied a very special position among them. He was not a grammarian, he was not a philologist in the strict sense of the word. In both respects Thurneysen is superior. Still one cannot imagine what Keltic studies would have been without him. He could not write bulky volumes, he could not stick for a long space of time to one and the same thing. Yet he did splendid work. Especially in the branch of lexicography. There he was a pioneer; he set the study of Irish lexicography – of primary importance in Irish! on a sound basis. Marstrander could not supersede him. The Contributions remain unequalled. His text-editions were exemplary. And what he published in his last years on the oldest poetry was his best work. There he was absolutely original. In the old poems he traced an evolution in the rules of poetic diction, which opened entirely new prospects. Thus his desultory way of working conduced to some results of the highest pitch at last.

I do not know how his wife will bear this loss, I never met her. I wrote to his sister, poor soul, to ask for some news about his end. Nobody there is to talk with me about him; thus I thought best to communicate with you about my present feelings. You will be also afflicted by his departure, I am sure. Best regards to your wife.

Ever yours
A.G. Van Hamel[11]

We have no evidence that Florence Meyer was present at her husband's funeral. Had she been, Toni Meyer would almost certainly have mentioned it. That she was affected by his death cannot be in doubt, no matter how much her feelings may have been qualified by the unhappiness in which her husband and herself had lived together. Gertrude

Schoepperle, now married to the mediaeval scholar Roger Loomis, wrote her a letter of sympathy, to which she sent a reply that indicates she was not unmoved by the tragedy, besides being attended by other worries. This is it:

Länggass str 26
Bern Schweiz
Febr 22 [1920]

My dear Mrs Loomis

Do forgive me for not answering your letter for so long but I have been so deep in the depths if one can say such a thing that life didn't seem worth bothering about. I am feeling better now both mentally and physically but Europe has left a sore spot in my heart that will be long healing I am afraid.

It has been so interesting and so tragic at the same time. And then the blow of my husband's death. Yes, life is a funny thing. Who would have thought that a simple girl born in a cabin in the prairies would have ended or at least spent part of her life in Germany with a great man such as my husband was. Yes, my husband received the announcement of your marriage and he was very glad for you. He often spoke of you and sent some of his works from Switzerland to you. I wonder if they ever arrived?

I have been in Bern some time trying to get a passport to come home but I am very much afraid by the time it is settled I shall not have money enough to use it. I am translating for newspapers and such work to keep my head above water for the time being. I do not want to go back to my profession as a nurse here. It is too poorly paid and too much drudgery. I would love to continue my lessons (singing) but it costs so much. I hope in spite of all the horrible things the world is doing today that you will be apportioned some part of the happiness you deserve. A few roses and not all thorns, just one now and then to make us appreciate the roses. Do write when you have time and cheer me up. I am so lonely.

Sincerely
Florence Meyer[12]

Florence Meyer, handicapped by lack of funds, did succeed in returning with her daughter to America. Toni Meyer, out of her kindness of heart and the loyalty due to the wife of her dead brother, assumed her worries as her own and did everything in her power to obtain the necessary finance for her maintenance and passage to America.

For Gertrude Schoepperle the United States was no woman's world. Her correspondence offers clear evidence of this. We remember Meyer's remark that she had been driven from Urbana and that America was not the country for her. Tragedy struck her too, her brilliant life cut tragically short by peritonitis. In Paris she felt that Joseph Vendryes was unfriendly because of her association with Kuno Meyer. It is possible she might have been mistaken. He wrote a gracious necrologue in her memory in *Revue Celtique*.

It may be appropriate to set out fully Osborn Bergin's evaluation of what Meyer meant to Irish scholarship, as printed in the *Freeman's Journal*:

There are many types of scholars in the world. There is the hermit type of well-nigh inhuman detachment, represented by the German philologist in Paris at the time of Napoleon's escape from Elba, who noticed nothing particular between that and the battle of Waterloo, so absorbed was he in the study of Sanskrit. Compared with him Meyer was a man of the world. He was keenly interested in art and letters, fond of travel, fond of club life, with a genius for writing letters, and a wide circle of friends. He had hosts of admirers who had little or no under-standing of his learning. Yet he was a true scholar, with a passion for research.

The earliest of his contributions to Celtic scholarship known to me is an edition of the text of the 'Boyish Exploits of Fionn', which appeared in the *Revue Celtique*, dated 1881. From that time up to a week ago he worked steadily at the rich, untilled field of Old and Middle Irish language and literature. In the index to Best's *Bibliography of Irish Philology and Printed Literature* to the end of 1912, there are 140 entries under the name of Kuno Meyer, not counting scores of short pieces published under the title 'Mitteilungen' or 'Contributions'. He wrote on many subjects, linguistic and literary – etymology, lexicography, personal names, placenames, law, saga, romance, metrics and poetry. But it was the literature that most attracted him. His heart was not in that microscopic investigation of sound-laws which arouses the fierce enthusiasm and the fierce controversies of the born philologist. When I was in Germany a fellow-countryman of mine, consulting the dean of his faculty about a course of study, protested that it would be useless to examine him on the fate of Indo-European short 'i' in Irish. The learned professor (whose real interest was in Shakespeare) replied with a smile that such questions were only put to natives of Germany. I am sure that Kuno Meyer's interest in pre-historic sound-changes was very slight, though he knew enough to appreciate other men's work in that line. His own work, especially in recent years, lay in the study of the structure of Irish verse, and in the interpretation of early Irish poetry..

When Meyer began to make his name as Celtic scholar, Whitley Stokes, after-wards his life-long friend, was in his prime, and had already started his great plan of editing and translating the greater part of our historic tales and romances. But when Stokes edited Irish verse, he turned, like O'Donovan and O'Curry before him, to 'the festologies, chronological, topographical and historical poems, which were composed for didactic purposes by learned professors at the monastic schools of Ireland.' Many years work at these lifeless compositions had made Stokes think there was little or no genuine poetry in Irish.

Meyer's researches proved to Stokes and others that ancient Ireland possessed not only an abundant storehouse of charming prose narrative, but a body of exquisite lyric poetry. He had a wonderful instinct for discovering gems of verse which earlier scholars had missed or misunderstood. As he says in the introduction to his Selections from Ancient Irish Poetry, published eight years ago: 'In nature poetry the Gaelic muse may vie with that of any other nation. Indeed, these poems occupy a unique position in the literature of the world. To seek out and watch and love Nature, in its tiniest phenomena as in its grandest, was given to no people so early and fully as to the Celt. Many hundreds of Gaelic and Welsh poems attest to this fact.' I may mention that only a few weeks ago Meyer edited, with translation and notes, the first part of a new series containing 167 fragments of early Irish lyrics.

But even a condensed review of his published works would fill several columns. He was not merely a productive scholar himself, but stimulated others to work, and supplied the necessary outlet. In 1896 he founded, with the late Professor Stern, the *Zeitschrift für celtische Philologie*, of which since 1911 he has been sole editor. In 1903 he founded the School of Irish Learning in Dublin, and until the outbreak of the war he was one of the editors of its journal *Ériu*. These journals are indispensable to all who are working at Middle Irish texts. Above all, an Irish student must have within reach of his hands Meyer's *Contributions to Irish Lexicography*.

The first volume, comprising the letters A-C, which appeared in 1906, was the fruit of many years reading of published and unpublished texts, and in spite of its defects, it is the book of reference most often consulted. The last time I saw Meyer, in the spring of 1914, he spoke of the enormous vocabulary of Middle Irish. 'We shall make crowds of mistakes', he said. He never claimed to be omniscient or impeccable. He had none of the absurd *amour propre* which makes certain scholars look upon criticism as a mortal insult. No one could be more grateful for a correction. But he had the natural human delight in the appreciation of his work shown by his fellow-workers. I think nothing pleased him more than the Miscellany published in his honour in 1912, shortly after his appointment to the Chair of Celtic in Berlin.

While other scholars surpassed Meyer in particular branches of his subject, no one else had so much influence on public opinion. By his enthusiasm, by the charm of his popular lectures, by his noble renderings of Irish lyrics – for he wrote English with an ease and grace that Englishmen might envy – he had convinced the public that the study of Early Irish literature was a fitting subject of higher education. When prejudicial opponents assumed without investigation that, being the product of a barbarous age, it must be rude and savage, he was able to point to compositions of a grace and dignity implying a high stage of refinement. To the charge recently made that his work was done for the glory of Germany and German scholarship, it may be answered that he never lost an opportunity of urging Irishmen and Welshmen to edit their own literature, and not to leave the work to be done by Germans.

Since 1914 Kuno Meyer's fame has been under a cloud. As a Berlin professor he had tasks thrust upon him from which he did not shrink, but which must surely have been uncongenial. He felt, and said at the time, that his lifework was ruined. During his American mission he endeavoured, under unpromising circumstances, to interest some students at least in Irish literature, and we have from his hand a *Miscellanea Hibernica* published by the University of Illinois. Since his return to Germany in 1917 he has produced, under growing privations and anxieties, an astonishing amount of good work. Cut off from the manuscripts of Dublin, Edinburgh, London and Oxford, he fell back on old transcripts and photographs. Though never in good health – he has been a martyr to rheumatism for the last twenty years – he worked and planned up to the end, and some of his most delightful contributions to the subject he loved so much saw the light this autumn. It is hard to realise that his wide learning, his ready sympathy, and his kindly criticism are no more. To the small band of Celtic scholars his sudden death is an incalculable loss.

Finally we might add the opinion of one of the most distinguished of modern Celtic scholars, Professor Kenneth Jackson, who has written of Meyer:

> He was one of the greatest Celtic scholars of his day. He belonged to the Heroic Age of Celtic, along with men like Stokes, Rhys, Loth and Strachan. His fertility in publication was absolutely outstanding, and most of his work is as important today as it ever was.[13]

For the rest of her life Toni Meyer mourned. For all that, she was a resolute and practical person and her innate strength of character came to her aid in the tasks that needed to be done. She now took the place of Kuno as correspondent with the Bests and other friends and loyally undertook the responsibilities towards Kuno's widow and daughter which circumstances demanded, keeping in touch with them and contributing as much as possible to their welfare and advantage. In this difficult time as in the years that followed Edith and Richard Best were her steadfast friends.

Toni told Richard that she wanted an urn with Celtic design made in Ireland to hold Kuno's ashes. As there were difficulties in the way of doing this she decided to have it made in Germany and have the Celtic design engraved on it. She wrote to Richard Best on 3 December 1919:

As to the urn, I wonder whether you could send me a design and we could have it made here. The ashes are sealed up in a heart-shaped metal vessel with the name and dates on it. ... Since I wrote you last, I received the very last impression of my beloved taken on his deathbed by one of the medical men who were present at the post mortem. It only shows the head and one might think he was asleep, yet there is the majesty of death about it. I look at it every night and my tears flow freely. I hope to secure it for you; it is so precious and sacred to me that I do not want to give it to many, but I know you will prize it and feel its wonderful charm.[14]

She was deeply grateful for the support of the Bests, and one of her letters to Richard reads:

You have been such a help to me all along and I acknowledge full of gratitude that I could not have a truer and better friend; ... Do you know that I like to think of you as a younger brother who is doing all he can to make me feel less the frightful gap which October 11th has rent in my life? Kuno was such a splendid correspondent and he hardly ever left me without news for a week. Now that voice is silent, but he often visits me in my dreams which I am most thankful for. Alas, if one could do without the rude awakening! I am to have the urn quite soon now.

With fondest greetings to you both.[15]

This was written on 5 September 1920. On the following month the urn was ready and she went to Halle to collect it, going from there to Leipzig where on 12 October she visited the Krematorium to place it, with Kuno's ashes inside, in the allotted niche. On the following day she wrote to Richard Best:

My dear friend,
I have just been to the cemetery again in most perfect weather – yesterday we deposited the urn, it looks beautiful. I am sure K. would have loved the sight of it. I adorned the niche with heather and fir which will last through the winter. Now I shall have to leave the noble champion at rest on time-honoured battle-ground. The colossal monument overlooks the whole place – an earnest of better times to come although I may not live to see them any more. I am leaving for Berlin this afternoon and shall be back in Templin on Sunday night.... My sister-in-law sailed from Liverpool on the 9th. I trust she and Margaret will have an agreeable passage in this beautiful weather. With fondest greetings to you both.

Yours
T.M.[16]

Toni Meyer kept up a regular correspondence with the Bests until the advent of the second world war, perhaps even later did we know, sending Richard from time to time letters of Celtic scholars which Kuno had preserved as well as various memorabilia of her brother. Like Edith Best she was an accomplished pianist and they shared a passion for music which for Toni very often provided a refuge from the harsh realities of life. But at all times her comments on musical events, composers and conductors make her a delightful correspondent. She visited Ireland twice after Kuno's death, in 1925 and 1936, as the much cherished friend of the Bests. Grief was renewed for her in 1930 with the death of her brother Eduard who was, in the words of Hugh Lloyd-Jones, "perhaps the most learned ancient historian who has ever lived'.[17] He was buried in Lichterfelde. Toni had planned to remove Kuno's ashes from Leipzig in

1934, when the lease of its location expired, and bring them to be buried beside Eduard, her wish being that the two brothers should be together like the two Grimms and the two Humboldts. This design was not carried out then. Kuno's ashes were finally transferred by his nephew Hans Eduard Meyer, and buried on 14 July 1971 at the Parkfriedhof, Berlin Lichterfelde. But the urn had been removed and could not be found. Toni, who had been living in the Johannesstift in Hamburg, died in the Summer/Autumn of 1945 and was buried on 9 November of that year.[18] Brave, talented and loyal, she deserves with her brother Kuno the honour of two nations, Germany and Ireland. Their two Dublin friends died, Edith Best in 1950, Richard in 1959.

NOTES

1. Meyer to Best, postcard addressed to National Library Dublin from Berlin-Lichterfelde, Mommsenstr. 7/8, dated, in error, 1/11/1919. Date corrected to 1/10/1919, probably by Best. On top of the card is a pencilled note in Best's handwriting: *'Received Saturday 11 Octr. the day of his death'*. NLI Ms No. 11002.

    The occasion of the dinner at which Stephen Gwynn, M.P. and his two parliamentary colleagues entertained Meyer and Schiemann is referred to in the following letter.

    Endsleigh Palace Hotel
    4/4/1914

    My dear Best
        ... I dined with Stephen Gwynn the other night who had invited Dillon and O'Connor, fresh from a very fine speech which I heard, to meet Schiemann and me. I also had some talk with Redmond, who said that one of the first things they would have to do was to bring me permanently to Dublin! Dillon told me how disappointed he was with my not accepting a post in the National University. I never heard such a wicked speech as that of Balfour's – but all this does not matter now ...'

    NLI Ms No. 11002 (38)

2. Toni Meyer to Edith and Richard Best. NLI Ms No. 11002.
2a. Toni Meyer to Best, 24 Nov. 1919, from Joachimsthaler Gymnasium, Templin. NLI Ms No. 11002.
3. H.G.S. in the *European Press, A Journal devoted to the furtherance of international understanding* (published semi-weekly, Berlin) Friday October 17, 1919, p. 2. In the issue of 13 October there is a poem *For Kuno Meyer* by Ethel Talbot Scheffauer. H.G.S. may have been her husband.
4. *Freeman's Journal* (Dublin) Saturday 18 October 1919. The remainder of the tribute appears towards the end of this chapter.
5. *Studies,* June 1920, 297-98.
6. Flower to Best, 13 June 1920. NLI Ms No 11000 (22). Seán Ó Lúing: 'Robin Flower (1881-1946)' in *Studies* Summer/Autumn 1981, p. 132.
7. J. Pokorny: Kuno Meyer in *Zeitschrift für celtische Philologie* XIII (1920) 283-85.
8. R. Thurneysen: Kuno Meyer in *Indogermanisches Jahrbuch* (1919) 164-67.
9. J. Vendryes: Kuno Meyer in *Revue Celtique* XXXVII (1919) 425-28.
10. Eleanor Hull: Kuno Meyer. By a pupil, in *Irish Book Lover* XI (1919) 35-36.
11. NLI Ms No. 11004 (7).
12. NLI Ms No. 11002.
13. Cf. Thomas Kelly: *For advancement of learning* (Liverpool 1981) 112. Students of Celtic will regret the death of Kenneth Jackson in February 1991. See the tribute to his work and memory by Muiris Mac Conghail in the *Irish Times* 18 Mar. 1991.

14. NLI Ms No. 11002 (46). Toni Meyer, postcard to R.I. Best, 3 Dec. 1919.
15. NLI Ms No. 11002.
16. *Ibid.*
17. Introduction xvi to U. von Wilamowitz-Moellendorff, *History of Classical Scholarship,* translated from the German by Alan Harris. London 1982.
18. The author is indebted for these details to Eduard Meyer's biographer, Dr. Christhard Hoffmann, Technische Universität Berlin.

Chapter 23

KUNO Meyer's premier service to Ireland was the establishment of the School of Irish Learning, the achievements of which in Celtic scholarship were original, extensive and of the highest creative importance. The School remained in existence until 1924 when it was merged in the Royal Irish Academy. Its lineal successor is the present Dublin School of Celtic Studies for which it was the model, and this later School, founded in 1940 as a constituent part of the Dublin Institute for Advanced Studies by an Act of the Oireachtas, carries on in its fine premises at 10 Burlington Road, Dublin, the work projected and begun by Kuno Meyer.

Meyer put Irish learning on the path of self-help and self-reliance. He introduced into Irish studies the concept of *Altertumswissenschaft,* of investigating and recording the early civilisation of Ireland from all its aspects, language, metrics, archaeology, poetry, history, customs and literature. The learned journal, *Ériu,* which he founded, and along with his colleague, John Strachan, edited, still flourishes, and was the precedent for others, like *Gadelica* (shortlived), *Celtica* the Journal of the Dublin School of Celtic Studies, and *Éigse,* a Journal of Irish Studies of the National University of Ireland. So too the celebrated *Zeitschrift für celtische Philologie* which he founded and edited with his fellow-celtollogue Ludwig Christian Stern continues brillantly to enlighten the domain of Celtic studies. He edited many early and mediaeval Irish texts to which he provided illuminating introductions.

He accomplished pioneer and essential groundwork in Irish lexicography. The variety and extent of his contributions to Celtic learning may be seen from his Bibliography which takes up forty-seven pages of the *Zeitschrift für celtische Philologie* and justifies the tribute he has earned from the most distinguished modern Celticist, Kenneth H. Jackson. His life and labours make up a large and important chapter in the history of Celtic scholarship. More perhaps than any other scholar he was at home in the unexplored maze of early Irish literature and could identify an obscure character mentioned in the manuscripts and point unerringly to his place and era. We may call Robin Flower as witness to this, whose own great Catalogue is a forest of information, but pays tribute to the pioneer researches of Meyer who had already been everywhere.

His familiarity with Irish texts to the point that enabled him to cull out and discuss a hidden personality may be exemplified from his correspondence with Wallace Lindsay, for instance, as when he discussed the identity of one Fethgna, of whom he says 'the best known person of that name is a bishop of Armagh, who died in 874. It was he who latinised his name Manonetus' adding that it was curious how the Irish in their etymologysing took no account of the quantity of vowels,[1] an observation characteristic of his inquiring mind.

He would take delight in noting an idiom in Greek or Latin literature and pointing out its exact parallel in Irish, which he would send off to Best with the advice to 'tell Bergin' or similarly extract a lingual secret from such a word as Old Ir. *fírinne*, a derivative from *fír* by the nominal suffix *-ine*, 'which in this case gets double *n* according to the law discovered by you' the recipient in this case being Eoin MacNeill, 'a little discovery which I am sure will please you,' and philological minutiae such as this were commonplace in his correspondence or conversation.

Meyer would have wished to redress the curiously indifferent attention, if not hostility, which his great predecessor Zimmer received in Ireland on account of the radical and independent views he put forward on aspects of early Christian Ireland.

The publication in 1911 of his *Ancient Irish Poetry* marks him as a man of high order in the ranks of literature. In this book Meyer revealed to the world the beauties of early Irish poetry. There is a certain literature which belongs to the realms of learning and linguistic discovery. We are introduced to a famous example of it in that first sentence of the *Grammatica Celtica* which, like a shaft of light in the darkness, dispels for ever the obscurities of Celtomania, just as we find it in Meyer's Introduction to his *Ancient Irish Poetry* no less than in the beautifully translated poems themselves, which are taken, as their gifted translator tells us, from 'a literature so little known that its very existence has been doubted or denied by some' and were being accepted in a growing recognition of the fact 'that the vernacular literature of ancient Ireland is the most primitive and original among the literatures of Western Europe, and that ... its importance as the earliest voice from the dawn of West European civilisation cannot be denied'.[2]

One of the great advantages possessed by Kuno Meyer in the milieu in which he worked was his perfect, and poetical, command of the English language. Frederick York Powell, a historian with a fine sense of literature, noted his talents as littérateur and historian at a Liverpool celebration in his honour.

> It is extraordinary that a man who was not born an Englishman should be able to give such an extremely beautiful rendering, such wonderful idiomatic translations, as he has given to us. Not only his good scholarship but his good English has astonished everyone. Further, not only is he a man with an artistic eye for everything that is beautiful, and suggestive, and stimulating, but he is also a judicious, and calm and reasoned historian.[3]

A striking appreciation of his merit as a poet came from Lascelles Abercrombie, himself a poet and critic of distinction, in the form of a letter written on receiving *King and Hermit* and *Four Songs of Winter and Summer:*

47 Greenpark Road,
Birkenhead
April 7 (19--)

Dear Mr. Meyer

I was at the University Club today for lunch and there found awaiting me a packet which, had I known it was there, would have brought me a considerable distance barefoot to get it. For my apparent rudeness in ignoring this delightful gift from you to me I must most humbly apologise; but, as I said, I was entirely unaware that to enter the Club would so enrich me. However, I hasten now to give you all the thanks I can for two books of a value, to me, quite immeasurable for what measure can be put to authentic poetry? It does not belong to dimensions. And in these translations of yours there is more than can be verbally appreciated. Please don't think I exaggerate their value to me: I wish I could. Without, I hope, impertinence, I want to tell you that your renderings strike me as most exquisite and genuine English poetry; for, unless I say that, I cannot indicate the extent of my gratitude. Only those to whom poetry is the main thing in this life can judge of the immoderate pleasure felt when their stores are increased as mine were today. Of one thing I am certain: I shall not learn Irish when I can get such versions as these.

I had already discovered 'King and Hermit' in the Picton library, and made much of my find; the Four Songs are new to me. It is quite impossible to particularize my enjoyments in these books. But ... such amazingly beautiful verses as 8 and 9 of King and Hermit, simply make me cry out with delight ...

Yours sincerely
Lascelles Abercrombie[4]

Thus Meyer used his talents in English as a vehicle to communicate to readers the beauties of Irish literature and to open up new and exciting perspectives of that literature, and in doing so, he and his Celtic fellow scholars brought into being original and creative performances in language and art.

What literature owes to Meyer and to his scholar-colleagues has received fine expression from a writer in the *Freeman's Journal* who had obviously followed closely, and with something like fervour, the unfolding of Celtic literature in the pages of the learned journals. The essay is unsigned, although one likes to think it might have been the work of Stephen MacKenna, translator of Plotinus, and one of the *Freeman's* brilliant journalists. It reads, in part:

The New Celtic Scholarship
'To every mind its own notion: many like to think of the work of the Celticists as a work of scholarship; to others, and especially in Ireland, it presents itself most decidedly as a work of literature.... But whatever may be the final verdict of the world upon the value of the old Irish literature, as compared with other languages and other civilisations, it remains an unquestionable fact that with the past twenty years or so there has sprung out a great stream of new thought and fancy, story and poem and estimation of life such as the intelligent must take count of, must value as a unique expression of mind and of art. Whitley Stokes, Standish Hayes O'Grady, Dr. Strachan, Dr. Kuno Meyer, and the diligent and brilliant band of professors and students who make *Ériu* for us, have been giving this generation, both in Irish of all periods and in singularly beautiful modern English, the first knowledge of a literature which – except for a few faithful scribes toiling in odd corners in their private devotion and for their private pleasure – has been buried for centuries. The formal scholarship of a slightly earlier generation was mainly concerned about linguistic technicalities ... but the newer scholarship has been

228

touched with the new humanistic spirit and works for delight as much as for information; it takes the wider scope and has a far deeper and more artistic spirit; it gives us the soul of beauty and the room of thought of the race and of the old times, not merely the dry bones of useful information.... And the story of Liadain and Curithir, with 'the fine poetry embedded in it', is an excellent example of the work being revealed for the first time to readers of English, work of which *Ériu* in its four volumes has already given a curious and fascinating assortment, sometimes mythological story, sometimes adventure tales such as might be from the 'boys' books' of the ancient Gael, sometimes pensive religious meditation, sometimes the prayer full of an intense spirituality, sometimes the lyric of love or of joy in the beauty of field and sea and mountain, the praise of verdure and waterfall, and of the quiet life of cattle and hens and bees. To people who talk – though, it must be admitted, with singular ignorance even of the English literature in which they live – as if the love of nature were a poetic discovery of the Lake School, this ancient Irish literature must come as a lovely surprise, with its passionate use of nature as a symbol or interpretation of the sorrow and joy and all the emotional experience of men.[5]

That what is called the Anglo-Irish literary movement profited from the rise and progress of Irish scholarship is patent enough. On the other hand, references in the correspondence of Meyer and Best to that stream of literature are few and far between and so far as they are concerned it might hardly be said to exist. There are brief and scattered references to W.B. Yeats, one of them being speculation as to the possibility of his being appointed to the chair of English in the new university. References to George Moore are more frequent, but these may be put down to his friendship, however deep, with R.I. Best and, for a while, with Meyer himself. There are minor asides about Lady Gregory. Meyer's favourite reading in English consisted of the works of Jane Austen, which he avers to have read 'for the nth time', but he was also familiar with R.L. Stevenson, Milton's sonnets, Boswell, and he kept abreast with what was modern in his time. He attended whenever possible the meetings of the Shakespeare Gesellschaft in Germany and his reading tastes lay in the broad stream of English literature. Amongst his favourite authors in French were Alphonse Allais and Anatole France. He was a good Classical scholar but to him Celtic literature was a wide and ample world, standing on its own quality and importance and dominating his interest and attention.

There is the comparison to be made between Johann Kaspar Zeuss and Kuno Meyer of having both set out on voyages of discovery which they traversed with brilliant success. Father Francis Shaw, S.J., has said of Zeuss that 'It must be rare for a nation to owe as much to one man as the Irish people owes to Johann Kaspar Zeuss ... no other has ever done, or will ever do as much to bring honour and recognition to the Irish language as Zeuss did'.[6]

About this there can be no argument. Zeuss comes first. Where then do we place Kuno Meyer in the roll of honour? In second, but in the words of an ancient critic, closer to the first than to the third. Robin Flower acknowledged his greatness in the midst of a war which had separated them: 'There are few men to whom I (and the studies I serve) owe more than to Meyer.' He paid further tribute to Meyer's indomitable spirit and in the *Times Literary Supplement* defended him against the animadversions of Dr. Norman Moore.

Meyer's work for the Irish language must be seen as part of the intellectual background to Ireland's struggle for liberty. Wilhelm Schulze stated this in his memorial lecture on Meyer and Professor Liam O'Briain's experience in the 1916 Rising, to be related in the next chapter, provides dramatic illustration of its actuality.

The collection of his correspondence which is centred not only in Dublin and Liverpool, but also doubtless in many German archives which have yet to be investigated, would document the progress of two or three decades of Celtic learning, besides illustrating the fellowship of those scholars working in the field of Celtic. He was a great letter writer, extensively in English, but also in German, in a clear miniscule hand which makes him a pleasure to read. His sister, Antonie, seems to have been the custodian of some of this correspondence. She refers to the interesting letters he wrote home during his early years in Edinburgh. He mentions keeping a diary. He must have received numerous letters from colleagues, and he mentions that he had letters from Whitley Stokes bound in two volumes, with enough left over to make a third. To seek out and assemble his correspondence would be a worthwhile task. It would make work for many research scholars. This task, and other similar work, will become part of the fellowship of studies which we hope will operate in future times between Germany and Ireland.

While his work for Celtic learning formed the over-riding interest of his life, there remains an important dimension relating to his twenty-seven years residence in England in the course of which he forged numerous personal links and friendships which it must have caused him distress to sunder in the grim circumstances of war. This dimension is given due importance in the appreciation by his friend who wrote in the *European Express*.

By a Liverpool writer who interviewed him[7] he was described as a man without affectation who did his work in a modest way. Perhaps he was weak in the domain of modern Irish though he made a genuine effort to remedy this, having gone with Eugene O'Growney to Aran in order to perfect his Irish conversation, though he failed to become proficient, not for want of application but because manifold duties always called him elsewhere. Through his energy and persuasion he made Liverpool an important centre in the growth and development of the Irish language movement. He was untiring in his appeals for the establishment of Celtic chairs in Glasgow, in Manchester where he called for a Celtic chair for John Strachan, in Cambridge where he hoped a chair would be made for Edmund Cosby Quiggin, and in London where he delivered many important and well attended lectures. Ella Young, who first saw him when he was lecturing for the Irish Literary Society, remembered him as passionately refuting attacks made on old Irish literature by critics of no knowledge. His indignation she noted to be curiously personal. He might have been a Celt defending his country's honour, rather than a German scholar.

Those who learned from him in the lecture room were high in their praise of his teaching qualities. 'He was a born teacher, vitalising, inspiring, encouraging, as no other teacher we have known has been' is the testimony of Eleanor Hull, one of his distinguished *alumni.*[8] He took an interest in his pupils and kept in touch with them by sending them copies of his work in Irish literature. His pupil, Maud Joynt, attesting to his love of knowledge for its own sake, points out, in a comparison with his eminent countryman Zimmer, that Zimmer, when possessed by one of his brilliant and startling hypotheses, would be inclined to find in every fact a proof of it whereas Meyer, by contrast, would view everything in the light of a calm, clear, passionless intellect, unswayed by bias.[9] His search for truth was made in the objective spirit of the Irish historian, *Beatha staraí fírinne.* His American student, Gertrude Schoepperle, who all but idolised him, saw him as a man of detached and impartial intellect, even in the middle of a great war which involved his country. Though the retiring disposition of Osborn Bergin inhibited him from expressing his feelings openly, he nevertheless could not hide his deep respect and friendship for Meyer. In saying that Meyer was under a cloud since the beginning of the war he may have had in mind academic circles in Britain and some in Ireland. Certainly Meyer's popularity in Gaelic Ireland was outstanding and Vendryes, in calling him *enfant chéri d'Irlande,* did not exaggerate, unfriendly in parts though Vendryes' recorded summing up of him was. The *Times* failed to notice his death. But his grateful student, David Evans, who as prisoner of war in Ruhleben camp appreciated Meyer's kindness, thought of him worthily and well: 'I uphold, defend and revere him and feel it my duty to state this to all his old friends. We Celts have lost part of our soul if some of us who knew him do not acknowledge him for the man that he was'.[10]

Anthologists have drawn upon his store, some liberally like David Greene and Frank O'Connor in *A Golden Treasury of Irish Poetry A.D. 600-1200,* others in a lesser degree, though no less significantly, like Myles Dillon in *Early Irish Literature,* where Meyer is acknowledged as easily the chief among translators of poetry, 'and one cannot do better than to borrow freely from his work' (p. 153). Helen Waddell signalized the first edition of her splendid book *The Wandering Scholars* with a keynote quotation in its prelims from Meyer's *Aislinge Meic Conglinne,* besides availing of his learned work, while Edward A. Armstrong has chosen aptly from his poetry and insight to illustrate his classic study of nature, *Birds of the Grey Wind* (pp. 114, 177). Austin Clarke's play *The Son of Learning* was inspired by *Aislinge Meic Conglinne,* and W. B. Yeats took his theme *The Crucifixion of the Outcast* from the same text, which he applauded in his review in *The Bookman* (February 1903). His publications feature in many learned bibliographies. The author of *Les Chrétientés Celtiques* (1911) refers to a host of texts of Old and Middle Irish from his hand (Introduction xxii) and scholars up to the present day have had recourse to his discoveries. In the 50th Anniversary Report of the School of Celtic Studies (1990) he is hailed as *Wegbereiter* – Forerunner.

Ireland honoured his memory by a symposium in the National Gallery in November 1969, attended by Éamon de Valera, when his work was reviewed by distinguished speakers. But Ireland has been negligent in allowing his works to go out of print. The Todd Lecture Series, to which he was a main contributor, included important texts like *Fianaigecht* and *Death-Tales of the Ulster Heroes* which were once on study courses of the universities but these, as well as his Ancient Irish Lyrics and Essay on Learning in Fifth Century Ireland, like many others, are long unavailable, unless in research libraries, to readers or students.

While the Dublin School of Celtic Studies in Burlington Road is the worthy physical monument to his memory, his revival as the progenitor of Celtic learning in Ireland is overdue and a reprint of a selection of his major studies might suitably become its prelude.

NOTES

1. Meyer to W.M. Lindsay, postcard from Charlottenburg, 19 Nov. 1912. c. 83, fol. 102, Bodleian Library Oxford. Other interesting correspondence in the Bodleian with Lindsay includes the following:
   'With regard to Dimma's curious *et,* have you looked at the Kilmalkedar Alphabet Stone, now alas illegible, but well drawn in Petrie and Stokes *Christian Inscriptions of Ireland?* Vol II plate V. What conclusions can you draw as to the age of the stone which is [in] one of the oldest Xian districts in Ireland, near Gallarus (i.e. Gall-árus 'settlement of Gauls')? Some of the other letters of this and other inscriptions are also very instructive.
   K.M.
   Just discovered a Dimma MacNathi, but he is too early. From his pedigree he must have died about 490! And yet Nathi at any rate is not such a common name.
   Postcard dated 10 June 1910 to W.M. Lindsay, 3 Howard Place, St. Andrews. Folio 336.
   My dear Lindsay,
   You deserve a monument! This is the best find – speaking in the name of Irish Philologie – you have made yet. No, the glosses were quite unknown. How came Stokes to miss them on his visit to Laon? But he was always in such a hurry. They are the prettiest scribal notes I know.
   [Meyer gives translations and explanatory notes:
   'Cold is this day. No wonder. It is winter'.
   'The light of the rush is not bright'
   Translated down to 27r]
   Altogether a fine haul, and pretty early too, say about 800.
   Could we get a photograph?
   ... I return to L'pool to-morrow. More power to your elbow!
   Yours always
   Kuno Meyer
   Letter 21 June 1910 on Shelbourne Hotel Dublin notepaper.
2. Kuno Meyer, *Selections from Ancient Irish Poetry,* London 1911 and 1928; Introduction vii.
3. A Celtic Chair for Professor Kuno Meyer (Liverpool Univ. Club 1903) 9.

4. Abercrombie to Meyer, April 7 (19-?) from 47 Greenpark Road, Birkenhead. TCD Ms No. 4224.
5. *The Freeman's Journal* (Dublin) 28 Dec. 1910.
6. Composite quotation from *Studies* (Summer 1954) 194; *Irish Press* (Dublin) 10 Nov. 1956.
7. 'A Celtic Chair for Liverpool University', in *Catholic Times* (Liverpool) 17 March 1911.
8. *Irish Book Lover* XI (Dec. 1919) 35.
9. *The Gaelic Churchman* (Dec. 1919) 16.
10. David Evans to R.I. Best 7 March 1920. NLI Ms No. 11002.

Chapter 24

THE last report but one of the School of Irish Learning covered the period 1915-1923.[1] Looking back over its twenty years of existence from its foundation in 1903 it was justly able to claim that the advancement in Celtic Studies which it was set up to promote had been phenomenal. Many of the great scholars who had served it generously during that time had died. John Strachan's unexpected death in 1907 was a major loss. He was a force in building up the School from the first day and worked for it loyally as teacher and editor. In April 1909 Whitley Stokes died. Far and away the greatest of the scientific Irish Celtic scholars, he gave the School the prestige of his name as governor and made important contributions to its journal *Ériu*. The improved second edition of his *Félire Oengusso* published in 1905 was designed by him for the use of the School's students. Edmund Hogan, S.J. died in November 1917 at the venerable age of eighty-six. Best known for his monumental *Onomasticon Hibernicum* he supplied for the placenames of Irish literature a companion to what Alfred Holder with his massive *Alt-Celtischer Sprachschatz* had done for Celtic Europe. Though he did not contribute to *Ériu*, his wise counsel as governor was availed of when most needed.

The death of Kuno Meyer in October 1919 was an irreparable loss, for though separated from the School for many years by war, he had remained in a symbolic way its very sheet anchor. Without him it was almost impossible to envisage the School's survival. Some months later, in January 1920, Edmund Cosby Quiggin of Caius College, Cambridge, a talented investigator of living Irish dialects, was struck down in his prime. And so the roll of honour continues, recording the deaths of other gifted students, Thomas P. O'Nolan (1913), Maura Power (July 1916) whose scholarly edition of *An Irish Astronomical Tract*[2] gave promise of a brilliant future, Edward Lucius Gwynn (August 1919) and Gertrude Schoepperle (Mrs Roger Loomis) in December 1921, well-known as a Romance scholar and through her co-editorship with Andrew Kelleher of Manus O'Donnell's classic Life of Columcille. Twice she crossed the Atlantic to attend the School's summer courses and afterwards worked to set up a library and school of Irish studies in the University of Illinois. Victim of prejudice against women, she had come up against difficulties in the course of her career. Another loss was Robin Flower's colleague, the mediaevalist William Paton Ker, who took a warm interest in the

School during its early years, generously providing scholarships for Welsh and Scottish students.

The shadows of war, and their pernicious effects on learning, could not be ignored. The report states:

> The period which has elapsed since the publication of our last report has not been favourable to the calm pursuit of learning. Owing to the troubled state of the country and the restrictions so long in force, the annual summer courses which used to attract students from distant parts of the country and from abroad, could not always be held.

All things considered, the Report puts up a brave front, but it could not conceal the fact that the School's outside links were severed, that it was approaching a crisis and that the odds against it were increasing to a degree that threatened its survival. What had all the appearance of a rescue operation was carried out during September 1920 by the devoted Osborn Bergin, who gave a second course of lectures on Irish Bardic poetry, of which his knowledge was unrivalled, earning, as he deserved, the cordial thanks of the Governors and Trustees. Through the generosity of Mrs. John Richard Green the School was enabled in 1923 to invite the cooperation of Dr Alf Sommerfelt of Christiania (Oslo) University to lecture on phonetics as related to the study of Irish Dialects. He was the last great linguist from outside the Irish shores to lecture in the school.[3]

Of the School premises, which in its latter period was located in 122A St. Stephen's Green, at the end of York St., on the other corner from the Royal College of Surgeons, not a stone upon a stone remains, being obliterated by modern commercial architecture. It has found mention in a striking volume of 1916 literature, *Cuimhní Cinn* (Recollections), by Liam Ó Briain, a pupil of the School and later Professor of Romance Languages in University College Galway. At Easter 1916 he had joined the Irish Citizen Army in the occupation of the College of Surgeons and was instructed by his officer Bob de Coeur to check the rooms opposite, from York Street to Proud's Lane, for materials useful to the insurgents.

One of these rooms, on the first floor, Liam Ó Briain knew well, although, arriving at it from overhead, he did not recognise it at once. The heavy door was locked. One of the men peered through the keyhole and reported to Bob de Coeur that the room was full of immense books, larger than he ever saw, ideal for making a barricade. Nothing better, said Bob de Coeur, for stopping bullets, break in and get them. Wait! said Liam Ó Briain, let me look in there. He saw, and recognized, the books. They were, the Book of Leinster, the Book of the Dun Cow, the Yellow Book of Lecan, the Book of Ballymote, Rawlinson B 112, all facsimiles of the old Irish codices published by the Royal Irish Academy. This was the School of Irish Learning, established by Liam Ó Briain's old teacher Kuno Meyer, where he had listened to many lectures from Kuno, Bergin, Marstrander, and, with Éamon de Valera by his side, from Pedersen. He addressed the men. Do you know what these books in there are? They are the old Irish books of Ireland, standing for four thousand years of civilisation. These, in a way, are what we are fighting for.

Whereupon they swore they would die before touching one of them. The room remained locked, its contents untouched, safe and secure until called into use again.[4]

By the time its Final Report, covering the years 1924-1925, was issued, the School had ceased to exist as a separate institution. It will be recalled that when it was founded in 1903, the cost of renting its rooms was paid by a liberal American sympathiser, Thomas Kelly of New York. This continued to be the case until 1919 when Mr. Kelly's help came to an end, leaving the School thereafter faced with a heavy rent which it could not meet. The universities had long ago robbed it of its teaching functions. What income the School was now earning came from subscriptions for *Ériu*, the sale of the School's publications and donations from private individuals. The Governors and Trustees met to consider the School's future. They felt they could not apply for an annual grant to the new Free State government, seriously overburdened as it was with other problems. The only course open was to merge with the body whose objects were most closely related to the School's own, namely the Royal Irish Academy. After negotiation with the Academy a union was accomplished. The School's valuable library of upwards of three hundred volumes, along with furniture and bookcases, were transferred to the Academy, which for its part undertook to continue the publication of *Ériu* to the same high standards as before and to promote the objects of the School. The Governor and Trustees met for the last time on 28 April 1926 when the Hon. Treasurer, Professor Thomas F. O'Rahilly, reported that the effects of the School had been transferred in accordance with the agreement and its incorporation with the Academy become a fact.

It was the end of a great chapter in the history of Celtic scholarship. There was a word of praise for Best from the lady whose munificence had been a constant support, Alice Stopford Green who, writing to him on 24 February 1924, paid him tribute for that 'the whole story is most creditable for you and those who helped you in the management of the School. I am afraid you had the most laborious part of it all, but the result is that we are handing over something remarkably good to the Academy, and I am sure they see that'.[6]

Wars are unkind to scholarship. It was perfectly true for Richard Best, who was the author of the above reports, to say that the years from 1915 to 1923 had not been favourable for the calm pursuit of learning, and this state of affairs was little alleviated in the ten or fifteen years which followed. True, there seemed to be a lull in the unsettlement of the period, in the course of which W.B. Yeats in his essay 'Ireland 1921-1931,'[7] praised the Free State government for producing the situation where 'the musician, the artist, the dramatist, the poet, the student' found they could give their whole heart to their work. But the times remained nervous and unquiet for some years to follow and Celtic learning suffered a decline.

236

It was not until 1936 that a move was made to continue, in effect, where the School of Irish Learning had left off. In that year there was drafted, on instructions from the Government, a 'Report on the present position of Irish Studies and suggestions for future developments', which was signed by Dr. Daniel A. Binchy on behalf of the Irish Studies Committee of the Royal Irish Academy. This Committee included Eoin MacNeill and R.I. Best, and the influence of the latter can be clearly traced in the document. There is a copy, running to 11¼ typed pages, foolscap size, amongst the Best papers in the National Library of Ireland.[8]

The Report recommended setting up 'A national Institute exclusively devoted to Irish studies' (page 8) and gave details of the shape which it should take:

'We are convinced that the cause of scholarship in Irish can best be served by an independent Institute, wholly devoted to this cause, and functioning under the guidance and control of experienced Irish scholars. In the following paragraphs we submit detailed proposals for an Institute of this kind.

Of all the institutions which have contributed in the past to our knowledge of the Irish Language the School of Irish Learning easily holds pride of place. Although it was in active existence for less than 20 years, and during all that time was gravely handicapped by lack of funds, it managed to issue an imposing list of scholarly publications some of which are now standard works in all universities where Irish is studied. In addition, nearly every scholar who has attained eminence in Celtic Studies in Ireland or abroad was associated with the School either as a teacher or a pupil. Its public courses, conducted by experts on various branches of Irish, and available to everyone interested on payment of a slight fee, created a new standard of Irish scholarship which it should be the aim of present and future generations to maintain.

We propose that the Government should revive the School of Irish Learning but on a much vaster scale. The former School had to exist almost entirely on donations from private individuals (apart from a grant of £100 per annum from the British Treasury, which was withdrawn after five years), and thus its activities were not merely limited, but largely dependent on the self-sacrificing devotion of Irish and foreign scholars working for nominal remuneration, and sometimes for none at all. We suggest that the new School be constituted by the Government as a national Institute by an annual Government grant such as is at present made to each of the constituent Colleges of the National University. Like the Collège de France, it should be primarily an Institute for research and publication but courses of lectures should also be given on specialised and advanced departments of Irish scholarship which would not normally be included in the programmes of the ordinary teaching bodies. These courses should, as in the Collège de France, be free, and open to any member of the public who can satisfy the lecturer that he possesses sufficient preliminary knowledge to be able to follow the lectures with profit.

The School should be given the status of a chartered public corporation, something like University College, with powers of regulating its domestic arrangements by internal statutes ... (page 9)

If the Government decides to carry through the big scheme, it will have the consolation of knowing that it has done everything humanly possible to ensure that future generations of Irishmen will not grow up strangers to the language and the civilisation of their ancestors. (page 12)

The recommendations of the Irish Studies Committee were put before the Government, cast into legal form and submitted for discussion and approval by both Houses of the Oireachtas under the title of the Institute for Advanced Studies Bill, 1940. The Bill in fact was one of dual intent, providing for 'The establishment and maintenance in Dublin of an Institute for Advanced Studies consisting of a School of Celtic Studies and a School of Theoretical Physics'. Only the School of Celtic Studies concerns us here.

The Taoiseach, Éamon de Valera, when seeking the approval in principle of Seanad Éireann for the Bill, explained that 'One of the immediate reasons for founding an institute of this kind is the obvious need to deal with a very considerable body of manuscript material which is available and which can be worked through only if it is systematically attacked'.[9]

He hoped that the School, when started, would be the great centre of Celtic Studies in the world, embracing Old, Middle and Modern Irish and including in its field of interest the sister Celtic languages, Welsh, Scottish, Manx, Cornish and Breton.[10] In the debates on the Bill which took place in Dáil and Seanad Éireann the names of Kuno Meyer or John Strachan or of any of the great Celtic masters were not mentioned, not because they were deliberately disregarded but because, except to a few scholars, they were in that day and to the legislators of that time totally unknown. Mr. de Valera hoped that one of the Houses of the Institute would be called Hamilton House, in honour of Sir William Rowan Hamilton, and the other some name 'like that of the patriot O'Curry or O'Donovan', which would inspire the workers of the Institute with the spirit of these men. As regards the School of Celtic Studies, which was at first located in Merrion Square, the title of Teach Uí Chomhraidhe or O'Curry House was given to it but this title lapsed, it appears, on the School being rehoused in its present imposing premises of 10 Burlington Road, Dublin 4. Maurice Moynihan, the editor of Mr. de Valera's *Speeches,* refers to Kuno Meyer as 'the founder and father of the Irish scholarly renaissance'.[11] If and when a name is to be conferred on the School of Celtic Studies, that of Kuno Meyer must come up for consideration.

The Institute for Advanced Studies Act was signed by the President on 19 June 1940 and passed into law. No more appropriate hand could have been put to its signature, for the President was Dr. Douglas Hyde who was on the Board of Governors of the School of Irish Learning on its foundation in 1903. Dr. Daniel A. Binchy became the first Chairman of the Governing Board of the School of Celtic Studies on its establishment in 1940. The first Senior Professors were Osborn J. Bergin (Director of the School), Thomas F. O'Rahilly and Richard Irvine Best. In the persons of Bergin and Best the link with the School of Irish Learning was maintained.

Best sent Robin Flower a copy of the *Irish Press* containing news of the Institute. 'I was delighted' wrote Flower, 'to see from the *Irish Press* that you sent me that the Institute has really got going, with you, Bergin and O'Rahilly in charge. It is a good omen for the future of Irish Studies in Ireland, a guarantee of the carrying on of the original work of the School of Irish Learning that did so much for us all'.[12]

NOTES

1. Printed in *Ériu* IX (1921-1923) 187-190.
2. Irish Texts Society Vol. XIV.
3. An extract from the Report reads:
   Dr. Sommerfelt gave a course of lectures during September (1923) on 'Practical Irish Phonetics and the study of Irish Dialects', which was attended by over twenty-five students, and aroused the keenest interest in circles outside. In his preliminary lectures he dealt with the general characteristics of a phonetic system and the salient features of Irish phonetics in particular. These were followed by a study of the sounds of Munster Irish ... It is hoped that the results of this the first scientific investigation of the rich phonology of West Munster dialects will shortly be published, when it will form a valuable addition to the studies of Donegal and Aran Irish which have hitherto received more attention.
   In his concluding lecture Dr. Sommerfelt dwelt on the importance of the study of dialects and the light they throw on the historical development of a country. He alluded to the splendid linguistic atlases brought out in France, Spain, Italy, Denmark and Romania, and expressed the hope that the Irish Government would soon inaugurate a dialect survey. The Governors are greatly indebted to Dr. Sommerfelt for carrying out this strenuous course, involving so long a journey and no little personal inconvenience.
4. Liam Ó Briain, *Cuimhní Cinn* (Baile Átha Cliath 1951) 120-121.
5. Printed in *Ériu* X (1926-1928) i-iv.
6. Quoted in Seán Ó Lúing, *Saoir Theangan* (Baile Átha Cliath 1989) 53.
7. W.B. Yeats, *Uncollected Prose*, II. Ed. John P. Frayne and Colton Johnson (London 1975) 486-490.
8. NLI Ms No. 11005. A pencilled annotation describes it as '2nd edition'.
9. *Speeches and Statements by Éamon de Valera 1917-73*. Ed. Maurice Moynihan (Dublin 1980) 437. According to Senator Professor Michael Tierney, the 'plan for an Institute of Celtic Studies arose from a memorandum submitted to the Taoiseach by the Irish Studies Committee of the Royal Irish Academy.' (Seanad Debates 24, 1332, 15 May 1940). This memorandum had been prepared by Daniel A. Binchy. *De Valera, Speeches,* p. 439, footnote 6.
10. *Ibid,* 440.
11. *Ibid,* 440, footnote 7.
12. Flower to Best, 13. XI. 1940, from 12 South Marine Terrace, Aberystwyth. NLI Ms No. 11000. The genesis and fortunes of the School are related in detail in its *Fiftieth Anniversary Report 1940/1990* which also includes personal essays by a variety of scholars on Aspects of Celtic Studies. Published by the School of Celtic Studies, Dublin Institute for Advanced Studies, 1990.

Appendix

(from *Celtia*, May-June 1903)

A SCHOOL OF IRISH RESEARCH

LECTURE BY PROFESSOR KUNO MEYER, PH.D.

On Thursday, May 14, Dr. Kuno Meyer delivered a lecture in the Large Concert Hall of the Rotunda. The lecturer chose as his subject, 'The Necessity for Establishing a School of Irish Literature, Philology, and History.' Dr. Douglas Hyde, President of the Gaelic League, occupied the chair, and there was a large attendance.

The President addressed the audience first in Irish, continuing in English, said that Dr. Kuno Meyer's lecture would not be in Irish, as some people feared. (Laughter.) The lecture would be delivered in English, and would be on the necessity of establishing a School of Irish Philology. History, and Literature here in Dublin. (Applause.) He then introduced the distinguished philologist, amidst loud applause.

Dr. Kuno Meyer then delivered his lecture, in the course of which he said – The Gaelic revival, one of the most remarkable and unexpected national movements of our time, is an event of such recency that even the youngest amongst us can remember its beginnings. It is one of those almost elemental phenomena, the suddenness and force of which seems to carry everything before it, while it astonishes no one more, perhaps, that those who have started it. (Applause.) Nor can the calmest and most sceptical onlooker remain indifferent, for the object at stake is the salvation of a nationality at the eleventh hour. (Applause.) Will this object be attained? Or will the movement come to a standstill as suddenly as it has sprung up? No one, I venture to say, can foretell, and I least of all. Friends, both in England and in Ireland, often ask me as one who has watched the movement from its beginning, and one who, as an outsider, may be supposed to have kept his head cool, what I think of it all, and whether I regard it as likely to be lasting. I can only answer that it has taken me completely by surprise. (Applause.) When I remember the apathy which existed but yesterday with regard to the Irish language and literature, to Irish art, and, indeed everything genuinely Irish, both among the people and the educated classes; when I call to mind that twenty years ago, when I first knew Ireland, under one of the most grotesque educational systems the world has ever seen – (applause) – children were thrashed for talking Irish within the hearing of the schoolmaster; or when I remember the pathetic endeavours of the men who then rallied to the rescue of an apparently dying language, the men who founded the Society for the Preservation of the Irish Language, and those who started the *Gaelic Journal*; when I recollect that we looked upon Hennessy, Standish Hayes O'Grady, and John Fleming as the last native Irish scholars whom the world would ever know – and then see what is going on around us now, I have to rub my eyes like one awaking from a dream to daylight and reality. (Applause.) But, for all that, I would not venture to prophesy. Not long ago Principal Rhys, the eminent Welsh scholar, told me that some time during the seventies of the last century he had predicted that the Welsh language would linger on for a

240

generation or two, and then die out. No one had better opportunities to know than he: no one could have been less prejudiced; there is no more ardent lover of his nationality and of his native language; and yet see how false his prediction has been. Some hidden fire still smouldered unnoticed among the ashes, a fresh breeze springs up, and almost in a moment the whole country from end to end is in a blaze. The Welsh language is now more firmly established than it has been for centuries. (Applause.) It is spoken and written by a young generation in a purity which has been unknown since the days of Goronwy and Lewis Morris in the eighteenth century. It is taught in the schools, recognised by the National University as ranking by the side of Greek and Latin; papers and periodicals abound; a national press is issuing the classics of the nation in splendid editions; a national library has been founded; the Eisteddfod – the Welsh Oireachtas – flourishes. (Applause.) A similar development seems to be taking place in Ireland under our eyes. (Applause.) Wherever one goes now one finds men and women, young and old, able to speak and read and write Gaelic; it is taught in the schools; ancient customs are revived; papers are springing up; Irish literature is being printed; the interest in the history and traditions of the country and the race is widening and deepening – (applause) – scholars are encouraged in their work. And, over and above this, the lives of thousands have been transfigured, and a new zest and spirit has entered into a nation whose despondency, whose listless, hopeless attitude towards itself and its interest used to be the saddest feature in its character. (Applause.) But I need not dwell on this wonderful transformation, familiar as it is to you all. I believe that its beneficial effects will not be confined to Ireland. I do not mean to refer to the advantage which must inevitably accrue to the best interests of the Empire from a strengthening of the Irish nation – there is the history of many centuries to prove that the policy to keep it weak was disastrous – (applause) – I desire to speak of a much humbler sphere, which the Gaelic revival is sure to influence most favourably – Celtic scholarship at home and abroad. (Applause). One of the discouraging phenomena to the foreign student hitherto was the curious indifference that in what should have been the home of Irish and Celtic studies prevailed among the learned as well as among the general public and the people at large. Another no less discouraging circumstance was the difficulty of acquiring, either through books, or by an easy intercourse with the people, the necessary knowledge of the spoken language in all its idiomatic force, and with all its dialectical varieties. Anyone who has followed the development of modern philology knows that its greatest achievements are derived from a minute study of the living languages, not from that of the more or less artificial language of literature. It would have been an irreparable loss to Celtic research for all time if the Irish language, which the German philologist, Schleicher, rightly called the Gothic of the Celtic family of speech – that is, the most primitive and original of all Celtic languages – had been suffered to die without having been studied exhaustively at the source, and on the spot, without having been chronicled down to the minutest details of sound, grammar, and idiom. There is no fear of that now. (Applause.) Ireland is in the fortunate position of having retained her dialects, while in other countries like England, they are now rapidly disappearing before a colourless and artificially polite standard, on the one hand, and the vulgar and debased speech of the great cities on the other. (Applause.) Let me here express the hope that nothing will be done to discourage the dialects as the spoken language of the home and everyday life. (Applause). They are the rich source from which the literary language will continue to draw its best inspiration. The literary language can take care of itself. It will develop with the taste, the culture, the learning of the individual writers. As the language spreads and grows, great writers will come to set the standard, to serve as models, as Keating has done now, for many generations. Now, while this is the hopeful prospect of the movement, there yet remain two important and essential things to be done, and the sooner they are done the better. One is to broaden and strengthen the movement at the root, by rousing those districts in which Irish is still the mother tongue to a better realisation of their importance and responsibility. (Applause.) That, I understand, is already part of the programme of the Gaelic League. The second requirement will form the chief subject of my address to-day. It is the necessity of bringing the movement into direct and intimate relations with scholarship, to provide an avenue for every student of Irish to the higher regions of study and research, to crown the whole edifice by a revival of native scholarship, and thus to bring about a second golden age of Irish learning. (Applause.) The aims of the Gaelic revival and those of scholarship are not incompatible; it would be deplorable for either if they were. The scholar's task is to study and elucidate the same past in which the roots of the movement lie – the same past, the chasm between which and a degenerate, modern Ireland you have succeeded in bridging over. This chasm threatened to sever for all eternity the Ireland of the past from an Ireland rapidly becoming wholly Anglicised. (Applause.) In 1851 Dr. O'Donovan, writing to a correspondent who had asked where the best speakers of Irish might be found, answered: 'In the poorhouse.' You have altered this. You have placed the best speakers of Irish in a seat of honour. (Applause.) But, remember, that you have also to fill a void – the gap which, through the death of O'Donovan and O'Curry, was cleft in native scholarship. The work which those two men achieved has never yet met with full recognition. (Hear, hear.) Apart from the work they did themselves, it was their knowledge and their original research which enabled scholars like Petrie, Todd, and Reeves to achieve great results in Irish archaeology, history, and literature. When O'Donovan and O'Curry were dead, further progress was rendered difficult, and almost impossible. The work which they left behind them has been, in Ireland at least, almost at a complete standstill since then in what I may call academic and official scholarship. You have all heard of the severe criticism which scholars at home and abroad have directed against the five volumes published under the auspicies of the Brehon Law Commission. The fact is that the bulk of the five volumes of laws is merely work done by O'Donovan and O'Curry over forty years ago. O'Donovan died in 1861, O'Curry in 1862; the fifth volume was published in 1901. It seems that the Brehon Laws Commissioners consider their work ended now that the excerpts and translation prepared and left by O'Donovan and O'Curry have come to an end. I gather this, in the first place, from the fact that a glossary to the five volumes has been published, a glossary again based upon faulty impressions of O'Donovan and O'Curry's extracts, not upon the original MSS.; and, secondly, from the rumour which has come to my ears that the Commissioners entertained the idea of sending an Irish scholar abroad to search for unpublished manuscripts of Brehon Laws in the libraries of the Continent. This would have been a wild-goose chase, for the MSS. do not exist – for every scholar knows that if O'Donovan and O'Curry had lived they would have told them that, with the exception of a few fragments of a legal treatise at Copenhagen, which has already been published by Stokes, of which there is a copy in the Royal Irish Academy, there are no law tracts in any of the Continental libraries. When I tell you, further, that all the time there are the most valuable legal documents lying unused and unpublished in the libraries of Trinity College, of the Royal Irish Academy, of the British Museum, and of the Bodleian, you will have some information as to the value of Royal Commissioners. Am I not right, then in saying that Irish scholarship, academical and official, is extinct since the time of O'Donovan and O'Curry? The question seems to me of such great importance that I may mention that it is my intention to address an open letter to the Commissioners on the whole subject. (Applause.) I am not, of course, unaware of the fact that there are excellent and hardworking Irish scholars in Ireland, but these scholars are isolated. They are working single-handed, and in the positions in which they are placed have no chance of creating a School of Irish Philology or History. There is the crux of the whole matter. If O'Donovan and O'Curry had but left a school behind, and in every other country they would have been enabled to do so, we should not complain of the standstill of Irish scholarship in Ireland. (Applause.) But the fault was not theirs. They met with little encouragement, except from a few enthusiasts. There was not, and there is not now any proper organisation for the academic pursuit of these studies. There was, and there still is, little interest in research and higher scholarship. I know that O'Donovan held for a time a Professorship in Belfast, but he seems to have had no pupils. At least, so I gather from a letter of his which has come into my hands. In the letter, written in 1851, O'Donovan says: 'I shall be in Belfast very soon again to deliver some lectures on the Celtic dialects. I do not believe that you or any other friends there will be able to procure me any pupils, and I am, therefore, afraid I cannot live among you.' I venture to say that if he were to come to Belfast now he would not be left without pupils, but that hundreds would flock to his classes. It has not always been so in Ireland. As late as the 17th century there existed throughout the country bardic schools, in which the Irish language and Irish literature, supported by liberal contributions from chiefs, were taught and studied, just as law schools and medical schools were kept up and supported in a similar way. These were the academies and universities of ancient Ireland. As you turn over the pages of the Four Masters you come again and again upon the obit of one of the professors of these schools. Now it is absolutely necessary, if there is to emanate from Ireland work of first-rate importance in history, philology, literature, archaeology, that there should be established a school in which the foundation for these studies would be laid by a study of the Irish language and literature. Without a knowledge of the Irish language in all its stages – old Irish, middle Irish, modern Irish – no real advance in our knowledge of the various subjects mentioned above is possible, because the source, the documents, are written in Irish. I need not here again dwell on the wealth and variety of Irish literature in all branches, or reiterate what I have said elsewhere, that no one is in a position to speak with authority of it as a whole. The facts are not yet before us. But let us consider for one moment the magnitude of the task that has yet to be accomplished. Let me begin with the language. To trace the history of the language from the oldest available records to modern times, to establish the laws which govern it, to follow its changes from period to period, from dialect to dialect, then, when all this has been done, to date and locate every piece of prose or poetry with exactness – these are some of the tasks which await the student of Irish philology. As to literature, the amount and variety of the work to be done is even greater. Here is the oldest vernacular poetry and prose of Western Europe – (applause) – handed down in hundreds of manuscripts, very few of which have been edited, many of which have hardly been opened for centuries, while the majority have only been hastily glanced at. What a task for generations of students! Who can say what revelations await us, what revolutions in our knowledge may be in store here? Every new publication comes as a surprise. The general reading public and the majority of the learned would almost refuse to credit the wealth, the age, the beauty, of this literature. Only the other day I sent a copy of a few old Irish nature poems to a well-known French scholar, who was delighted with them, but would not believe that I had not, in my translation, "*brodé*" – faked – the most part of them. This is characteristic of the ignorance and credulity prevailing even in the circles of the learned. The truth is that my poor reading labours in vain to express the beauty of the Irish original. Scholars and the public will judge differently when once the Irish classics, from the earliest times down to the eighteenth century, will be before the world in critical editions. This is a task essentially for Irishmen to perform. The difficulties for a foreign student are often too great and numerous, quite apart from the language, and, to be surmounted, demand an intimate knowledge of native lore that few foreigners can hope to attain. When we next consider the purely historical documents, whether of Church history or secular history – first those bearing upon pagan times, then those dating from the golden age of Ireland before the Norse invasion, next those of the Viking age of the ninth and tenth centuries, then those of the renaissance during the eleventh century, and so on in unbroken tradition to the eighteenth century – you will realise that it is idle to attempt to write the general history of Ireland, or the history of any special period, before they have all been published and made the subject of critical study. It would take me too long to continue this sketch of the work awaiting the hand of the historian, archaeologist, and topographer. I will say once more that, whatever the foreign student may achieve, he cannot hope to cope with its difficulties so successfully as the native student. It is a task which must be accomplished by Irishmen and Irishwomen essentially. Instead of further enlarging on this, let me illustrate what I have said by one single example, which must stand for hundreds that I might give. Among the priceless Stowe MSS. which were deposited by the British Government with the Royal Irish Academy in 1885, there is the "Book of Hy-Many' You may remember the pathetic indignation of O'Curry when he was denied access to the MSS, by their former owner, that churlish nobleman, Lord Ashburnham; O'Curry knew what their contents were, and ate his heart out. Now the MSS. have come back to Ireland; but there they have lain in the Academy unutilised, uncatalogued, for nearly twenty years, and yet what treasures they contain! There are to be found, among other things, the poems of MacLiag – the bard of Tadhg Mor O'Reilly – the follower of Brian na Boroimhe – all unedited. Imagine what might happen if it became known that an old English MS. existed containing poems by a bard attached to King Alfred, who had sung his battles, and the warriors who had fought under him. The news would spread like wildfire throughout the world of letters, and editions, learned and popular, would follow in rapid succession. (Applause.) Now, where are those Irish scholars to lift these and hundreds of similar treasures? They will not be found until a school of Irish philology has given them the necessary instruction and training, and has taught them the proper methods of study and research. (Applause.) The field is there, the materials are abundant, the laboratories, so to speak, are fully equipped, the workers alone are wanting. (Applause.) This is a national concern. To provide such students with the necessary instruction, to initiate them into the study of the older stages of the language, is, in my opinion, a question of national importance. (Hear, hear.) How is it to be done? At present there is no provision of this kind. If we could rely on the foundation of a National University in the immediate future, of a Celtic University – (loud applause) – if I may so call it, the solution would be easy. In such a University there should be chairs for Irish Philology, for Irish History, and Archaeology, and a well-equipped library, and we might look forward then to a flourishing school of Irish research; but these things lie on the knees of the god's, and meanwhile valuable time is being lost. It is necessary also to train scholars who can take their places as teachers in that University when the time for it comes. (Applause.) Can we expect anything from Trinity College? (Laughter, and "No.") No, I think not. I see no sign of it. Trinity College is modelled upon the obsolescent system of the older English Universities, in which the instruction is given almost exclusively in certain recognised subjects, while the time of instruction is controlled by prescribed curricular examinations, so that the true object of learning is lost sight of. Such a system is concerned almost exclusively with the acquisition of knowledge which is already common property, instead of widening, increasing, and advancing knowledge and learning. The question next arises whether the Royal Irish Academy can be expected, or can be induced, to organise such a school. Not unless the Gaelic League were to storm it, reorganise it on scholarly lines, and make it what it ought to be – the home and centre and the workshop of Irish studies and research. (Applause.) No; I think little or no support is to be looked for from these quarters. If it were really alive to the progress and to the needs of Celtic scholarship, if it were really the home and centre of Irish studies, no institution would be more suited to take up such a scheme. But it cannot be called so. It has founded no school, it trains no scholars, it has published no catalogues of its MSS. When its President was approached some time ago to co-operate in inducing the government to make a grant for the cataloguing of Irish MSS., he declined to do so. (Shame). Since the days of O'Curry, it has, I believe, not bought a single MS. What, then, are we to do? At this point, perhaps, you will bear with me if I tell you an old story, which may be new to some of you. One day during the end of the eighth century, when Charlemagne sat upon the Throne, a British merchant ship landed upon the coast of France having two great Irish scholars and divines on board as passengers. While the merchants put forth their wares and were busy proclaiming them, these two Irishmen cried out to the people: 'If there is anyone in search of wisdom and knowledge, let him come to us; we have some to dispose of.' (Applause.) The rumour of their arrival spread throughout the land, and reached the ears of the Emperor. He sent for them, and asked them what they required for their merchandise. They declared they needed nothing but a suitable place to teach in, intelligent students to teach, and for themselves food and dress. Charles immediately placed one of them, Clement by name, at the head of the school at his own Court, and placed the other, whose name was Dungal, at Pavia. (Applause.) Such is the story told by the chronicler of St. Gall. I think its application to our case is evident. Secure but the necessary scholars, able and willing to teach; furnish a place for them to teach in, and provide them with earnest and intelligent students, and the thing is done. (Hear, hear.) The question of funds is not the first and only consideration in such matters. The determination to carry the scheme through, co-operation, organisation, are infinitely more important. (Hear, hear.) I venture, then, to suggest the following simple scheme. Begin in the simplest, humblest way. I feel sure that men like Father Hogan, Father Dineen, Douglas Hyde, Prof. Strachan,

Dr. Joyce, Mr. Coffey – to mention only a few whose names occur to me – will one and all give their help and their services, each in his own province of learning. (Applause.) As for myself, I am ready to begin to-morrow – (applause) – if you provide me but with a room and a blackboard and the students. (Renewed applause.) Liverpool is but a few hours' pleasant sail from here, and I can come over often. Let the Gaelic League take the matter in hand. Hire a room or two somewhere in the centre of the city; furnish them with the nucleus of an Irish working library. As for the necessary money – and very little will be needed to start – use your organisation, approach the Corporation, the rich men and women in sympathy with the movement, open a subscription list to-night. (Applause.) Then we will found a periodical devoted to Irish research, and exchange it with the great libraries and academies of the world. Perhaps when you have achieved so much, the eyes of the Government will be opened, and they will bestow their money where they will get better value for it. (Applause.) Do not, I beseech you, regard my little scheme as Utopian. Its success depends upon one thing, and upon one thing only – the enthusiasm and application of the students. (Hear, hear.) But I must have gauged the Gaelic movement wrongly if we cannot depend on this. I believe there are hundreds of young men and women who have already acquired a scholarly knowledge of the modern language, eager to avail themselves of every opportunity of becoming better acquainted with the ancient language of their native land, of equipping themselves with the necessary knowledge for independent research in the vast mines of its literature, and of swelling the ranks of a small band of Celtic students. There I leave the matter for the present, in the full conviction that I have not spoken in vain. (Loud applause.)

Dr. Douglas Hyde, on his own behalf, and on behalf of those present, wished to thank Dr. Kuno Meyer for his interesting and useful lecture, and for suggesting a scheme for establishing a school of Irish literature, philology, and history. Since the lecturer first became acquainted with the Gaelic movement, he had consistently championed it in quarters where it was most unpopular. They owed the lecturer a deep debt of gratitude. (Applause.)

The proceedings then ended.

SOURCES CONSULTED
(other sources indicated in text)

1. Bibliographies, Dictionaries etc.: General

Hayes, Richard James, ed: *Manuscript sources for the history of Irish civilisation.* 11 vols, Boston, Mass.: G. K. Hall, 1965. *First supplement 1965-1975.* 3 vols. Boston, Mass.: G. K. Hall, 1979.
Ed., *Sources for the history of Irish civilisation. Articles in periodicals.* 9 vols. Boston, Mass.: G. K. Hall, 1970.
De Hae, Risteárd [Richard James Hayes], agus Brighid Ní Dhonnchadha, do chuir in eagar: *Clár Litridheacht na Nua-Ghaedhilge 1850-1936.* 3 Iml.
I. Na leabhra.
II. Filidheacht i dTréimhseacháin.
III. Prós i dTréimhseacháin.
Baile Átha Cliath: Oifig Dhíolta Foillseacháin Rialtais, 1938-1940.

Best, Richard Irvine: *Bibliography of Irish Philology and of Printed Irish Literature.* Dublin: Printed under the authority of His Majesty's Stationery Office by Browne and Nolan, Ltd., 1913.
Bibliography of Irish Philology and Manuscript Literature. Publications 1913-1941. Dublin: The Dublin Institute for Advanced Studies, 1969.
Dictionary of the Irish Language. Based mainly on Old and Middle Irish Materials. Royal Irish Academy 1913-76. With special reference to the original Fasciculus 1, D-degoir, published in August 1913 under the editorship of Carl J. S. Marstrander, and the *Historical Note* iii-vi, provided by E. G. Quin, General Editor, 1953-75.
British Museum: *Catalogue of the Irish Manuscripts in the British Museum Vol I-III.* Vol 1 by Standish Hayes O'Grady, 1926. Vol II by Robin Flower, 1926. Vol III by Robin Flower, revised by Myles Dillon, 1953. London: The Trustees of the British Museum, 1926-53.

Meyer, Kuno: *Contributions to Irish Lexicography.* Volume I, Part I, A-C. Halle a. S.: Max Niemeyer; London: David Nutt, 1906. Part II, D-dno. Halle a.S.: Max Niemeyer, 1906-[1907].
Cf.p.150 of this biography in which Meyer states he left his interleaved copies of A-DNO and all his other lexicography material to Hans Hessen.

Hessen, Hans: *Hessen's Irish Lexicon. A Concise Dictionary of Early Irish.* Edited by Séamus Caomhánach, Rudolf Hertz, Vernam E. Hull and Gustav Lemacher, S.J. Halle (Saale): Max Niemeyer Verlag, 1933-40. [Only Vol. I, fasciculi 1-2 and Vol. II, fasciculi 1-3 published].
Cf. p. xiv '... it was not possible to wait until the unpublished letters of Kuno Meyer's *Contributions* were edited'.

Kenney, James F.: *The sources for the early history of Ireland: Ecclesiastical.* Dublin: Pádraic Ó Táilliúir, 1979. (Reprint. Originally published 1929 by Columbia University Press).

Zeuss, Johann Kaspar: *Grammatica Celtica e monumentis vetustis tam Hibernicae linguae quam Britannicarum dialectorum Cambricae Cornicae Aremoricae comparatis Gallicae priscae reliquiis construxit I. C. Zeuss. Editio altera curavit H. Ebel.* Berolini: Apud Weidmannos, MDCCCLXXI.

Holder, Alfred: *Alt-Celtischer Sprachschatz.* 3 vols. Leipzig: Teubner, 1891-1913.

2. Bibliography and writings of Kuno Meyer

(a) Bibliography of the publications of Kuno Meyer in *Zeitschrift für celtische Philologie* XV, I, 1-47, plus Index of Words 48-65. Compiled by R.I. Best, it sets out his works chronologically, year by year, from 1879 to 1923, the items relating to 1920, 1921 and 1923 being from his *Nachlass* edited by Julius Pokorny. Dr. Best points out in his introductory paragraph that Meyer's interest was widely distributed, leaving his mark on almost every section of Irish studies, but that poetry and lexicography would seem to have attracted him most. This extensive bibliography has the character of a reference book or index to the progress of Celtic studies in his time and gives an overview of his impressive achievement. Many of the items are headed *Mitteilungen aus irischen Handschriften,* Gleanings from Irish manuscripts; *zur keltischen Wortkunde,* on Celtic philology; *Erschienene Schriften,* notices of published writings. Meyer contributed five items to the Todd Lecture Series of the Royal Irish Academy. Strictly speaking these were not lectures. They were editions of texts, with introduction, translation, notes and glossary, which were presented at meetings of the Academy and spoken about in a general way by the editor. These were: No XIII, *The Triads of Ireland* (1906); XIV, *The Death-Tales of the Ulster Heroes* (1906); XV, *The Instructions of King Cormac Mac Airt* (Tecosca Cormaic) (1909); XVI, *Fianaigecht* (1910); XVII, *Betha Colmáin Mac Lúacháin. Life of Colmán son of Lúachán* (1911); *Imram Curaig Mailedúin,* read on 30 Nov. 1910 and proposed to appear with other texts as No. XVIII, but not published, was reprinted in *ZCP* XI, 148ff.

(b) Besides the Todd Lecture series, other writings of Meyer from the foregoing Bibliography consulted include –
Eine irische Version der Alexandersage. Leipzig: Druck von Pöschel & Trepte, 1884.
The Cath Finntrága, or Battle of Ventry. Oxford: Clarendon Press, 1885.
Merugud Uilix maicc Leirtis. The Irish Odyssey. London: David Nutt, 1886.
Aislinge Meic Conglinne. The Vision of Mac Conglinne. London: David Nutt, 1892. Reprint New York 1974 (Lemma).
The Voyage of Bran Son of Febal to the Land of the Living [Vol. 1] London: David Nutt, 1895. (Grimm Library No. 4).
The Voyage of Bran, Vol. II, comprising the Celtic Doctrine of Re-birth, by Alfred Nutt. With Appendices: the transformations of Tuan mac Cairill, the Dinnshenchas of Mag Slecht, edited and translated by Kuno Meyer. London: David Nutt, 1897. (Grimm Library No. 6).
King and Hermit. A colloquy between King Guaire of Aidne and his brother Marbán. Being an Irish poem of the 10th century. London: David Nutt, 1901.
Liadain and Curithir. An Irish love-story of the 9th century. London: David Nutt, 1902.
Four Old-Irish songs of summer and winter. London: David Nutt, 1903.
Cáin Adamnáin. An Old-Irish treatise on the Law of Adamnán. Oxford, Clarendon Press, 1905.
A primer of Irish metrics. Dublin: School of Irish Learning, Hodges Figgis & Co.; London: David Nutt, 1909.
Selections from Ancient Irish Poetry. London, Constable and Company Ltd., 1911. Notes on the sources of the poems pp 111-114. In his Bibliography of Meyer's works, R. I. Best states that a second edition containing several addi-

tional poems was issued in 1913 (ZCP XV, 31). Constable's 1928 reprint does not mention this.

Hail Brigit. An Old-Irish poem on the Hill of Alenn. Halle a. S.: Max Niemeyer; Dublin: Hodges Figgis & Co. Ltd., 1912.

Learning in Ireland in the fifth century and the transmission of letters. Dublin: School of Irish Learning, 1913.

Otia Merseiana. The publication of the Arts Faculty of University College Liverpool. 4 Vols. 1899-1904. London: Longmans, Green & Co. for the University Press of Liverpool. Contains several contributions by Meyer.

(c) *Reports of Lectures by Kuno Meyer.*

A survey of Celtic Philology. *The Gael,* XX (N.S. 297-301), New York, 1901.

Early Irish Literature. Delivered in Central Hall, Rosemary Street, Belfast, 25 March 1902. Reports in *Irish News* (Belfast) and *News-Letter* (Belfast) 26 March 1902.

An appeal for a Gaelic Academy. An address delivered to the Liverpool Branch of the Gaelic League on 26 October 1904. Copy in R. I. Best papers, National Library of Ireland.

The making of the Irish Language. Lecture by Kuno Meyer. Report in *United Irishman* (Dublin), 15 July 1905, p. 1.

The University and the teaching of Celtic. Lecture delivered on 4 July 1908 in the Leinster Lecture Hall, Molesworth Street, Dublin. Report in *Freeman's Journal,* 6 July 1908.

The influence of Celtic literature on the literature of Europe. *Gaelic American* (New York), 9 January 1909.

The relations of Ireland with Great Britain and the Continent in the early centuries of our era. – Margaret Stokes Memorial Lecture, 1910, delivered at Alexandra College, Dublin, 10 May 1910. Report in *Freeman's Journal,* 11 May 1910.

Ancient Irish Literature. Delivered in Queen's University, Belfast. Report in *Northern Whig,* 22 October 1910.

Ancient Irish Language and Literature. At same venue. Report in *Northern Whig,* 24 October 1910.

Heinrich Zimmer. Brief report in *Manchester Guardian,* 6 February 1911; reprint in *Revue Celtique,* xxxii (1911), 219-220.

Interview with Dr. Kuno Meyer. Report in *Catholic Times* (Liverpool), 17 March 1911.

Learning in Ancient Ireland. *Weekly Freeman* 28 September 1912.

The City and University of Liverpool in retrospect, with an appeal for the founding of a chair of Celtic Philology in the University. Address given by Kuno Meyer to the Liverpool Welsh National Society at the celebration of St. David's Day in the Adelphi Hotel, Liverpool, 1913. Report in the *Liverpool [----?],* 3 March 1913. Copy in R. I. Best papers, National Library of Ireland.

(d) *Journals, periodicals, etc., edited by Kuno Meyer with others.*

Zeitschrift für celtische Philologie. Vols. I-VII edited by Kuno Meyer and Ludwig Christian Stern. Vols. VIII-XIII edited by Kuno Meyer. Halle a. S.; Max Niemeyer, 1896-1919.

Archiv für celtische Lexicographie. Edited by Whitley Stokes and Kuno Meyer. Vols. I-III. Halle a. S.; Max Niemeyer, 1900-1907.

Ériu: The Journal of the School of Irish Learning. Vols. I-III edited by Kuno

Meyer and John Strachan; Vol. IV ed. by Meyer and Osborn Bergin; V-VI ed. by Meyer and Carl Marstrander; VII by Meyer and R. I. Best. Dublin 1904-1914.

Anecdota from Irish Manuscripts. Edited by Osborn J. Bergin, Richard I. Best, Kuno Meyer, James G. O'Keeffe. Halle a. S.: Max Niemeyer; Dublin: Hodges, Figgis & Co., Ltd. Vols. I-V, 1907-1913.

3. Books, pamphlets, articles in periodicals etc.

Bergin, Osborn and Marstrander, Carl, eds.: *Miscellany presented to Kuno Meyer by some of his friends and pupils on the occasion of his appointment to the chair of Celtic Philology in the University of Berlin.* Halle a. S.: Max Niemeyer Verlag, 1912.

Conway, Stanley: *The University Club, Liverpool: its history from 1896-1956.* Liverpool, 1969.

Dillon, Myles: *Early Irish Literature.* Chicago: University of Chicago Press, 1948.

Ehrenberg, Victor: *Aspects of the Ancient World.* Oxford: Basil Blackwell, 1946.

Easton, Malcolm and Holroyd, Michael: *The Art of Augustus John.* London: Secker and Warburg, 1974.

E[lton], O[liver], ed. *A Miscellany presented to John Macdonald Mackay LL.D.* July 1914. Liverpool: At the University Press; London: Constable and Company Ltd., 1914.

Frayne, John P. and Johnson, Colton, eds.: W. B. Yeats, *Uncollected Prose.* 2 vols. London: Macmillan, 1970-75.

Gilbert, Rosa Mulholland: *Life of Sir John T. Gilbert.* London: Longmans, Green, and Co., 1905.

Hoffmann, Christhard: 'Eduard Meyer' in *Classical Scholarship. A biographical encyclopedia.* New York & London: Garland Publishing, 1990.

Holroyd, Michael: *Augustus John, a biography.* 2 vols., London: Heinemann, 1974-75.

Hone, Joseph: *The life of George Moore.* London: Gollancz, 1936.

Intermediate Education (Ireland) Commission. Appendix to the Final Report of the Commissioners. Part II. Miscellaneous Documents. Dublin: printed for Her Majesty's Stationery Office by Alexander Thom & Co., 1899.

Kelly, Thomas: *For advancement of learning. The University of Liverpool 1881-1891.* Liverpool: Liverpool University Press, 1981.

Kessler, Harry Clemens Ulrich, Count: *The diaries of a cosmopolitan. Count Harry Kessler, 1918-1937.* Translated and edited by Charles Kessler, etc. London: Weidenfeld and Nicolson, 1971.

McDowell, R. B.: *Alice Stopford Green. A passionate historian.* Dublin: Allen Figgis, 1967.

Merriman, Brian: *Cúirt an mheadhóin oidhche.* Ein komisches Epos in vulgäririscher Sprache ... herausgegeben von Ludwig Christian Stern. (Sonderabdruck aus der ZCP. Band V. 1905). Halle a. S.: Max Niemeyer, 1904.

Meyer, Kuno: *Kunonis Meyeri quem vocant tón Kúna Musarum Munuscula ...* Hamburgi: ex typographia Ferdinandi Schlotkii, anno MDCCCLXXIX.

A Celtic chair for Professor Kuno Meyer. Liverpool: Liverpool University Club, 1903.

Kuno Meyer Symposium at National Gallery. Report in *Irish Times* p. 5, *Irish Press, Irish Independent,* Friday, 28 Nov. 1969.

Schulze, Wilhelm: Kuno Meyer, 1858-1919. An oration delivered in Berlin on 28 Jan. 1920, before the Fichte-Hochschulgemeinde. *Studies,* June 1920. 291-97.

Moore, George: *Hail and Farewell.* 3 vols. London: Heinemann, 1911-1914.

Moynihan, Maurice, ed.: *Speeches and Statements by Éamon de Valera 1917-73*. Dublin: Gill and Macmillan, 1980.

Murphy, William M., *Prodigal Father*. Ithaca and London: Cornell University Press, 1978.

Muir, Ramsay: *An autobiography and some essays*. Ed. by Stuart Hodgson. London: Lund Humphries, 1943.

Muspratt, Edmund Knowles: *My Life and Work*. London, New York: John Lane, 1917 [1916].

Ó Briain, Liam: *Cuimhní Cinn*. Baile Átha Cliath: Sáirséal agus Dill, 1951.

O'Connor, Frank and David Greene, eds.: *A Golden Treasury of Irish poetry: A.D. 600 to 1200*. London: Macmillan, 1967. (Reprint: Dingle: Brandon, 1990).

Ó Domhnaill, Mártan, An tAth. *Oileáin Árann*. [Baile Átha Cliath]: C.S. Ó Fallamhain, Teo, 1930.

O'Kelleher, Andrew and Gertrude Schoepperle: *Betha Colaim Chille. Life of Columcille* compiled by Manus O'Donnell in 1532. Urbana, Illinois: (Published by the University of Illinois), 1918.

Ó Lúing, Seán: Robin Flower (1881-1946) *Studies* Summer/Autumn 1981, 121-134.
    Carl Marstrander (1883-1965). *Cork Hist. & Arch. Journal*. Jan-Dec 1984, 108-124.
    Kuno Meyer by Augustus John. A brief history of a famous portrait. *Studies* Winter 1982, 325-343.

Ó Raifeartaigh, Tarlach, ed.: *The Royal Irish Academy. A bicentennial history 1785-1985*. Dublin: Royal Irish Academy, 1985.

Raleigh, Sir Walter: *Laughter from a cloud*. London: Constable and Company Limited, 1923.

Reid, B.L.: *The man from New York; John Quinn and his friends*. New York: Oxford University Press, 1968.
    The lives of Roger Casement. New Haven and London: Yale University Press, 1976.

Reilly, Charles Herbert: *Scaffolding in the sky*. London: Routledge, 1938.

Sampson, John. *In lighter moments*. Liverpool: University College Liverpool; London: Hodder and Stoughton, 1934.

Schoepperle, Gertrude: *Mediaeval studies in memory of Gertrude Schoepperle Loomis*. Various contributors, including Douglas Hyde, R. I. Best, J. Vendryes. Paris: Librairie Honoré Champion; New York: Columbia University Press, 1927.

Stockley, William Frederick Paul: *Essays in biography*. Cork: Cork University Press, 1933.

Stokes, Whitley and John Strachan: *Thesaurus Palaeohibernicus*. Vol. I, 1901. Vol. II, 1903. Cambridge: Cambridge University Press, 1901-03. 1975 reprint, with Supplement by Stokes, by Dublin Institute for Advanced Studies.

Stokes, Whitley: *A criticism of Dr. Atkinson's Glossary to Volumes I-V of the Ancient Laws of Ireland*. London: David Nutt, 1903.

Stokes, Whitley: *In Cath Catharda*. The Civil War of the Romans. An Irish version of Lucan's *Pharsalia*. Leipzig: S. Hirzel, 1909.

The Whitley Stokes Library. Presented to University of London, University College, by Miss Maive and Miss Annie Stokes. n.d. [1911].

Stokes, Whitley, ed.: *Irish Glosses. A Mediaeval Tract on Latin Declension*. Dublin: Irish Archaeological and Celtic Society, 1860.

Stokes, Whitley, ed.: *Félire Oengusso Céli Dé. The Martyrology of Oengus the Culdee*. London: Henry Bradshaw Society, 1905 (Vol. XXIX). Reprinted by Dublin Institute for Advanced Studies, 1984.

Scéala Scoil an Léinn Cheiltigh. Newsletter of the School of Celtic Studies. Ed. Rolf Baumgarten. No. 1, 1987 – No. 4, 1990. Dublin Institute for Advanced Studies.

Scoil an Léinn Cheiltigh. School of Celtic Studies. *Fiftieth Anniversary Report 1940-1990*. Dublin Institute for Advanced Studies, 1990.

Wade, Allan, ed.: *The letters of W. B. Yeats*. London: Rupert Hart-Davis, 1954.

Wilamowitz-Moellendorff, Ulrich Von: *History of Classical Scholarship,* translated from the German by Alan Harris. London: Duckworth, 1982.

Zimmer, Heinrich: *The Celtic Church in Britain and Ireland*. Translated by A. Meyer. London: David Nutt, 1902. Translated from *Realencyklopädie für protestantische Theologie und Kirche,* Vol X. Translation carried out under the constant supervision of Whitley Stokes, Alfred Nutt, Oliver Elton and Kuno Meyer.

4. Periodicals and Newspapers consulted

The Academy
The Athenaeum
The Bookman
British Academy *Proceedings*
Catholic Times and Catholic Opinion (Liverpool)
Catholic University Bulletin
Celtia
Celtic Review
Celtica
Cork Historical and Archaeological Society *Journal*
Dublin Magazine
Éigse
Études Celtiques
European Press
Folklore
Freeman's Journal
Weekly Freeman
The Gael (New York)
Gaelic American
The Gaelic Churchman
Indogermanisches Jahrbuch
Irish Book Lover
Irische Korrespondenz
Irish Educational Review
Irish Fireside
Irish Independent
Irish Press
Irish Review
Irish Times
The Irishman/An tÉireannach (London)
Irisleabhar Mhuighe Nuadhad
Irisleabhar na Gaedhilge/Gaelic Journal
Das Johanneum ·
Journal of the Gypsy Lore Society
Journal of the Royal Asiatic Association
Philological Society *Transactions*

Revue Celtique
Royal Irish Academy *Proceedings*
Saturday Review
Scríobh
Studies
Sunday Independent
The Times
Times Literary Supplement
United Irishman (Dublin) ed. Arthur Griffith
The Vital Issue
Westminster Gazette

5. Manuscript Sources

National Library of Ireland
Richard Irvine Best Papers

Ms No. 11000. Letters to R. I. Best, mainly from Celtic scholars, including Osborn Bergin, Robin Flower, Henri Gaidoz, Dom Louis Gougaud.

Ms No. 11001. Letters to R. I. Best, from Celtic scholars and others. Correspondents include Alice Stopford Green, Paul Grosjean, Douglas Hyde, J. Loth, Eoin MacNeill, Carl Marstrander.

Ms No. 11002. A substantial collection of letters and documents, ca. 500, in a metal box, containing three important elements – Meyer's correspondence with Richard Best, 1903-1919; Best's correspondence with Meyer (incomplete); Toni Meyer's correspondence with Edith and Richard Best, 1919-1939 (incomplete), with associated material. This is the most important single repository of which use has been made in this biography. It will be noted that some citations therefrom have sub-numbers, while most have not. The explanation is that, at a certain stage in the years during which this study was in progress, the collection was re-organised chronologically into convenient, numbered folders, thus making for more specific reference. However, as the references used have been dated in every instance possible, particular items can be checked.

Ms No. 11003. Letters to R. I. Best, mainly from Celtic scholars, including An tAth. Peadar Ua Laoghaire, T. F. O'Rahilly, C. Plummer, L. C. Purser, E. C. Quiggin, Sir John Rhys, M. L. Sjoestedt, AE. 1895-1955.

Ms No. 11004. Letters to R. I. Best from James Stephens, A. G. Van Hamel, J. Vendryes, J. C. Watson, etc. 1895-1955.

Ms. No. 11005. Letters, notes and memoranda relating to the state of Irish studies since the foundation of Saorstát Éireann, the foundation of the Dublin Institute for Advanced Studies etc., including memoranda of Osborn Bergin, T. F. O'Rahilly, D. A. Binchy, etc. 1936-1945.

Ms No. 11007. Transcripts and notes by Whitley Stokes and letters to R. I. Best concerning the papers of Stokes from his daughter, Maive Boothby, 1911.

Ms No. 11008. Notes by R. I. Best of lectures on Celtic topics by Marstrander, Stokes, Strachan, Bergin.

Ms No. 3890. Six letters from Meyer to John Smyth MacDonald (1898-1919) and letter from Jean MacDonald to Prof. H. G. Murphy.

Ms No. 5459. Sir Roger Casement to Kuno Meyer, 12 Nov. 1914.

Ms No. 8616. Letters from Meyer to Mrs Mary Hutton, 1900-1910.

Ms. No. 8607. Letters to Frances Geoghegan, from Kuno Meyer, York Powell, Charles Bonnier, 1898-1927.

Ms G. 685. Óráid do Chuno Meyer, 1915, ó Scoil Ghaedhilge Boston.

Ms No. 425A. Letters to Mario Esposito from Kuno Meyer and others. Early 20th Century.

Ms No. 15, 535. Letters from various correspondents to Mrs Mary Hutton.

Ms No. 18, 252. Meyer to Hyde re proposed School of Irish Learning.

Mss Nos 17465 and 17629. Correspondence of Meyer with Joseph McGarrity, Clan na Gael leader, Philadelphia, 1914-1917.

Ms No. 2113. Kuno Meyer to James George O'Keeffe on matters connected with Irish studies. 1904-1912.

Ms No. 2114. Charles Plummer and John Strachan to James George O'Keeffe, mainly on Irish studies. 1904-1924.

Ms No. 13336. Correspondence of John Strachan.

Eoin MacNeill papers, Ms No. 10, 882.

Alice Stopford Green papers. Mss Nos 9932, 10452,10457, 15077, 15091, 15122.

Royal Irish Academy. R.I.A. 12 0 21-24. Correspondence of Eleanor Knott with Irish scholars, including Meyer, Bergin, Best, Fraser, Marstrander, An tAth. Peadar Ua Laoghaire.
Photographs of Celtic scholars and of Staff and Students of the School of Irish Learning.

Bodleian Library, Oxford. Correspondence of Kuno Meyer with Edward Williams Byron Nicholson, Bodley Librarian; Gilbert Murray; Wallace Martin Lindsay.

University of Liverpool.
1.   Recollections of J. Glyn Davies: Liverpool University Archives, Box 159, No. 17.

2 (a) List (15 pp.) of letters and postcards to Professor J. Glyn Davies 1887-1919, with notes on the subjects of correspondence.

   (b) List (2 pp) of correspondence of Kuno Meyer held by the University Archives, other than correspondence with J. Glyn Davies, 1899-1902.

Xerox copies of this material kindly supplied by Adrian R. Allan, Assistant Archivist, University of Liverpool.

Trinity College Dublin: Manuscript Department. Mss Nos 4222-4224, 7970, 10085. An important collection of correspondence to, and from, Meyer. Letters from Celtic scholars, some in German from L. C. Stern, Windisch, Rudolf Thurneysen; letters from Douglas Hyde and others to Meyer; letters and postcards from Meyer to Whitley Stokes; notes and extracts from Stokes correspondence by R. I. Best; letters from various correspondents and miscellaneous items, presscuttings, photographs, etc.

Index

256

Finnbarr, Saint, 116.
Fischer, Emil, 204.
Fish Creek, 191.
Fisher, Gregory, 125.
Fitzgerald, T.A., O.F.M., 65, 117.
Fitzgeralds, from Ireland, 150.
Fitzmaurice-Kelly, James, 119.
Fleming, John (Seaghán Pléimion), 8, 23, 25, 33, 115, 240.
Florence, 108.
Florida, 192.
Flower, Robin, 65, 77, 119, 121, 129, 131, 133, 134, 135, 143, 145, 151, 155, 159, 160, 161, 165, 166, 172, 181, 182, 203, 204, 206, 207, 210, 217, 224, 226, 229, 234, 238, 239.
Fock, booksellers, 132, 133.
France, 105, 111, 160, 201, 203, 211.
France, Anatole, 151, 229.
Frankfurt, 216.
Franz Ferdinand, Archduke, 160.
Fraser, John, 65, 135.
Frayne, John P., 239.
Frazer, James George, 4.
Frederick (Friedrich) the Great, 107, 190.
Freiburg in Breisgau, 37, 42, 48, 63, 64, 85, 106, 111, 145, 150, 161.
Frenchpark, 17, 23, 36.
Freund, 180.
Friedel, 111.
Friedrich (Frederick) the Great, 107, 190.
Friedrichroda, 119, 127.
Fry, Elliot and Fry, photographers, 120.

Gaelic League, 1, 16, 18, 22, 26, 27, 28, 36, 74, 75, 77, 115, 169, 213, 240, 242, 245, 246.
Gaidoz, Henri, 14, 44, 49, 60, 84, 93, 110, 136, 151, 184, 185, 205, 209.
Gallárus, 62, 232.
Galway, 30, 44, 59, 60, 65, 69, 74, 76, 77, 135, 235.
Gaul, 119.
Gaulish scholars, 122.
Genoa, 83.
Geoghegan, Fanny, 184.
Geoghegan, Sam, 184, 206.
Geoghegan, Séamus, 184.
Geoghegan, William P., 34, 179, 206.
Geoghegan, Mrs William P., 184, 206.
George, David Lloyd, 5, 93, 106, 199, 209.
Gerhardt, Elena, 125.
Giessen, 103, 211, 216.
Gilbert, John T., 49.
Giles, p., 62.
Gissing, George, 108.
Gladstone, William Ewart, 62, 63, 217.
Glasgow, 230.
Glastonbury, 121.
Glück, Wilhelm, 14.

Gobineau, Joseph-Arthur de, 84.
Goethe, Johann Wolfgang von, 1, 76, 120, 134, 160, 204.
Goethegesellschaft, 118.
Gogarty, Oliver St. John, 58.
Gonne, Maud, 173.
Gonville and Caius College, 172.
Gort, 19, 23.
Gossensass, 48, 50.
Gotch, Francis, 96.
Gothenburg, 198.
Göttingen, 8, 120, 214.
Gougaud, Dom Louis, 165, 189.
Gower, George Leveson, 62.
Grant, James, 53.
Graves, Alfred Percival, 155.
Green, Alice Stopford (Mrs. John Richard Green), 26, 30, 32, 33, 34, 35, 37, 38, 39, 40, 41, 42, 45, 61, 64, 68, 70, 71, 72, 75, 76, 79, 80, 83, 90, 97, 106, 107, 110, 111, 112, 119, 120, 124, 127, 129, 130, 131, 133, 153, 154, 157, 159, 161, 163, 168, 176, 177, 178, 179, 180, 181, 188, 189, 190, 191, 192, 193, 194, 196, 201, 202, 204, 207, 210, 211, 212, 214, 235, 236.
Greene, David, 231.
Gregory, Augusta, 1, 19, 20, 23, 131, 229.
Grenville Place, 73.
Grey, Sir Edward, 159.
Greystones, 7, 131.
Griffith, Arthur, 37.
Grimm, Jacob, 165.
Grimms, Jacob and Wilhelm, 224.
Guenzel, L., 188.
Güterbock, Bruno G., 87.
Gwynn, Edward, 30, 31, 34, 45, 46, 58, 91, 113, 139, 140, 141, 142, 143, 145, 146, 150, 153.
Gwynn, Edward Lucius, 106, 111, 215, 234.
Gwynn, Stephen, M.P., 106, 114, 120, 123, 215, 224.

Hague, The, 161.
Hahnenklee, 85.
Haldane, Lord, 163.
Halle, 13, 43, 120, 127, 205, 223.
Hamburg, 2, 11, 88, 114, 117, 169, 201, 202, 203, 204, 205, 210, 211, 212, 216, 224.
Hamburg-Amerika Line, 155.
Hamilton, William Rowan, 238.
Hampstead, 137.
Hanover, 161, 164.
Harkampf, Miss, 159.
Harnack, Adolf, 88, 104, 123, 124, 160, 165.
Harris, Alan, 205.
Harrison, Damer, 10.
Harrison, Sarah, 117.
Harvard, 64, 136, 155, 167, 169, 174, 185.

Kuhn, Ernst, 31, 87.

Lake District, 143, 144, 150.
Lang, Andrew, 7.
Laon, 232.
Larkin, James, 197, 200.
Law, Bonar, 114.
Lawrence, Sir Edward, 20.
Leahy, Arthur Herbert, 61.
Leeds, 4, 20.
Lehmann, Lille, 154.
Lehmann-Haupt, Carl Friedrich Ferdinand, 97, 180, 183.
Leibnitz, 157, 158, 160.
Leigh, Austen, 62.
Leipzig, 13, 37, 43, 73, 84, 104, 105, 111, 115, 126, 128, 132, 133, 137, 150, 152, 153, 162, 165, 204, 205, 215, 217, 223.
Lennon, Councillor, 117.
Lepsius, 104.
Lessing, Gotthold Ephraim, 89.
Lever, of Port Sunlight, 83.
Lew Trenchard, Devon, 8.
Lewis, Florence Luella (Florence Youngblood), 195, 212.
Lewis, Margaret, 206, 215.
Lewis, Timothy, 59.
Leyden, 122.
Lichterfelde, 164, 209, 211, 214, 223, 224.
Limerick, 12, 189, 191.
Lincolnshire, 61.
Lindsay, Wallace Martin, 14, 131, 226, 232.
Liszt, Abbé Franz, 76, 160.
Liverpool, 3, 4, 6, 7, 10, 16, 20, 21, 23, 24, 28, 32, 38, 39, 40, 46, 49, 53, 54, 56, 60, 65, 67, 77, 79, 82, 84, 86, 88, 89, 93, 94, 95, 97, 98, 99, 100, 101, 104, 109, 113, 117, 118, 122, 123, 124, 126, 127, 129, 130, 151, 152, 153, 154, 155, 160, 164, 171, 172, 174, 178, 183, 190, 203, 205, 208, 223, 227, 230, 232, 233, 246.
Llanbedr, 9.
Lloyd George, David, 93, 100, 106.
Lloyd-Jones, Hugh, 223.
Lloyd, Joseph Henry (Seosamh Laoide), 61, 62, 64, 65.
Lodge, Oliver J., 99.
Lohne, 161.
London, 4, 9, 14, 20, 21, 24, 31, 45, 49, 61, 73, 74, 84, 88, 90, 91, 92, 93, 94, 95, 101, 106, 109, 117, 118, 119, 121, 122, 125, 127, 129, 130, 131, 133, 136, 143, 151, 155, 156, 160, 162, 170, 174, 181, 191, 194, 202, 204, 232.
Long Island, 170.
Long, William, 63.
Los Angeles, 116.
Losty, M.J., Sword Bearer, 117.
Loth, Joseph, 14, 52, 60, 84, 133, 135, 136, 143, 153, 184, 222.
Lucan (Marcus Annaeus Lucanus), 43, 46, 73.
Lucerne, 145.
Luders, 104.
Lyall, Sir Charles, 90.
Lynch, 44.
Lyon, 54.
Lyster, T.W., 152, 160.
Macalister, Robert Alexander Stewart, 36, 67, 76, 78, 113, 132, 133, 140, 148.
McClelland, 47, 105.
McColl, D.S., 130.
Mac Conghail, Muiris, 224.
Mac Cuarta, Séamus Dall, 184.
Mac Cuilennáin, Cormac, 146.
Mac Curtin (Andrew or Hugh), 184.
MacDonald, Jean, 208, 213.
MacDonald, John Smyth, 10, 208, 213.
MacDonnell, Sir Antony, 31, 32, 34, 36.
McDowell, R.B., 33, 80, 174.
McGarrity, Joseph, 187, 188, 189, 190, 191, 192, 193, 195, 198, 199, 200.
Mackay, John MacDonald, 99, 151, 152, 154, 160, 189.
MacKenna, Stephen, 65, 288.
MacKinnon, Donald, 60.
MacNaughton, Lord, 131.
MacNaughton, Miss, 131, 151.
MacNeill, James G. Swift, 131.
MacNeill, Eoin (John), 17, 29, 34, 46, 55, 57, 58, 60, 67, 68, 70, 72, 74, 88, 89, 131, 132, 133, 142, 154, 179, 197, 203, 210, 213, 227, 237.
Macran, Henry Stewart, 167, 168, 185.
Magdalen College, 96.
Magee, William Kirkpatrick (John Eglinton), 94, 121.
Mahaffy, John Pentland, 15, 17, 18, 75, 83, 105, 111, 167, 168, 185.
Maidstone, 152, 161.
Mair, Alexander, 28, 208.
Majuba Hill, 105.
Manchester, 4, 15, 20, 29, 38, 40, 41, 42, 49, 51, 52, 53, 59, 61, 230.
Manchester Guardian, 116.
Manitius, Max, 125, 128.
Manners, Victoria, 62.
Mannix, Monsignor Daniel, 115.
Marburg, 3.
Marin, John, 23.
Marstrander, Carl Johan Sverdrup (C. M.; Ó Uaimhín), 43, 46, 56, 65, 66, 73, 75, 78, 79, 81, 82, 83, 85, 86, 94, 95, 96, 97, 100, 106, 107, 108, 109, 110, 111, 113, 114, 118, 119, 120, 122, 123, 126, 127, 130, 131, 132, 133, 134, 137, 138, 139, 140, 141, 142, 143, 144, 145, 146, 147, 148, 149, 150, 151, 152, 154, 155, 158, 163, 164, 166, 168, 184, 185, 201,

265